AF567196

Peripheral Nerve Stimulation

Progress in Neurological Surgery

Vol. 24

Series Editor

L. Dade Lunsford Pittsburgh, Pa.

Peripheral Nerve Stimulation

Volume Editor

Konstantin V. Slavin Chicago, Ill.

59 figures, 4 in color, and 10 tables, 2011

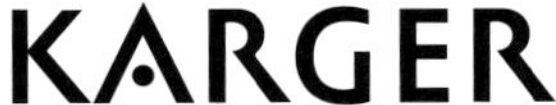

Basel · Freiburg · Paris · London · New York · Bangalore · Bangkok · Shanghai · Singapore · Tokyo · Sydney

Prof. Konstantin V. Slavin, MD
University of Illinois at Chicago
Department of Neurosurgery
Chicago, Ill., USA

Library of Congress Cataloging-in-Publication Data

Peripheral nerve stimulation / volume editor, Konstantin V. Slavin.
p. ; cm. -- (Progress in neurological surgery, ISSN 0079-6492 ; vol. 24)
Includes bibliographical references and index.
ISBN 978-3-8055-9488-2 (hard cover : alk. paper) -- ISBN 978-3-8055-9489-9 (e-ISBN)
1. Chronic diseases--Treatment. 2. Pain--Treatment. 3. Neural stimulation. 4. Nerves, Peripheral. I. Slavin, Konstantin V. II. Series: Progress in neurological surgery ; v. 24.
[DNLM: 1. Chronic Disease--therapy. 2. Pain--therapy. 3. Electric Stimulation Therapy. 4. Peripheral Nerves--physiology. W1 PR673 v.24 2011 / WL 704]
RC108.P47 2011
616'.044--dc22

2011003657

www.karger.com
Printed in Switzerland on acid-free paper by Reinhardt Druck, Basel
ISSN 0079–6492
ISBN 978–3–8055–9488–2
e-ISBN 978–3–8055–9489–9

Contents

VII **Series Editor's Note**
Lunsford, L.D. (Pittsburgh, Pa.)

IX **Preface**
Burchiel, K.J. (Portland, Oreg.)

1 **History of Peripheral Nerve Stimulation**
Slavin, K.V. (Chicago, Ill.)

16 **Central Mechanisms of Peripheral Nerve Stimulation in Headache Disorders**
Bartsch, T. (Kiel); Goadsby, P.J. (San Francisco, Calif.)

27 **Peripheral Nerve Stimulation for Chronic Neurogenic Pain**
Al-Jehani, H.; Jacques, L. (Montreal)

41 **Percutaneous Peripheral Nerve Stimulation**
Aló, K.M. (Houston, Tex./Monterrey); Abramova, M.V.; Richter, E.O. (New Orleans, La.)

58 **Peripheral Nerve Stimulation for the Treatment of Truncal Pain**
Cairns, K.D.; McRoberts, W.P. (Fort Lauderdale, Fla.); Deer, T. (Charleston, W.Va.)

70 **Peripheral Subcutaneous Stimulation for Intractable Abdominal Pain**
Barolat, G. (Denver, Colo.)

77 **Subcutaneous Occipital Region Stimulation for Intractable Headache Syndromes**
Weiner, R.L. (Dallas, Tex.)

86 **Peripheral Nerve Stimulation for Occipital Neuralgia: Surgical Leads**
Kapural, L.; Sable, J. (Cleveland, Ohio)

96 **Occipital Nerve Stimulation: Technical and Surgical Aspects of Implantation**
Trentman, T.L.; Zimmerman, R.S.; Dodick, D.W. (Phoenix, Ariz.)

109 **Peripheral Neuromodulation for Migraine Headache**
Ellens, D.J.; Levy, R.M. (Chicago, Ill.)

118 **Occipital Neuromodulation for Refractory Headache in the Chiari Malformation Population**
Vadivelu, S.; Bolognese, P.; Milhorat, T.H.; Mogilner, A.Y. (Manhasset, N.Y.)

126 **Peripheral Nerve Stimulation in Chronic Cluster Headache**
Magis, D.; Schoenen, J. (Liège)

133 **Peripheral Nerve Stimulation for Fibromyalgia**
Plazier, M.; Vanneste, S.; Dekelver, I. (Antwerp); Thimineur, M. (Derby, Conn.); De Ridder, D. (Antwerp)

147 **'Hybrid Neurostimulator': Simultaneous Use of Spinal Cord and Peripheral Nerve Field Stimulation to Treat Low Back and Leg Pain**
Lipov, E.G. (Hoffman Estates, Ill.)

156 **Stimulation of the Peripheral Nervous System for the Painful Extremity**
McRoberts, W.P.; Cairns, K.D. (Fort Lauderdale, Fla.); Deer, T. (Charleston, W.Va.)

171 **Sphenopalatine Ganglion Interventions: Technical Aspects and Application**
Oluigbo, C.O.; Makonnen, G. (Columbus, Ohio); Narouze, S. (Cuyahoga Falls, Ohio); Rezai, A.R. (Columbus, Ohio)

180 **Spinal Nerve Root Stimulation**
Kellner, C.P.; Kellner, M.A.; Winfree, C.J. (New York, N.Y.)

189 **Technical Aspects of Peripheral Nerve Stimulation: Hardware and Complications**
Slavin, K.V. (Chicago, Ill.)

203 **Peripheral Nerve Stimulation: Definition**
Abejón, D. (Madrid); Pérez-Cajaraville, J. (Pamplona)

210 **The Future of Peripheral Nerve Stimulation**
Stanton-Hicks, M. (Cleveland, Ohio); Panourias, I.G.; Sakas, D.E. (Athens); Slavin, K.V. (Chicago, Ill.)

218 **Author Index**

219 **Subject Index**

Series Editor's Note

The 24th volume of *Progress in Neurological Surgery* brings an excellent analysis of the state of the art of peripheral nerve stimulation for a wide variety of chronic pain states. Konstantin Slavin has assembled an international cadre of physicians and surgeons with extensive experience in the use of stimulation for these steadily increasing indications. The authors clearly demonstrate that this technology is a mainstream management strategy for a group of conditions that are often misdiagnosed and undertreated. This volume provides much needed technical know-how based on the extensive experience of the authors. Indications, methods, results and complications are covered in detail. As with many chronic pain conditions, high-level evidence-based medicine studies are difficult to design and perform. For many conditions such as the management of chronic pain states, we must rely on the accumulated experience of practitioners from across the world. This new volume should be an excellent resource for both students and chronic pain specialists. Hopefully, it will also assist others to realize that peripheral nerve stimulation is a valuable procedure that deserves recognition and reimbursement. I am indebted to Dr. Slavin for his efforts to bring this volume to fruition and to Karger Publishers for their superb work to edit, set and illustrate this important monograph.

L. Dade Lunsford, MD
Pittsburgh, Pa.

Preface

Since the introduction of dorsal column stimulation by Shealy, and soon thereafter peripheral nerve stimulation (PNS) by Sweet, the use of neurostimulation has become the foundation of the field of neuromodulation. The concept that paresthesia-inducing electrical stimulation could be analgesic was revolutionary, and was based largely on the gate control theory of Melzack and Wall and earlier work by Noordenbos. What follows this preface is literally the first chapter of this excellent monograph, presenting a detailed history of the field. I would encourage readers not to skip over that rendition of what is almost certainly one of the most interesting and successful epochs in the history of clinical neuroscience. Given this, I will not dwell further on this fascinating background.

PNS has given us ready access to the central systems of pain modulation. Our knowledge of these systems has certainly advanced since the first publication of the gate theory, yet this knowledge remains rudimentary. Physiologic studies at the level of the periphery, spinal cord, brainstem, basal ganglia, and cortex have begun to paint a picture of a complex ascending influence of PNS on sensory processing. Positron emission tomography (PET) and functional MRI (fMRI) have complemented these insights and hold tremendous promise for further understanding of the central effects of PNS.

While neurostimulation has played an undeniably important role in the development of clinical neuromodulation, realistically, we cannot be satisfied with the level of evidence that supports its clinical use. The inception of spinal cord stimulation (SCS) as a clinical tool came well before our current concepts of evidence-based medicine had matured. Although many of us believe SCS can be an effective measure for the control of neuropathic pain, it may, to some degree, be too late to produce convincing evidence of its efficacy. Because SCS is an established (and funded) procedure, the best clinical studies that can now be performed on SCS are compromised by the current standards of practice, and both patient and surgeon expectations. The actual evidence that neurostimulation works is, at best, modest. This is a parable we cannot ignore.

I believe that we are now at a point when we can begin to answer fundamental questions regarding the mechanism of PNS-induced analgesia. Going forward, we should hold ourselves to a high standard of understanding before venturing into new applications of PNS. Given the deceptive ease of application, the temptation to apply this approach nonspecifically is great. Clinical outcome data acquired by the most rigorous methodology and vetted by contemporary analytical standards will be crucial to the vitality of this field.

It is for this reason that I congratulate Dr. Slavin for assembling this important monograph. In the evidence presented herein, he has set a high bar for authoritative exposition and a basis for clinical practice. I think this book will provide a landmark in our progress in PNS therapy, and a reference for both veterans and neophytes.

Kim J. Burchiel, MD, FACS
Portland, Oreg.

Slavin KV (ed): Peripheral Nerve Stimulation.
Prog Neurol Surg. Basel, Karger, 2011, vol 24, pp 1–15

History of Peripheral Nerve Stimulation

Konstantin V. Slavin

Department of Neurosurgery, University of Illinois at Chicago, Chicago, Ill., USA

Abstract

Peripheral nerve stimulation (PNS) is an established neuromodulation approach that has been successfully used for the treatment of various painful conditions since the early 1960s. This review provides a comprehensive summary of relevant publications on PNS dividing its history into three distinct periods. The milestones of the field are related to the development of procedures, equipment and indications. As the most rapidly growing segment of operative neuromodulation, PNS continues to evolve as current and emerging clinical indications become matched by basic and clinical research, technological developments and procedural refinements.

Whenever a new patient in my practice is considered for a peripheral nerve stimulation (PNS) procedure, the same questions inevitably come up in conversation with the patient and family, and then again with the referring/primary physician, and finally with the insurance company where the procedure is reviewed – how new and experimental PNS is and how different it is from other neuromodulation approaches. This situation reflects the current state of PNS and indicates several important issues. First of all, there is a significant shortage of information regarding this approach, partly due to lack of awareness in the medical community at large, and, to a major degree, to lack of commercial support from the device-manufacturing companies – in stark contrast with an abundance of educational materials for more established neuromodulation approaches of spinal cord stimulation and intrathecal drug delivery. Second, and probably just as important, is the paucity of scientific clinical and basic research work in support of the PNS approach, its safety, efficacy, and cost-effectiveness. Last and probably intimately related to the first two issues, is the lack of regulatory approval for PNS as a technical application for existing devices that are used for it in routine practice.

Unfortunately, this situation represents a somewhat vicious cycle – there are no marketing efforts from device manufacturers and distributors due to the lack of regulatory approval, and this approval will never be given unless the manufacturers apply for it. Lack of marketing efforts, low awareness and lack of educational materials have, for a long time, resulted in a low volume for this particular device application – and its off-label status and unlikely chance of getting insurance approval made the situation worse since low volumes translate into lack of clinical experience and difficulty in collecting sufficient clinical data to come up with any scientific information that would be needed to get the regulatory approval.

Despite all these hurdles, the field is developing rapidly, and the increasing number of publication regarding the use of the PNS approach supports its gradual acceptance by the neuromodulation community. The goal of this chapter is to briefly review the PNS history and to track the 40 some year long path from the original introduction to clinical practice to its current state.

Invention of PNS

For many centuries electricity has been used to treat a variety of human ailments. Therapeutic effects of electric shocks from torpedo fish were known in antiquity, and pain relief from electrical discharges of this Mediterranean ray was described by Scribonius Largus in patients with gout and headaches. The pain would get better when these patients touched the electric fish or when they put their feet into a pool with torpedo fish [1]. This approach to pain control apparently persisted for a very long time – and there is mention of the electric fish being used for pain control in early American plantations [2].

A more modern approach to peripheral electrical stimulation was introduced at the beginning of the 20th century when a consumer electrical device called Electreat was introduced for the treatment of pain and many other conditions [3]. This technology was later translated into a transcutaneous electrical nerve stimulation (TENS) that continues to be widely available today.

Before this, however, there was a very interesting description of electricity being used for pain control when directly applied to the peripheral sensory ('sentient') nerve. In 1859, Julius Althaus wrote the following [4]:

> . . .'a direct reduction of sensibility in a nerve can be accomplished in the following way: if a continuous, or a rapidly interrupted induced current of medium intensity is sent through the trunk of a nerve – say the ulnar, or the sciatic. . . and the action of the current be kept up for a quarter of an hour or more, the pain which is excited by this proceeding becomes much less, after a certain time, than it was at the beginning of the operation, and a feeling of numbness is produced in the limb. I do not mean to say that sensibility can be entirely destroyed by this local application of electricity, but I am quite satisfied that it is notably diminished by it. The result is much more striking if there is a morbid increase in sensibility in a nerve, as in the case in neuralgia, than if a nerve in its normal state is acted upon.'

He then went on to describe differential effects of cathodal and anodal stimulation on patients' perception, as well as the effect of increasing the frequency of stimulation, up to a certain limit, that produces a stronger decrease in nerve sensitivity – a surprising depth of observations with mid-19th century technology.

The true beginning of clinical PNS application or treatment of pain started in the 1960s. The creators of the 'gate control' theory of pain, Drs. Melzack and Wall, postulated in their article published in *Science* in 1965 that innocuous sensory information may suppress the transmission of pain [5]. Nonpainful information is delivered to a secondary afferent neuron (or the first central transmission cell) that also receives information from nociceptive afferents. The same large fibers that carry non-nociceptive information excite cells in the substantia gelatinosa that inhibit transmission of painful signals from the periphery.

Although this theory was based on serious experimental findings, clinical confirmation was needed to check its validity. In a follow-up paper called 'Temporary abolition of pain in man' published in 1967, Wall and Sweet demonstrated that nonpainful electrical stimulation of the peripheral nerve does indeed suppress pain perception in the area that it innervates. In a true spirit of science, they did it by inserting electrodes into their own infraorbital foramina [6].

Later, this was described in a book 'Pain and the Neurosurgeon' [7]:

> 'Turning from their animal studies to man, Wall and one of us (WHS) asked ourselves if artificially intense stimulation confined to the low-threshold A fibers could produce a clinically demonstrable reduction of pain. We first tested ourselves, using 0.1-ms square waves at 100 cps, sticking into our own infraorbital nerves needle electrodes insulated except for the tip. Tingling, buzzing or vibrating sensations were evoked in some portion of the sensory domain of our nerves at a voltage near the threshold. These were not unpleasant feelings and were always tolerable for an indefinite period. Moreover, we each had analgesia to pinprick in this area of paresthesia during the stimulation. But both the objective sensory loss and our subjective sensations returned rapidly to normal when the stimulus stopped.'

Soon thereafter, an implantable device was created and used in patients with chronic pain [8]. The first PNS surgery was done on a 26-year-old woman with clinical presentation consistent with a complex regional pain syndrome (CRPS) [7]:

> 'On October 9, 1965, Dr. Wall and one of us (Dr. W.H. Sweet) implanted a pair of silastic split-ring platinum electrodes around the ulnar and another pair around the median nerve in the arm carrying the wires out of the skin at the mid-forearm. On the median nerve 0.1-ms pulses at 100/s and 0.6 V provoked a pleasant tingling in the lateral three fingers and corresponding hand and stopped the pain in the medial three fingers and hand as well as tenderness in the third finger and palm.'

This quote clearly breaks the myth of PNS being a 'novel' modality as its clinical application for treatment of pain preceded, albeit by only a year or two, the introduction of spinal cord stimulation (SCS) by Shealy et al. [9].

PNS Progress: Early Years

The 50-year history of the clinical use of PNS may be divided into several distinct periods. The first period, a period of semi-experimental PNS use, started with the pioneering experience of Wall, Sweet, and others, and lasted for 15–20 years. That was a time when PNS surgery could be done only in a few leading centers – primarily due to the lack of commercially available equipment. Even before publication of the first series of 8 patients with neuropathic pain in whom stimulation resulted in lasting pain suppression as long as the stimulator was 'on' [6], Shelden [10] implanted PNS electrodes around the mandibular branch of the trigeminal nerve and stimulated them through an implanted receiver at 14 kHz achieving temporary relief of severe facial pain.

As a matter of fact, subsequent publications revealed that these implantations were performed as early as 1962, even before the 'gate control' theory of pain was introduced [11]. Shelden and colleagues in Pasadena, Calif., operated on 3 patients with third-division trigeminal neuralgia using a technique 'based on nerve depolarization'. Stimulation parameters allowed delivering up to 10 V of electricity at 14.5 kHz using a receiving unit connected to the mandibular division with platinum electrodes. The device was intended to be turned on when the patients experienced their pain attacks at frequent intervals throughout the day. The first of these 3 patients had complete relief of his pain with numbness in the sensory distribution of the stimulated nerve and after several weeks of stimulation experienced prolonged remission and then successfully used the device again when the pain recurred 7 years later. The second patient never used the device and remained pain free for more than 10 years. The third patient was pain free for 5 years but the device malfunctioned when the pain recurred. This was thought to be due to excessive fluid absorption by the silastic covering of the implant [11].

Over the following 10 years, multiple reports appeared in the literature dealing with various applications of PNS, summarizing experience with various types of equipment, and describing different surgical techniques for PNS electrode implantation. The articles that appeared in the 1970s and 1980s [12–27] mostly represented single-institution series with use of different electrodes that were implanted in direct contact or in close vicinity of the peripheral nerve, the same nerve that was thought to be responsible for the generation of pain either as a result of direct traumatic or iatrogenic injury or as a part of CRPS.

The use of 'cuff-type' electrodes, later supplemented or replaced by 'button-type' electrodes, was generally associated with good outcomes. In most series, good (more than 50%) pain relief was observed in the majority of patients. Longer follow-up showed a decrease in the percentage of patients experiencing significant improvement in pain intensity. For example, in 1976 Sweet [17] reported an overall long-term success rate of 25%, and in 1982, Nashold et al. [24] reported successful outcomes in 53% of patients with upper extremity nerve implants and only 31% of patients with sciatic nerve implantation, making a total success rate of less than 43%. The problems, however, included the need in surgical exposure of the nerve to be stimulated and difficulty in achieving adequate positioning of contacts for optimal paresthesia coverage [21]. In addition, multiple reports of nerve injury from electrode insertion or stimulation-related fibrosis made PNS less attractive [14, 28], particularly since the SCS approach became widely accepted as a means of long-term treatment of medically intractable neuropathic pain of various etiologies. Interestingly enough, the very-long-term follow-up of patients implanted with these cuff electrodes showed that the beneficial effects of PNS may last for longer than 20 years in a cohort of patients [29].

To overcome the need in surgical exposure of the peripheral nerve, a percutaneous trans-spinal technique of electrode insertion was developed where a cylindrical electrode was inserted through a downward-directed epidural needle and then advanced into the foramen next to the exiting nerve root [30]. The original report suggested using this approach for the combination of SCS and PNS, but later this technique was adapted for dedicated spinal root stimulation [31, 32].

A wealth of important information was gathered during the first two decades of PNS use. One of the phenomena reported at that time was increased responsiveness to stimulation in some of the stimulated patients. One of the reports noted that about third of PNS patients may reduce the amount of stimulation required to relieve pain after 6 months of stimulation [16]. Patients with peripheral nerve injuries treated with PNS described a decrease in their need for stimulation, and this took on average 1 year to occur. By then, the pain relief was satisfactory and the stimulator use infrequent [23].

Even during early PNS development, an importance of psychological evaluation and its value in patient selection was clearly identified. In addition to secondary gains, economical and noneconomical [15], various psychological and psychiatric conditions, such as depression, conversion disorder, hypochondriasis, and personality disorders were noted to be associated with poor prognosis [24]. It became clear that only formal psychiatric and psychological testing can reveal nonorganic issues, such as fear of failure, marital conflicts, financial gain, employment-related conflicts, all of which may affect the outcome of the patient's treatment [24].

PNS Progress: Maturation Stage

During the second period, starting in the mid-1980s, PNS was treated as an established surgical procedure. The electrode implantation involved surgical exploration of the peripheral nerve and placement of a flat plate ('paddle'-type) multi-contact electrode immediately next to it. Since these electrodes (such as Resume and Symmix, manufactured by Medtronic, Minneapolis, Minn., USA) were already widely used for SCS, there was no need in using cuff-like devices, and introduction of implantable pulse generators rather than previously used radiofrequency-coupled devices made long-term stimulation easier for the patients who did not have to carry an external stimulator and keep attaching the transmitting antennae to the skin above the internal receiver. After the first report by Racz et al. [33] in 1988 that illustrated details of this approach based on experience with 2 patients with CRPS type 2 (causalgia) due to electric burns 6 and 3 years earlier, multiple enthusiastic centers worldwide continued using PNS for various neuropathic pain syndromes [34–43], but the relative lack of interest among the majority of the implanters resulted in little effort from the device manufacturers in getting appropriate FDA approval for use of their implantable generators in PNS. Even now, according to the manufacturers' manuals, the only devices specifically approved for peripheral nerve stimulation are the radiofrequency systems made by Medtronic and the neuromodulation division of St. Jude Medical (formerly Advanced Neuromodulation Systems, Plano, Tex., USA). To make a more straightforward implantation of a paddle electrode next to the peripheral nerve to be stimulated, it was suggested to attach a special mesh to the paddle base [44]. This eventually resulted in development of a dedicated PNS paddle electrode with mesh integrated into the paddle (OnPoint, Medtronic).

Elimination of cuff-type electrodes resulted in decreasing the risk of perineural fibrosis, but did not make the implantation procedure less invasive and the entire process more conducive for a full-scale pre-implantation trial, similar to what is being done in the SCS field. As a matter of fact, the lack of predictability and true testability of the PNS approach was a major obstacle for wide acceptance of the technique. Early on, it was noted that a local anesthetic nerve block is not a predictor of pain relief with stimulation [17].

Later, an initial optimism regarding the use of TENS in the selection of PNS candidates [15] was cooled down by a larger and longer experience of the same group showing that the long-term success rate was essentially equal among those who did and did not respond to TENS prior to the PNS procedure [19]. The same conclusions were reached by another group of implanters earlier [14].

A slightly different approach was advocated by Long [12] in 1973 who suggested using a percutaneous electrical nerve stimulator with 18-gauge thin wall needles and cordotomy electrodes for the screening of PNS applicability. This practical suggestion, along with the initial experience of Wall and Sweet with infraorbital nerve stimulation [6], may be considered a prototype for the subsequently developed separate technique of percutaneous electrical nerve stimulation (PENS) reviewed later in this paper. To the best of our knowledge, however, the PENS approach did not become an accepted means of PNS screening although some centers continued using it on a regular basis [27].

The main accomplishments of the second period in PNS history were the definition of PNS indications and the stimulation parameters. Despite some concerns, PNS did not get completely replaced by the SCS approach, but remained a preferred option for those neuropathic conditions where a single and relatively easily reachable nerve was thought to be a culprit of pain generation. A larger series of patients with

CRPS type 1 (reflex sympathetic dystrophy) [36] and painful nerve injuries [39–42] summarized the experience with more than 150 patients and confirmed a relatively consistent pattern of long-term effectiveness in 55–78% of the patients without any major adverse events or complications.

Use of paddle electrodes for PNS application remains an accepted clinical approach. In addition to stimulation of large peripheral nerves in the extremities, paddle electrodes are used for occipital nerve stimulation for the treatment of occipital neuralgia and transformed migraines [45–47]. The main benefits of this approach are the unidirectional nature of stimulation as the contacts of each paddle are shielded by the insulated plastic base of the paddle, and the lower incidence of electrode migration due to geometry of the paddle. These very qualities, however, may become disadvantages, as for example in those situations where electrode position requires omnidirectional stimulation. Similarly, higher tissue resistance around the paddle electrode provides higher electrode stability but is associated with a higher incidence of electrode fractures. The most important issue, however, is the invasiveness of paddle electrode insertion that may be overcome once devices for percutaneous insertion of narrow paddle electrodes become available. An example of this may be an Epiducer device that accommodates a narrow paddle Lamitrode S series electrodes (both manufactured by St. Jude Medical) if it is ever adapted for extraspinal application.

PNS Progress: Percutaneous Era

The most recent, third period in PNS history started with the pioneering work of Weiner and Reed [48] that described a percutaneous technique of electrode insertion in the vicinity of the occipital nerves in order to treat occipital neuralgia. Although previously described for the treatment of occipital neuralgia and various headache disorders [19, 23, 27], PNS of the occipital nerve(s) did not become widely accepted due to discouraging initial results and a cumbersome process of the occipital nerve dissection needed for the application of wrap-around PNS electrode(s). Weiner's ingenious innovation was in showing that placing a PNS electrode in the proximity of the nerve is just as effective for pain relief and also more technically simple and less invasive.

Although percutaneous electrode insertion for PNS was mentioned as early as 1982 by Urban and Nashold [30] when the authors used an epidural needle to reach the contralateral intervertebral foramen and advanced a stimulating electrode toward the selected spinal nerve, this technique was used in conjunction with SCS but never took off as an accepted modality. But soon after Weiner's publication in 1999, Burchiel and others [49–56] described the use of this technique in both the occipital and trigeminal areas, and after that the approach was modified by many implanters in terms of electrode type, insertion procedure, indications, etc.

The original PNS indication of occipital neuralgia, both idiopathic and post-traumatic, used by Weiner in a cohort of 13 patients over a 6-year interval (1992–1998), evolved over time and subsequently included so-called cervicogenic headaches [52], pain due occipital neuroma [53] and craniofacial neuropathic pain [50]. Following this flurry of brief mentions, anecdotal reports and preliminary experiences, several larger series and detailed technical reports were published further establishing the practice of PNS with percutaneous electrodes [57–65]. Use of PNS for migraines, suggested by Popeney and Aló [57] based on experience with 25 patients in an uncontrolled study, was supported by subsequent clinical publications [66–69] and in-depth imaging study [70]. Subsequently, three neuromodulation device manufacturing companies (Medtronic, St. Jude Medical and Boston Scientific) launched prospective randomized studies to determine the benefits of occipital PNS for migraine patients; the high prevalence of migraines in the general population and a large number of medically intractable cases make this indication potentially the largest in PNS applications. In addition to occipital PNS with percutaneous electrodes, occipital PNS paddles [46] and a combination of supraorbital and occipital PNS [68, 69] have been tried for migraine treatment and prevention.

A rarer, usually just as disabling, and perhaps much more resistant to medical treatment, problem of cluster headaches became another indication for occipital PNS [71–75]. Here, occipital PNS is an alternative or a complement to hypothalamic deep brain stimulation, and much lower invasiveness with associated lower procedural risks make occipital PNS a preferred or initial surgical modality for cluster headache management. In addition to PNS aimed at the occipital nerves, supraorbital PNS has also been tried for cluster headache patients [76].

Supraorbital PNS has been used for a variety of indications – originally, it was suggested for ophthalmic postherpetic neuralgia [54, 58] and trigeminal neuropathic pain [50, 59, 64]. Larger series described the use of supraorbital PNS for supraorbital neuralgia [77], and more recently it was tried for migraines [68, 69] and cluster headaches [76].

The procedure was not limited to the upper neck and face area – other reports detailed the use of PNS in other parts of the body. For example, percutaneously inserted PNS electrodes were used for control of inguinal pain after herniorrhaphy [78], and paraspinal electrodes have been used for the treatment of low back and sacroiliac pain [79], thoracic postherpetic pain [80], scapular pain [81], as well as coccydynia [82]. Even the more traditional PNS indication – CRPS type 2 of the arm – has been successfully treated with percutaneous PNS [83]. In addition, a concept of stimulating the area that hurts culminated in development of modified PNS technique – subcutaneous neuromodulation targeted at the site of pain [84]. This approach has been refined in treatment of abdominal [85], low back [86–88] and neck pain [88, 89]. In addition to percutaneous electrodes, this subcutaneous/epifascial PNS application for localized pain syndromes was recently described with paddle leads as well [90].

Finding peripheral nerve for percutaneous PNS application may be challenging. In cases of supraorbital and infraorbital PNS, this does not seem to be a problem as the anatomical variability is rather minimal [59]. But in case of peripheral nerves in extremities, it may require real-time ultrasound guidance. After initial cadaver-based evaluation [91, 92], this approach was successfully used in clinical practice [93, 94]. Moreover, ultrasound guidance was suggested for the insertion of occipital PNS electrodes in order to reduce the distance between the stimulating electrode and the targeted nerve(s) [95].

Percutaneous Nerve Stimulation

A slightly different direction that employs a similar principle has been explored in the last few decades for the treatment of pain. If the initial experience of Shelden and colleagues [10, 11] with implanted electrodes and receivers became a prototype for true PNS, the experiments of Wall and Sweet [6] that used temporary electrodes for the temporary suppression of pain may be considered a prototype of so-called percutaneous electrical nerve stimulation (PENS).

PENS treatment is performed with bipolar needle-like electrodes that are inserted into the tissues (as opposed to TENS where electrical stimulation is delivered through the skin) and then removed at the end of the treatment session. This approach was used in the treatment of low back pain [96–99], sciatica [100], diabetic neuropathic pain [101], and headaches [102, 103]. It was also tried in the treatment of acute herpetic pain [104] and pain due to bone metastases [105].

Despite thorough analysis of all the stimulation parameters (duration, frequency, electrode montage and location) and their effects on treatment results [106–109], PENS did not become widely accepted – although the recent introduction of a commercially available PENS apparatus (Algotech Ltd., West Sussex, UK) may change the level of interest to this relatively noninvasive neuromodulation approach.

PNS Progress: Recent Advancements

The newest trends in PNS have to do with new indications, new devices, new techniques and new terminology. As the field of PNS rapidly evolves, all of these aspects translate into a large number of publications and research projects stimulating individual investigators and multidisciplinary collaboration.

One of the most fascinating developments with PNS was the discovery of its global pain-relieving effect on patients with fibromyalgia [110, 111]. A larger study of this particular indication for occipital PNS is currently underway. A similar study of neuromodulation in fibromyalgia evaluates the effects of vagal nerve stimulation on this disabling condition [112]. Interestingly enough, the vagal nerve stimulation procedure that is widely used for the treatment of epilepsy and has some potential in the treatment of refractory depression has also been tried for the treatment of migraines and cluster headaches [113].

The general trend for lowering invasiveness and reducing surgical trauma became the reason for the development of a new PNS device that may potentially revolutionize the entire PNS field. Introduced about 10 years ago [114, 115], this miniaturized rechargeable stimulation device (Bion, Boston Scientific, Valencia, Calif., USA) has been tested in variety of clinical applications. In its current shape and size, it was used in the treatment of urinary incontinence [116] and subsequently tried for the treatment of severe headaches [117, 118]. In a series of patients with hemicrania continua, the Bion stimulator provided significant pain reduction (80–95%) in 4 of 6 patients at the latest follow-up [117]. A different group of implanters documented sustained improvement in headache intensity in a majority of patients treated with Bion [118]. Neither report showed any major complication, such as infection, erosion or migration of the microstimulator device.

With wider acceptance of PNS in the neuromodulation community, multiple reports focused on surgical and device-related complications associated with PNS use [119, 120]. The high frequency of electrode migrations, erosions and disconnections prompted the development of surgical techniques aimed at a minimization of operative mishaps and refinement of the implantation procedure [121–123].

Finally, the issues regarding the exact procedural meaning and variations in PNS spectrum of interventions stirred discussion and controversy. Some of the recent publications address this in a constructive manner [124, 125], but there is a good chance that this discussion will continue as newer approaches emerge in addition to or instead of existing traditional interventions.

Conclusion

Despite almost a half-century-long history, PNS appears to be both understudied and underutilized in modern neuromodulation practice. As the most rapidly growing segment of operative neuromodulation, PNS will continue to evolve as current and emerging clinical indications become matched by basic and clinical research, technological developments and procedural refinements.

References

1 Rode J: Scribonius (Largus). Padua, Compositiones Medicae, 1655, pp 23–24.
2 Kellaway P: The part played by electric fish in the early history of bioelectricity and electrotherapy. Bull Hist Med 1946;20:112–137.
3 Gildenberg PL: History of electrical neuromodulation for chronic pain. Pain Med 2006;7:S7–S13.
4 Althaus J: A Treatise on Medical Electricity, Theoretical and Practical; and Its Use in the Treatment of Paralysis, Neuralgia, and Other Diseases. Philadelphia, Lindsay & Blakiston, 1860, pp 163–170.
5 Melzack RA, Wall PD: Pain mechanisms: a new theory. Science 1965;150:971–979.
6 Wall PD, Sweet WH: Temporary abolition of pain in man. Science 1967;155:108–109.
7 White JC, Sweet WH: Pain and the Neurosurgeon: A Forty-Year Experience. Springfield, Thomas, 1969, pp 894–899.
8 Sweet WH, Wepsic JG: Treatment of chronic pain by stimulation of fibers of primary afferent neuron. Trans Am Neurol Assoc 1968;93:103–107.
9 Shealy CN, Mortimer JT, Reswick JB: Electrical inhibition of pain by stimulation of the dorsal columns: preliminary clinical report. Anesth Analg 1967;46:489–491.
10 Shelden CH: Depolarization in the treatment of trigeminal neuralgia: evaluation of compression and electrical methods; clinical concept of neurophysiological mechanism; in Knighton RS, Dumke PR (eds): Pain. Boston, Little, Brown, 1966, pp 373–386.
11 Shelden CH, Paul F, Jacques DB, Pudenz RH: Electrical stimulation of the nervous system. Surg Neurol 1975;4:127–132.
12 Long DM: Electrical stimulation for relief of pain from chronic nerve injury. J Neurosurg 1973;39:718–722.
13 Cauthen JC, Renner EJ: Transcutaneous and peripheral nerve stimulation for chronic pain states. Surg Neurol 1975;4:102–104.
14 Kirsch WM, Lewis JA, Simon RH: Experiences with electrical stimulation devices for the control of chronic pain. Med Instrum 1975;9:217–220.
15 Picaza JA, Cannon BW, Hunter SE, Boyd AS, Guma J, Maurer D: Pain suppression by peripheral nerve stimulation. II. Observations with implanted devices. Surg Neurol 1975;4:115–126.
16 Nashold BS Jr, Goldner JL: Electrical stimulation of peripheral nerves for relief of intractable chronic pain. Med Instrum 1975;9:224–225.
17 Sweet WH: Control of pain by direct electrical stimulation of peripheral nerves. Clin Neurosurg 1976; 23:103–111.
18 Campbell JN, Long DM: Peripheral nerve stimulation in the treatment of intractable pain. J Neurosurg 1976;45:692–699.
19 Picaza JA, Hunter SE, Cannon BW: Pain suppression by peripheral nerve stimulation: chronic effects of implanted devices. Appl Neurophysiol 1977–1978;40:223–234.
20 Nashold BS Jr, Mullen JB, Avery R: Peripheral nerve stimulation for pain relief using a multicontact electrode system: technical note. J Neurosurg 1979;51: 872–873.
21 Law JD, Sweet J, Kirsch WM: Retrospective analysis of 22 patients with chronic pain treated by peripheral nerve stimulation. J Neurosurg 1980;52:482–485.
22 Nashold BS: Peripheral nerve stimulation for pain. J Neurosurg 1980;53:132–133.
23 Long DM, Erickson D, Campbell J, North R: Electrical stimulation of the spinal cord and peripheral nerves for pain control: a 10-year experience. Appl Neurophysiol 1981;44:207–217.
24 Nashold BS Jr, Goldner JL, Mullen JB, Bright DS: Long-term pain control by direct peripheral-nerve stimulation. J Bone Joint Surg Am 1982;64:1–10.
25 Goldner JL, Nashold BS Jr, Hendrix PC: Peripheral nerve electrical stimulation. Clin Orthop Relat Res 1982;163:33–41.
26 Long DM: Stimulation of the peripheral nervous system for pain control. Clin Neurosurg 1983;31: 323–343.
27 Waisbrod H, Panhans C, Hansen D, Gerbeshagen HU: Direct nerve stimulation for painful peripheral neuropathies. J Bone Joint Surg (Br) 1985;67:470–472.
28 Nielson KD, Watts C, Clark WK: Peripheral nerve injury from implantation of chronic stimulating electrodes for pain control. Surg Neurol 1976;5:51–53.
29 Van Calenbergh F, Gybels J, Van Laere K, et al: Long term clinical outcome of peripheral nerve stimulation in patients with chronic peripheral neuropathic pain. Surg Neurol 2009;72:330–335.
30 Urban BJ, Nashold BS Jr: Combined epidural and peripheral nerve stimulation for relief of pain. Description of technique and preliminary results. J Neurosurg 1982;57:365–369.
31 Aló KM, Yland MJ, Redko V, Feler C, Naumann C: Lumbar and sacral nerve root stimulation (NRS) in the treatment of chronic pain: a novel anatomic approach and neurostimulation technique. Neuromodulation 1999;2:23–31.
32 Haque R, Winfree CJ: Spinal nerve root stimulation. Neurosurg Focus 2006;21:E4.

33 Racz GB, Browne T, Lewis R Jr: Peripheral stimulator implant for treatment of causalgia caused by electrical burns. Tex Med 1988;84:45–50.

34 Strege DW, Cooney WP, Wood MB, Johnson SJ, Metcalf BJ: Chronic peripheral nerve pain treated with direct electrical nerve stimulation. J Hand Surg Am 1994;19:931–939.

35 Heavner JE, Racz G, Diede JM: Peripheral nerve stimulation: current concepts; in Waldman SD, Winnie AP (eds): Interventional Pain Management. Philadelphia, Saunders, 1996, pp 423–425.

36 Hassenbusch SJ, Stanton-Hicks M, Schoppa D, Walsh JG, Covington EC: Long-term results of peripheral nerve stimulation for reflex sympathetic dystrophy. J Neurosurg 1996;84:415–423.

37 Stanton-Hicks M, Salamon J: Stimulation of the central and peripheral nervous system for the control of pain. J Clin Neurophysiol 1997;14:46–62.

38 Shetter AG, Racz GB, Lewis R, Heavner JE: Peripheral nerve stimulation; in North RB, Levy RM (eds): Neurosurgical Management of Pain. New York: Springer, 1997, pp 261–270.

39 Ebel H, Balogh A, Volz M, Klug N: Augmentative treatment of chronic deafferentiation pain syndromes after peripheral nerve lesions. Minim Invasive Neurosurg 2000;43:44–50.

40 Novak CB, Mackinnon SE: Outcome following implantation of a peripheral nerve stimulator in patients with chronic nerve pain. Plast Reconstr Surg 2000;105:1967–1972.

41 Eisenberg E, Waisbrod H, Gerbershagen HU: Long-term peripheral nerve stimulation for painful nerve injuries. Clin J Pain 2004;20:143–146.

42 Mobbs RJ, Nair S, Blum P: Peripheral nerve stimulation for the treatment of chronic pain. J Clin Neurosci 2007;14:216–223.

43 Jeon IC, Kim MS, Kim SH: Median nerve stimulation in a patient with complex regional pain syndrome type II. J Korean Neurosurg Soc 2009;46: 273–276 .

44 Mobbs RJ, Blum P, Rossato R: Mesh electrode for peripheral nerve stimulation. J Clin Neurosci 2003; 10:476–477.

45 Jones RL: Occipital nerve stimulation using a Medtronic Resume II® electrode array. Pain Physician 2003;6:507–508.

46 Oh MY, Ortega J, Bellotte JB, Whiting DM, Aló K: Peripheral nerve stimulation for the treatment of occipital neuralgia and transformed migraine using a C1–2–3 subcutaneous paddle style electrode: a technical report. Neuromodulation 2004;7:103–112.

47 Kapural L, Mekhail N, Hayek SM, Stanton-Hicks M, Malak O: Occipital nerve electrical stimulation via the midline approach and subcutaneous surgical leads for treatment of severe occipital neuralgia: a pilot study. Anesth Analg 2005;101:171–174.

48 Weiner RL, Reed KL: Peripheral neurostimulation for control of intractable occipital neuralgia. Neuromodulation 1999;2:217–221.

49 Slavin KV, Burchiel KJ: Peripheral nerve stimulation for painful nerve injuries. Contemp Neurosurg 1999;21:1–6.

50 Slavin KV, Burchiel KJ: Use of long-term nerve stimulation with implanted electrodes in the treatment of intractable craniofacial pain. J Neurosurg 2000;92:576.

51 Weiner RL: The future of peripheral nerve stimulation. Neurol Res 2000;22:299–304.

52 Weiner RL, Aló KM, Reed KL, Fuller ML: Subcutaneous neurostimulation for intractable C-2–mediated headaches. J Neurosurg 2001;94:398A.

53 Hammer M, Doleys DM: Perineuromal stimulation in the treatment of occipital neuralgia: a case study. Neuromodulation 2001;4:47–51.

54 Dunteman E: Peripheral nerve stimulation for unremitting ophthalmic postherpetic neuralgia. Neuromodulation 2002;5:32–37.

55 Aló KM, Holsheimer J: New trends in neuromodulation for the management of neuropathic pain. Neurosurgery 2002;50:690–704.

56 Weiner RL: Peripheral nerve neurostimulation. Neurosurg Clin N Am 2003;14:401–408.

57 Popeney CA, Aló KM: Peripheral neurostimulation for the treatment of chronic, disabling transformed migraine. Headache 2003;43:369–375.

58 Johnson MD, Burchiel KJ: Peripheral stimulation for treatment of trigeminal postherpetic neuralgia and trigeminal posttraumatic neuropathic pain: a pilot study. Neurosurgery 2004;55:135–142.

59 Slavin KV, Wess C: Trigeminal branch stimulation for intractable neuropathic pain: technical note. Neuromodulation 2005;8:7–13.

60 Rodrigo-Royo MD, Azcona JM, Quero J, Lorente MC, Acín P, Azcona J: Peripheral neurostimulation in the management of cervicogenic headaches: four case reports. Neuromodulation 2005;4:241–248.

61 Slavin KV, Nersesyan H, Wess C: Peripheral neurostimulation for treatment of intractable occipital neuralgia. Neurosurgery 2006;58:128–132.

62 Johnstone CS, Sundaraj R: Occipital nerve stimulation for the treatment of occipital neuralgia: eight case studies. Neuromodulation 2006;9:41–47.

63 Weiner RL: Occipital neurostimulation (ONS) for treatment of intractable headache disorders. Pain Med 2006;7:S137–S139.

64 Slavin KV, Colpan ME, Munawar N, Wess C, Nersesyan H: Trigeminal and occipital peripheral nerve stimulation for craniofacial pain: a single-institution experience and review of the literature. Neurosurg Focus 2006;21:E5.
65 Schwedt TJ, Dodick DW, Hentz J, Trentman TL, Zimmerman RS: Occipital nerve stimulation for chronic headache – long-term safety and efficacy. Cephalalgia 2007;27:153–157.
66 Rogers LL, Swidan S: Stimulation of the occipital nerve for the treatment of migraine: current state and future prospects. Acta Neurochir Suppl 2007; 97:121–128.
67 Hagen JE, Bennett DS: Occipital nerve stimulation for treatment of migraine. Pract Pain Managem 2007;7:43–45, 56.
68 Reed KL, Black SB, Banta CJ II, Will KR: Combined occipital and supraorbital neurostimulation for the treatment of chronic migraine headaches: initial experience. Cephalalgia 2010;30:260–271.
69 Burns B: 'Dual' occipital and supraorbital nerve stimulation for primary headache. Cephalalgia 2010;30:257–259.
70 Matharu MS, Bartsch, Ward N, Frackowiak RSJ, Weiner R, Goadsby PJ: Central neuromodulation in chronic migraine patients with suboccipital stimulators: a PET study. Brain 2004;127:220–230.
71 Schwedt TJ, Dodick DW, Trentman TL, Zimmerman RS: Occipital nerve stimulation for chronic cluster headache and hemicrania continua: pain relief and persistence of autonomic features. Cephalalgia 2006; 26:1025–1027.
72 Burns B, Watkins L, Goadsby PJ: Treatment of medically intractable cluster headache by occipital nerve stimulation: long-term follow-up of eight patients. Lancet 2007;369:1099–1106.
73 Magis D, Allena M, Bolla M, De Pasqua V, Remacle JM, Schoenen J: Occipital nerve stimulation for drug-resistant chronic cluster headache: a prospective pilot study. Lancet Neurol 2007;6:314–321.
74 Leone M, Franzini A, Cecchini AP, Broggi G, Bussone G: Stimulation of occipital nerve for drug-resistant chronic cluster headache. Lancet Neurol 2007;6:289–291.
75 Burns B, Watkins L, Goadsby PJ: Treatment of intractable chronic cluster headache by occipital nerve stimulation in 14 patients. Neurology 2009; 72:341–345.
76 Narouze SN, Kapural L: Supraorbital nerve electric stimulation for the treatment of intractable chronic cluster headache: a case report. Headache 2007;47: 1100–1102.
77 Amin S, Buvanendran A, Park K-S, Kroin JS, Moric M: Peripheral nerve stimulator for the treatment of supraorbital neuralgia: a retrospective case series. Cephalalgia 2008;28:355–359.
78 Stinson LW Jr, Roderer GT, Cross NE, Davis BE: Peripheral subcutaneous electrostimulation for control of intractable post-operative inguinal pain: a case report series. Neuromodulation 2001;4:99–104.
79 Paicius RM, Bernstein CA, Lempert-Cohen C: Peripheral nerve field stimulation for the treatment of chronic low back pain: preliminary results of long-term follow-up: a case series. Neuromodulation 2007;10:279–290.
80 Yakovlev AE, Peterson AT: Peripheral nerve stimulation in treatment of intractable postherpetic neuralgia. Neuromodulation 2007;10:373–375.
81 Theodosiadis P, Samoladas E, Grosomanidis V, Goroszeniuk T, Kothari S: A case of successful treatment of neuropathic pain after a scapular fracture using subcutaneous targeted neuromodulation. Neuromodulation 2008;11:62–65.
82 Kothari S: Neuromodulatory approaches to chronic pelvic pain and coccygodynia. Acta Neurochir Suppl 2007;97:365–371.
83 Monti E: Peripheral nerve stimulation: a percutaneous minimally invasive approach. Neuromodulation 2004;7:193–196.
84 Goroszeniuk T, Kothari S, Hamann W: Subcutaneous neuromodulating implant targeted at the site of pain. Reg Anesth Pain Med 2006;31:168–171.
85 Paicius RM, Bernstein CA, Lempert-Cohen C: Peripheral nerve field stimulation in chronic abdominal pain. Pain Physician 2006;9:261–266.
86 Krutsch JP, McCeney MH, Barolat G, Al Tamimi M, Smolenski A: A case report of subcutaneous peripheral nerve stimulation for the treatment of axial back pain associated with postlaminectomy syndrome. Neuromodulation 2008;11:112–115.
87 Falco FJE, Berger J, Vrable A, Onyewu O, Zhu J: Cross talk: a new method for peripheral nerve stimulation: an observational report with cadaveric verification. Pain Physician 2009;12:965–983.
88 Reverberi C, Bonezzi C, Demartini L: Peripheral subcutaneous neurostimulation in the management of neuropathic pain: five case reports. Neuromodulation 2009;12:146–155.
89 Lipov EG, Joshi JR, Sanders S, Slavin KV: Use of peripheral subcutaneous field stimulation for the treatment of axial neck pain: a case report. Neuromodulation 2009;12:292–295.
90 Ordia J, Vaisman J: Subcutaneous peripheral nerve stimulation with paddle lead for treatment of low back pain: case report. Neuromodulation 2009;12: 205–209.
91 Huntoon MA, Huntoon EA, Obray JB, Lamer TJ: Feasibility of ultrasound-guided percutaneous placement of peripheral nerve stimulation electrodes in a cadaver model: Part one, lower extremity. Reg Anesth Pain Med 2008;33:551–557.

92 Huntoon MA, Hoelzer BC, Burgher AH, Hurdle MF, Huntoon EA: Feasibility of ultrasound-guided percutaneous placement of peripheral nerve stimulation electrodes and anchoring during simulated movement. II. Upper extremity. Reg Anesth Pain Med 2008;33:558–565.
93 Narouze SN, Zakari A, Vydyanathan A: Ultrasound-guided placement of a permanent percutaneous femoral nerve stimulator leads for the treatment of intractable femoral neuropathy. Pain Physician 2009;12:E305–E308.
94 Huntoon MA, Burgher AH: Ultrasound-guided permanent implantation of peripheral nerve stimulation (PNS) system for neuropathic pain of the extremities: original cases and outcomes. Pain Med 2009;10:1369–1377.
95 Skaribas I, Aló K: Ultrasound imaging and occipital nerve stimulation. Neuromodulation 2010;13:126–130.
96 Ghoname EA, Craig WF, White PF, et al: Percutaneous electrical nerve stimulation for low back pain: a randomized crossover study. JAMA 1999;281:818–823.
97 Weiner DK, Rudy TE, Glick RM, et al: Efficacy of percutaneous electrical nerve stimulation for the treatment of chronic low back pain in older adults. J Am Geriatr Soc 2003;51:599–608.
98 Yokoyama M, Sun X, Oku S, et al: Comparison of percutaneous electrical nerve stimulation with transcutaneous electrical nerve stimulation for long-term pain relief in patients with chronic low back pain. Anesth Analg 2004;98:1552–1556.
99 Weiner DK, Perera S, Rudy TE, Glick RM, Shenoy S, Delitto A: Efficacy of percutaneous electrical nerve stimulation and therapeutic exercise for older adults with chronic low back pain: a randomized controlled trial. Pain 2008;140:344–357.
100 Ghoname EA, White PF, Ahmed HE, Hamza MA, Craig WF, Noe CE: Percutaneous electrical nerve stimulation: an alternative to TENS in the management of sciatica. Pain 1999;83:193–199.
101 Hamza MA, White PF, Craig WF, et al: Percutaneous electrical nerve stimulation: a novel analgesic therapy for diabetic neuropathic pain. Diabetes Care 2000;23:365–370.
102 Ghoname EA, Craig WF, White PF: Use of percutaneous electrical nerve stimulation (PENS) for treating ECT-induced headaches. Headache 1999;39:502–505.
103 Ahmed HE, White PF, Craig WF, Hamza MA, Ghoname ES, Gajraj NM: Use of percutaneous electrical nerve stimulation (PENS) in the short-term management of headache. Headache 2000;40:311–315.
104 Ahmed HE, Craig WF, White PF, et al: Percutaneous electrical nerve stimulation: an alternative to antiviral drugs for acute herpes zoster. Anesth Analg 1998;87:911–914.
105 Ahmed HE, Craig WF, White PF, Huber P: Percutaneous electrical nerve stimulation (PENS): a complementary therapy for the management of pain secondary to bony metastasis. Clin J Pain 1998;14:320–323.
106 Hamza MA, Ghoname EA, White PF, et al: Effect of the duration of electrical stimulation on the analgesic response in patients with low back pain. Anesthesiology 1999;91:1622–1627.
107 Ghoname ES, Craig WF, White PF, et al: The effect of stimulus frequency on the analgesic response to percutaneous electrical nerve stimulation in patients with chronic low back pain. Anesth Analg 1999;88:841–846.
108 White PF, Ghoname EA, Ahmed HE, Hamza MA, Craig WF, Vakharia AS: The effect of montage on the analgesic response to percutaneous neuromodulation therapy. Anesth Analg 2001;92:483–487.
109 White PF, Craig WF, Vakharia AS, Ghoname E, Ahmed HE, Hamza MA: Percutaneous neuromodulation therapy: does the location of electrical stimulation affect the acute analgesic response? Anesth Analg 2000;91:949–954.
110 Thimineur M, De Ridder D: C2 area neurostimulation: a surgical treatment for fibromyalgia. Pain Med 2007;8:639–646.
111 Slavin KV: Peripheral neurostimulation in fibromyalgia: a new frontier. Pain Med 2007;8:621–622.
112 http://clinicaltrials.gov/ct2/show/NCT00294281.
113 Mauskop A: Vagus nerve stimulation relieves chronic refractory migraine and cluster headaches. Cephalalgia 2005;25:82–86.
114 Loeb GE, Peck RA, Moore WH, Hood K: BION™ system for distribute neural prosthetic interfaces. Med Eng Physics 2001;23:9–18.
115 Carbunaru R, Whitehurst T, Jaax K, Koff J, Makous J: Rechargeable battery-powered Bion microstimulators for neuromodulation. Conf Proc IEEE Eng Med Biol Soc 2004;6:4193–4196.
116 Groen J, Amiel C, Bosch JL: Chronic pudendal nerve neuromodulation in women with idiopathic refractory detrusor overactivity incontinence: results of a pilot study with a novel minimally invasive implantable mini-stimulator. Neurourol Urodyn 2005;24:226–230.
117 Burns B, Watkins L, Goadsby PJ: Treatment of hemicrania continua by occipital nerve stimulation with a Bion device: long-term follow-up of a crossover study. Lancet Neurol 2008;7:1001–1012.

118 Trentman TL, Rosenfeld DM, Vargas BB, Schwedt TJ, Zimmerman RS, Dodick DW: Greater occipital nerve stimulation via the Bion microstimulator: implantation technique and stimulation parameters. Clinical trial: NCT00205894. Pain Physician 2009;12:621–628.
119 Falowski S, Wang D, Sabesan A, Sharan A: Occipital nerve stimulator systems: review of complications and surgical techniques. Neuromodulation 2010;13:121–125.
120 Jasper JF, Hayek SM: Implanted occipital nerve stimulators. Pain Physician 2008;11:187–200.
121 Gofeld M: Anchoring of suboccipital lead: case report and technical note. Pain Pract 2004;4:307–309.
122 Franzini A, Messina G, Leone M, Broggi G: Occipital nerve stimulation (ONS). Surgical technique and prevention of late electrode migration. Acta Neurochir (Wien) 2009;151:861–865.
123 Trentman TL, Slavin KV, Freeman JA, Zimmerman RS: Occipital nerve stimulator placement via a retromastoid to infraclavicular approach: a technical report. Stereotact Funct Neurosurg 2010;88:121–125.
124 Slavin KV: Peripheral nerve stimulation for neuropathic pain. Neurotherapeutics 2008;5:100–106.
125 Abejón D, Krames ES: Peripheral nerve stimulation or is it peripheral subcutaneous field stimulation; what is in a moniker? Neuromodulation 2009;12:1–4.

Konstantin V. Slavin, MD
University of Illinois at Chicago
Department of Neurosurgery, M/C 799
912 South Wood Street
Chicago, IL 60612 (USA)
Tel. +1 312 996 4842, Fax +1 312 996 9018, E-Mail kslavin@uic.edu

Slavin KV (ed): Peripheral Nerve Stimulation.
Prog Neurol Surg. Basel, Karger, 2011, vol 24, pp 16–26

Central Mechanisms of Peripheral Nerve Stimulation in Headache Disorders

Thorsten Bartsch[a] · Peter J. Goadsby[b]

[a]Department of Neurology, University Hospital of Schleswig Holstein, University of Kiel, Kiel, Germany; [b]Headache Group, Department of Neurology, University of California, San Francisco, San Francisco, Calif., USA

Abstract

The effect of peripheral neurostimulation has traditionally been attributed to the activation of non-noxious afferent nerve fibers (Aβ-fibers) thought to modulate Aδ and C-fiber-mediated nociceptive transmission in the spinal cord, compatible with the 'gate control theory of pain'. The concept has been extended since its initial description and more recent experimental evidence suggests that the analgesic effects of peripheral nerve stimulation in pain states such as in chronic headache require an interplay of multiple influences. Besides segmental pain-modulating mechanisms in the spinal cord involving various transmitter systems, experimental evidence suggests also a contribution of descending pain modulating pathways in mediating the analgesic effect of peripheral nerve stimulation. Beyond the concept of neuromodulation – decreasing excitation or increasing inhibition – a prerequisite of this arrangement is the convergence of different types of afferent activity and an intact descending modulatory network. In this review, we focus on the functional anatomy, pathophysiological mechanisms and neurophysiological and pharmacological findings elucidating the central mechanisms of peripheral nerve stimulation.

It is very well known that a non-painful stimulation of peripheral nerves can elicit analgesic effects [1, 2]. This phenomenon has been used in certain pain syndromes using non-invasive per- or transcutaneous electrical nerve stimulation (high- and low-frequency transcutaneous nerve stimulation; TENS), percutaneous electrical nerve stimulation (PENS/acupuncture-like TENS; AL-TENS) and spinal cord stimulation (SCS). The analgesic effect is critically dependent on the intensity of the electrical stimulation. In recent years, peripheral nerve stimulation (PNS) has been also applied to patients with medically intractable chronic headaches.

Gate Control Theory of Pain

Traditionally, the effect of peripheral neurostimulation has been attributed to the activation of non-noxious afferent nerve fibers (Aβ-fibers) which is thought to modulate Aδ and C-fiber-mediated nociceptive transmission in the spinal cord, compatible with the 'gate control theory of pain'. The understanding of pain – modulatory mechanisms in the spinal cord as well as in the supraspinal structures has been greatly advanced by the 'gate control theory' by Melzack and Wall [3]. Although considerably extended and modified since then, this framework in essence proposed that the transmission of pain in the spinal cord is modulated by excitatory and inhibitory influences [4]. These influences may arise from intrinsic factors within the spinal cord or from supraspinal projections onto the spinal cord, or both. This short- and long-lasting relay function of the spinal cord may play an important role in pathophysiological pain states, such as in persistent pain, central sensitization, hyperalgesia and allodynia [5]. The concept of modulation also implies a changeable, plastic transmission. Besides the concept of modulation – decreasing excitation or increasing inhibition –, a prerequisite of this arrangement is the convergence of different types of afferent activity. Another prerequisite of an adequate effect of PNS is an intact descending modulatory network. In accordance with the gate control theory outlined above, a similar interplay of multiple mechanisms of segmental spinal inhibiting effects and descending pain inhibitory pathways may mediate the analgesic effects of PNS.

Central Mechanisms of Pain Processing: Central Sensitization and Descending Inhibition

Nociceptive spinal cord neurons can be sensitized due to a strong afferent stimulation by small-fiber afferents. This hyperexcitability is reflected in a reduction of the activation threshold, an increased responsiveness to afferent stimulation, an enlargement of receptive fields or the emergence of new receptive fields and the recruitment of 'silent' nociceptive afferents. The clinical correlates of this central hypersensitivity in migraine patients include the development of spontaneous pain, hyperalgesia and allodynia [5, 6]. The hypersensitivity of the afferent synaptic input in the spinal cord is thought to be due to the stimulation-induced release of various neuropeptides, such as CGRP, or to augmented glutamate release and action at the NMDA receptor, but may also be due to decrease of local segmental spinal inhibition in response to the afferent stimulation [5, 7].

These stimulation-induced neuroplastic changes could also be found in the neural population of the trigeminocervical complex that received convergent synaptic input from the dura mater and the greater occipital nerve (GON) [8]. Noxious stimulation of the dura mater was eliciting facilitated responses in the GON and vice versa. These findings highlight the potential of dura-GON-sensitive neurons in the trigeminocervical complex to undergo a central sensitization with an increased excitability to converging synaptic inputs. This shows that dural afferents and GON afferents do not just represent an anatomical connection, but that these connections are functionally relevant in terms of mutual changes of excitability.

The above-described mechanisms of convergence and central sensitization are important to understand the clinical phenomena of spread and referral of pain by which pain originating from an affected tissue is perceived as originating from a distant receptive field that does not necessarily involve a peripheral pathology in the cervical innervation territory [9, 10].

It is now well established that the nociceptive inflow to second-order neurons in the spinal cord and the trigeminocervical complex is subject to a modulation by descending inhibitory projections from brainstem structures such as the periaqueductal gray (PAG), nucleus raphe magnus (NRM) and the rostroventral medulla (RVM) [11–14] as stimulation of these regions produces profound antinociception [15, 16]. In particular, recent findings suggest that the ventrolateral division of the PAG (vlPAG) has a pivotal role in trigeminal nociception as stimulation of the vlPAG modulates dural nociception and selectively receives input from trigeminovascular afferents [17–21] (fig. 1).

In recent years it emerged that the pain-modulating circuits in the brainstem are not only involved in antinociception but, under certain conditions, also in the facilitation of central sensitization and secondary hyperalgesia [22, 23]. These findings suggest the possibility that the level of excitability of dura-sensitive neurons in the trigeminocervical complex could be increased by, possibly dysfunctional, brainstem pain-modulatory structures.

Spinal Mechanisms

In accordance with the gate control theory outlined above, a similar interplay of multiple mechanisms on the spinal cord may contribute to the analgesic effects of PNS. Earlier studies in animals showed a decreased activity in dorsal horn cells in both, spontaneous activity and nociceptive evoked responses during TENS [24, 25]. However, despite similar effects as well as values of stimulation parameters in TENS and PNS, it is not entirely clear if both methods share the same neuromodulatory mechanisms. As in SCS, PNS may also decrease long-term potentiation of nociceptive wide dynamic range neurons in the spinal dorsal horn [26, 27]. With regard to the pathophysiological mechanisms involved in acute and persistent pain states, as outlined above, TENS may depotentiate central sensitization mechanisms in the dorsal horn including secondary hyperalgesia [28, 29].

In recent years, it emerged that several neurotransmitter systems are involved in segmental spinal cord effects of TENS (fig. 1). Low frequency TENS activates serotoninergic (5-HT2 and 5-HT3) synaptic transmission, probably reflecting the activation of descending serotoninergic pathways [30–32]. Inhibitory projections in the spinal cord are also activated via gamma-aminobutyric acid (GABA) (A) receptors as TENS increases extracellular GABA concentrations and the effect of PNS is prevented by the blockade of spinal GABA(A) receptors [30, 33]. Using spinal microdialysis in

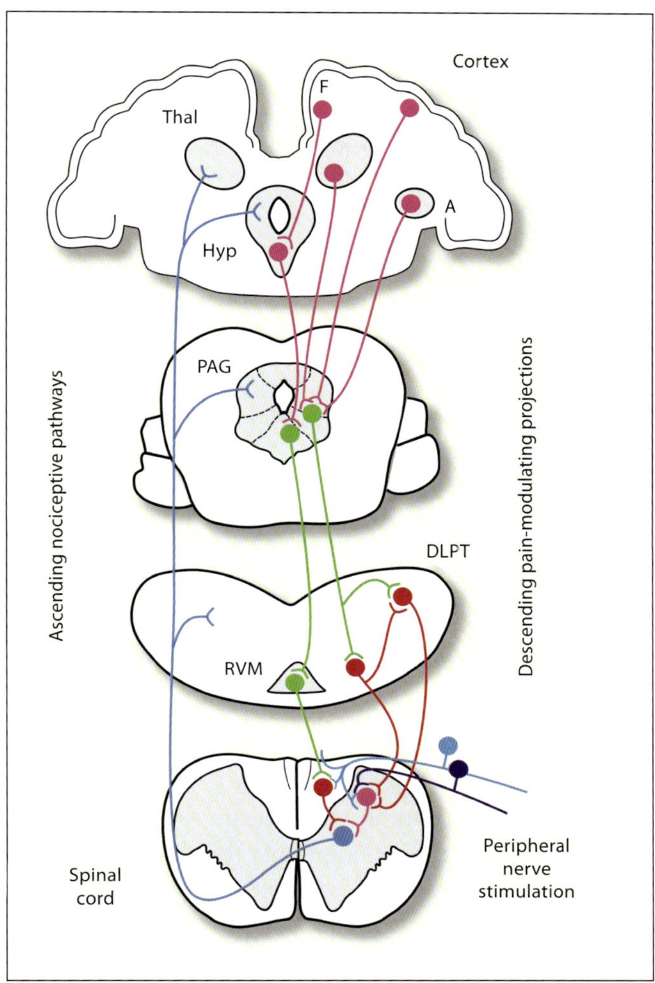

Fig. 1. Schematic drawing illustrating the functional anatomy of pain-modulatory pathways in the spinal cord and supraspinal structures. Nociceptive and non-nociceptive information is relayed in the spinal dorsal horn where it subject to segmental modulatory mechanisms either intrinsic or extrinsic from descending projections. The convergent neuron in the dorsal horn may be sensitized due to an increased afferent inflow into the spinal cord by strong noxious stimuli. The nociceptive input is transmitted to supraspinal relay sites, e.g. thalamus and cortex, and is subject to inhibitory anti-nociceptive projections by pain modulatory circuits in the brainstem. Pain processing on different levels may be modulated by neurostimulation of peripheral nerves. Modified after Fields [15], with permission. A = Amygdala; DLPT = dorsal lateral pontine tegmentum; F = frontal lobe; Hyp = hypothalamus; PAG = periaqueductal gray; RVM = rostral ventral medulla; Thal = thalamus.

arthritic rats, the role of the opiodergic-dependent glutamate and aspartate release in the spinal cord was studied. TENS led to a δ-opioidergic mediated blockade of the excitatory transmitter glutamate and aspartate [34, 35]. Similarly, TENS and SCS activate spinal muscarinic M1 and M3, but not spinal nicotinic receptors [35–37].

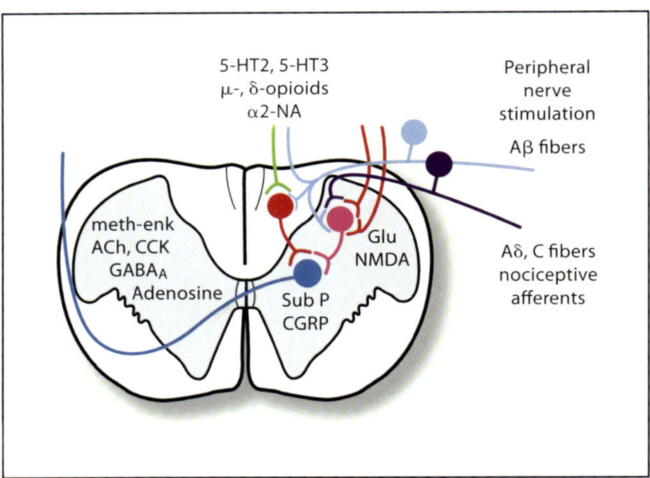

Fig. 2. Schematic section of the spinal cord indicating the intrinsic neuronal connections of afferent input, segmental interneurons and ascending pathways. Various neurotransmitter systems are putatively involved in the modulation of nociceptive and non-nociceptive information by means of peripheral nerve stimulation and by segmental and descending pathways. ACh = Acetylcholine; CCK = cholecystokinin; CGRP = calcitonin gene-related peptide; GABA = gamma-aminobutyric acid; Glu = glutamate; 5-HT = serotonin; meth-enk = methionine-enkephalin; NA = noradrenaline; NMDA = N-methyl D-aspartic acid; Sub P = substance P.

The involvement of α_2-noradrenergic receptors in the neuromodulatory effects of TENS was implied as the application of clonidine augments the analgesic effects of TENS [38]. Spinal blockade of α_2-noradrenergic receptors similarly decreases the analgesic effects of TENS [39, 40]. Using immunohistochemistry and RT-PCR, it was shown that percutaneous electrical nerve stimulation elicited an increased expression of somatostatin in the dorsal root ganglion (DRG) and spinal dorsal horn in rats [41]. Interestingly, pharmacological therapy combined with electrical neuromodulation may show an increased efficacy or delay an analgesic tolerance [38, 42].

Supraspinal Mechanisms of PNS

There is recent experimental evidence indicating that supraspinal structures, such as PAG, are also involved in mediating the antinociceptive effects of neurostimulation [43, 44]. A PET study investigating the effect of SCS in pain-free angina pectoris patients demonstrated increased blood flow in the vlPAG during neurostimulation [45]. Further effects were also observed at the thalamic level [46, 47].

A microdialysis study on transmitter release in the PAG of rats receiving spinal cord stimulation demonstrated that neurostimulation caused a decrease of GABA levels but not of serotonin or substance P [43, 44]. As GABA neurons in the PAG exert a tonic inhibitory effect on the activity in descending pain inhibitory pathways, including trigeminovascular inputs [48], it is suggested that a decreased GABA level in this region following repeated spinal cord stimulation may lead to activation of descending anti-nociceptive projections with subsequent pain reduction [49–51].

In an experimental arthritis animal model it was shown that in animals with joint inflammation, after inducing a central sensitization, application of TENS significantly increased withdrawal thresholds of the paw and knee joint in the group. Reversible functional inactivation of vlPAG prevented the effects of TENS in terms of increased withdrawal thresholds. However, blockade of neuronal pathways in the vlPAG after induction of an inflammation also transiently reversed the behavioral changes indicative of a mechanical hyperalgesia, thus suggesting a role for the vlPAG in the facilitated transmission of pain from deep somatic tissue [52]. Furthermore, blockade of μ- and δ-opioid receptors in RVM prevents the analgesic effects of TENS [53, 54]. In NRM, PNS modulates synthesis of orphanin FQ, an endogenous ligand for the opioid receptor-like-1 receptor and orphanin FQ peptide level [41].

Pharmacology

Since the early studies on PNS, opioidergic mechanisms have been suggested to be involved in the effects of PNS and, at least partly, contribute to the analgesic effect of PNS. In humans, experimental data show an increased concentration of β-endorphins and methionine-enkephalin in the cerebrospinal fluid after the application of high-frequency TENS [55, 56]. As discussed earlier, the involvement of pain-modulating structures in the midbrain such as PAG and RVM also suggests an involvement of its opioidergic projections [57]. Indeed, TENS elicit its analgesic effects by activation of μ- and δ-opioid receptors in the RVM and the spinal cord [52, 53, 58]. With regard to TENS, low-frequency TENS elicits an antihyperalgesic effect through μ-opioid receptor activation whereas high-frequency TENS leads to antihyperalgesia through delta opioid receptors in the spinal cord. Blockade of μ- and δ-opioid receptors in the spinal cord and rostral ventral medulla prevents the analgesic effect produced by TENS in arthritic rats [58].

Mechanisms of Analgesic Tolerance of PNS

A frequent problem with PNS and TENS is the emergence of an analgesic tolerance after repeated application. This analgesic tolerance to TENS is accompanied with a cross-tolerance to δ- and/or μ-opioid receptors [59]. This analgesic tolerance can be prevented by blocking spinal cholecystokinin (CCK) A and B as well as NMDA receptors and CCK receptors in the PAG, respectively [60–62]. Obviously, the vlPAG is critical for mediating the tolerance effect [15, 59, 63].

Peripheral Neurostimulation in Headache

It is very well known that a nonpainful stimulation of peripheral nerves can elicit analgesic effects [1]. This effect has also been used in certain chronic headache syndromes using TENS, SCS or subcutaneous stimulation [64].

The mechanisms of the analgesic effects of peripheral neurostimulation most likely involve multiple pain-processing circuits in the central nervous system [65]. Firstly, direct effects of electrical stimulation on peripheral nerve excitability have been described, including transient slowing in conduction velocity, increase in electrical threshold and decrease in response probability [66]. However, occipital nerve stimulation (ONS) did not significantly modify pain thresholds in cluster headache patients [67]. Secondly, projection fibers within the spinal ascending tracts represent only a minority whereas propriospinal neurons and interneurons of the spinal dorsal horn outnumber these projection neurons [68], so that the segmental neural network might represent the site of the neuromodulatory effect [32, 69]. Indeed, it has been suggested that the somatosensory neurostimulation of afferent A-β fibers blocks the nociceptive transmission on a segmental level, thus revisiting the 'gate control theory' by Melzack and Wall [25, 68, 70, 71].

Similar mechanisms, i.e. gate control at the segmental level as well as activation of descending pain inhibitory pathways, may be operative in ONS. However, the existence of a trigeminocervical complex adds an additional level of complexity. It has been shown that nociceptive input from afferents in the trigeminal nerve and cervical afferents (C2–C3) converge on to the same nociceptive second-order neuron in the trigeminocervical complex that extends as a functional unit from the level of the trigeminal nucleus caudalis to at least the C2 segment. The resulting loss of spatial specificity helps to explains why ONS may have an antinociceptive effect in the territory of the trigeminal as well as occipital nerves [65, 72–74].

Interestingly, recent evidence suggests that afferents from deep somatic tissue but not cutaneous afferents mediate the antihyperalgesic effect of peripheral nerve stimulation [75].

The role of supraspinal structures in mediating an antinociceptive effect in ONS has been recently been studied with functional brain imaging [76]. Eight patients with chronic migraine, who responded to a nonpainful high-frequency stimulation (50–120 Hz) of afferents in GON using bilaterally implanted neurostimulators, were PET scanned in different states: during stimulation when the patient was pain-free, during nonstimulation with pain and typical clinical features, and during partial activation of the stimulator with different levels of paresthesia [76]. Stimulation decreased the pain ratings of the patients by 75–100% within the first 30 min. Pain consistently reoccurred after turning off the device. The stimulation elicited a sensation of paresthesia within the cutaneous distribution of the GON that was used as a monitor of a valid stimulation. Changes in cerebral blood flow during the pain state were observed in the dorsal rostral pons, anterior cingulate cortex (ACC) and cuneus, sites that are known to be activated during migraine [77, 78]. The activation pattern in the dorsal rostral pons is highly suggestive of a role for this structure in the pathophysiology of chronic migraine. In the paresthesia state during neurostimulation, ACC and left pulvinar activation were observed indicating that ONS can modulate activity in the thalamus. Indeed, the pulvinar has been suggested to be involved in pain modulation as neurosurgical pulvinotomy has been performed in relieving intractable pain [79, 80]. Preliminary analysis of a PET study in chronic cluster headache treated with ONS suggests that the cerebral reward system, including the ventral striatum and nucleus accumbens, may mediate an additional effect [81].

The suboccipital stimulation in this study is similar to the stimulation of the dorsal columns of the spinal cord [64, 82] where segmental circuits and/or ascending tracts of the spinal cord are stimulated. Here, the therapeutic effect is mostly restricted to the spinal cord segment of the stimulated afferents [82].

The mechanisms of these analgesic effects within the trigeminocervical complex and supraspinal structures are not entirely clear. Propriospinal neurons and interneurons of the spinal dorsal horn outnumber projection neurons within the spinal ascending tracts [68], so that the segmental neural circuitry might be the site of this neuromodulatory effect [69].

Thus, future research on peripheral nerve stimulation should focus on the pharmacological mechanisms of the neuromodulatory effects and elucidating the neuroanatomy of the CNS structures involved using neuroimaging. Further studies are needed to define the predictors of an optimal treatment response and to describe the long-term outcome.

References

1 Woolf C, Thompson J: Stimulation-induced analgesia: transcutaneous electrical nerve stimulation (TENS) and vibration; in Wall P, Melzack R (eds): Textbook of Pain. New York, Churchill-Livingstone, 1994, pp 1191–2008.

2 Wall PD: The gate control theory of pain mechanisms: a re-examination and re-statement. Brain 1978;101:1–18.

3 Melzack R, Wall PD: Pain mechanisms: a new theory. Science 1965;150:971–979.

4 Dickenson AH: Gate control theory of pain stands the test of time. Br J Anaesth 2002;88:755–757.

5 Sandkühler J: Models and mechanisms of hyperalgesia and allodynia. Physiol Rev 2009;89:707–758.

6 Burstein R, Cutrer MF, Yarnitsky D: The development of cutaneous allodynia during a migraine attack clinical evidence for the sequential recruitment of spinal and supraspinal nociceptive neurons in migraine. Brain 2000;123:1703–1709.

7 Woolf CJ, Salter MW: Neuronal plasticity: increasing the gain in pain. Science 2000;288:1765–1769.

8 Bartsch T, Goadsby PJ: Increased responses in trigeminocervical nociceptive neurons to cervical input after stimulation of the dura mater. Brain 2003;126:1801–1813.

9 Ruch TC: Pathophysiology of pain; in Ruch TC, Patton HD (eds): Physiology and Biophysics. Philadelphia, Saunders, 1965, pp 345–363.

10 Arendt-Nielsen L, Laursen RJ, Drewes AM: Referred pain as an indicator for neural plasticity. Prog Brain Res 2000;129:343–356.

11 Behbehani MM: Functional characteristics of the midbrain periaqueductal gray. Prog Neurobiol 1995; 46:575–605.

12 Sandkuhler J, Fu QG, Zimmermann M: Spinal pathways mediating tonic or stimulation-produced descending inhibition from the periaqueductal gray or nucleus raphe magnus are separate in the cat. J Neurophysiol 1987;58:327–341.

13 Fields HL, Heinricher MM: Anatomy and physiology of a nociceptive modulatory system. Philos Trans R Soc Lond B Biol Sci 1985;308:361–374.

14 Ren K, Dubner R: Descending control mechanisms; in Basbaum AI, Bushnell MC (eds): Science of Pain. Oxford, Academic Press, 2008, pp 723–762.

15 Fields H: State-dependent opioid control of pain. Nat Rev Neurosci 2004;5:565–575.

16 Heinricher MM, Ingram SL: The brainstem and nociceptive modulation; in Basbaum AI, Bushnell MC (eds): Science of Pain. Oxford, Academic Press, 2008, pp 593–626.

17 Keay KA, Bandler R: Vascular head pain selectively activates ventrolateral periaqueductal grey in the cat. Neuroscience Lett 1998;245:58–60.
18 Hoskin KL, Bulmer DC, Lasalandra M, Jonkman A, Goadsby PJ: Fos expression in the midbrain periaqueductal grey after trigeminovascular stimulation. J Anat 2001;198:29–35.
19 Knight YE, Goadsby PJ: The periaqueductal grey matter modulates trigeminovascular input: a role in migraine? Neuroscience 2001;106:793–800.
20 Knight YE, Bartsch T, Kaube H, Goadsby PJ: P/q-type calcium-channel blockade in the periaqueductal gray facilitates trigeminal nociception: a functional genetic link for migraine? J Neurosci 2002;22:1–6.
21 Bartsch T, Knight YE, Goadsby PJ: Activation of 5-ht1b/1d receptors in the periaqueductal grey inhibits meningeal nociception. Ann Neurol 2004; 56:371–381.
22 Urban MO, Gebhart GF: Supraspinal contributions to hyperalgesia. Proc Natl Acad Sci USA 1999;96: 7687–7692.
23 Ren K, Dubner R: Descending modulation in persistent pain: an update. Pain 2002;100:1–6.
24 Garrison DW, Foreman RD: Decreased activity of spontaneous and noxiously evoked dorsal horn cells during transcutaneous electrical nerve stimulation (TENS). Pain 1994;58:309–315.
25 Garrison DW, Foreman RD: Effects of transcutaneous electrical nerve stimulation (TENS) on spontaneous and noxiously evoked dorsal horn cell activity in cats with transected spinal cords. Neurosci Lett 1996;216:125–128.
26 Wallin J, Fiska A, Tjolsen A, Linderoth B, Hole K: Spinal cord stimulation inhibits long-term potentiation of spinal wide dynamic range neurons. Brain Res 2003;973:39–43.
27 Yakhnitsa V, Linderoth B, Meyerson BA: Spinal cord stimulation attenuates dorsal horn neuronal hyperexcitability in a rat model of mononeuropathy. Pain 1999;79:223–233.
28 Sluka KA, Bailey K, Bogush J, Olson R, Ricketts A: Treatment with either high or low frequency TENS reduces the secondary hyperalgesia observed after injection of kaolin and carrageenan into the knee joint. Pain 1998;77:97–102.
29 Ma YT, Sluka KA: Reduction in inflammation-induced sensitization of dorsal horn neurons by transcutaneous electrical nerve stimulation in anesthetized rats. Exp Brain Res 2001;137:94–102.
30 Radhakrishnan R, King EW, Dickman JK, Herold CA, Johnston NF, Spurgin ML, Sluka KA: Spinal 5-HT(2) and 5-HT(3) receptors mediate low, but not high, frequency TENS-induced antihyperalgesia in rats. Pain 2003;105:205–213.
31 Sluka KA, Lisi TL, Westlund KN: Increased release of serotonin in the spinal cord during low, but not high, frequency transcutaneous electric nerve stimulation in rats with joint inflammation. Arch Phys Med Rehabil 2006;87:1137–1140.
32 Song Z, Ultenius C, Meyerson BA, Linderoth B: Pain relief by spinal cord stimulation involves serotonergic mechanisms: an experimental study in a rat model of mononeuropathy. Pain 2009;147:241–248.
33 Maeda Y, Lisi TL, Vance CG, Sluka KA: Release of GABA and activation of GABA(A) in the spinal cord mediates the effects of TENS in rats. Brain Res 2007;1136:43–50.
34 Sluka KA, Vance CG, Lisi TL: High-frequency, but not low-frequency, transcutaneous electrical nerve stimulation reduces aspartate and glutamate release in the spinal cord dorsal horn. J Neurochem 2005; 95:1794–1801.
35 Radhakrishnan R, Sluka KA: Spinal muscarinic receptors are activated during low or high frequency TENS-induced antihyperalgesia in rats. Neuropharmacology 2003;45:1111–1119.
36 Schechtmann G, Song Z, Ultenius C, Meyerson BA, Linderoth B: Cholinergic mechanisms involved in the pain relieving effect of spinal cord stimulation in a model of neuropathy. Pain 2008;139:136–145.
37 Song Z, Meyerson BA, Linderoth B: Muscarinic receptor activation potentiates the effect of spinal cord stimulation on pain-related behavior in rats with mononeuropathy. Neurosci Lett 2008;436:7–12.
38 Sluka KA, Chandran P: Enhanced reduction in hyperalgesia by combined administration of clonidine and TENS. Pain 2002;100:183–190.
39 King EW, Audette K, Athman GA, Nguyen HO, Sluka KA, Fairbanks CA: Transcutaneous electrical nerve stimulation activates peripherally located alpha-2a adrenergic receptors. Pain 2005;115:364–373.
40 Resende MA, Sabino GG, Candido CR, Pereira LS, Francischi JN: Local transcutaneous electrical stimulation (TENS) effects in experimental inflammatory edema and pain. Eur J Pharmacol 2004;504: 217–222.
41 Dong ZQ, Xie H, Ma F, Li WM, Wang YQ, Wu GC: Effects of electroacupuncture on expression of somatostatin and preprosomatostatin mRNA in dorsal root ganglions and spinal dorsal horn in neuropathic pain rats. Neurosci Lett 2005;385:189–194.
42 Wallin J, Cui JG, Yakhnitsa V, Schechtmann G, Meyerson BA, Linderoth B: Gabapentin and pregabalin suppress tactile allodynia and potentiate spinal cord stimulation in a model of neuropathy. Eur J Pain 2002;6:261–272.

43 Lindblom U, Tapper DN, Wiesenfeld Z: The effect of dorsal column stimulation on the nociceptive response of dorsal horn cells and its relevance for pain suppression. Pain 1977;4:133–144.

44 Garrison D, Foreman R: Decreased activity of spontaneous and noxiously evoked dorsal horn cells during transcutaneous electrical nerve stimulation (TENS). Pain 1994;58:309–315.

45 Hautvast RW, Ter Horst GJ, DeJong BM, DeJongste MJ, Blanksma PK, Paans AM, Korf J: Relative changes in regional cerebral blood flow during spinal cord stimulation in patients with refractory angina pectoris. Eur J Neurosci 1997;9:1178–1183.

46 Olausson B, Xu ZQ, Shyu BC: Dorsal column inhibition of nociceptive thalamic cells mediated by gamma-aminobutyric acid mechanisms in the cat. Acta Physiol Scand 1994;152:239–247.

47 Gildenberg PL, Murthy KS: Influence of dorsal column stimulation upon human thalamic somatosensory-evoked potentials. Appl Neurophysiol 1980; 43:8–17.

48 Knight YE, Bartsch T, Goadsby PJ: Trigeminal antinociception induced by bicuculline in the periaqueductal gray (PAG) is not affected by PAG p/q-type calcium channel blockade in rat. Neurosci Lett 2003;336:113–116.

49 Stiller CO, Linderoth B, O'Connor WT, Franck J, Falkenberg T, Ungerstedt U, Brodin E: Repeated spinal cord stimulation decreases the extracellular level of gamma-aminobutyric acid in the periaqueductal gray matter of freely moving rats. Brain Res 1995;699:231–241.

50 Duggan AW, Foong FW: Bicuculline and spinal inhibition produced by dorsal column stimulation in the cat. Pain 1985;22:249–259.

51 Stiller CO, Cui JG, O'Connor WT, Brodin E, Meyerson BA, Linderoth B: Release of gamma-aminobutyric acid in the dorsal horn and suppression of tactile allodynia by spinal cord stimulation in mononeuropathic rats. Neurosurgery 1996;39: 367–374; discussion 374–375.

52 DeSantana JM, Da Silva LF, De Resende MA, Sluka KA: Transcutaneous electrical nerve stimulation at both high and low frequencies activates ventrolateral periaqueductal grey to decrease mechanical hyperalgesia in arthritic rats. Neuroscience 2009; 163:1233–1241.

53 Kalra A, Urban MO, Sluka KA: Blockade of opioid receptors in rostral ventral medulla prevents antihyperalgesia produced by transcutaneous electrical nerve stimulation (TENS). J Pharmacol Exp Ther 2001;298:257–263.

54 Ainsworth L, Budelier K, Clinesmith M, Fiedler A, Landstrom R, Leeper BJ, Moeller L, Mutch S, O'Dell K, Ross J, Radhakrishnan R, Sluka KA: Transcutaneous electrical nerve stimulation (TENS) reduces chronic hyperalgesia induced by muscle inflammation. Pain 2006;120:182–187.

55 Han JS, Chen XH, Sun SL, Xu XJ, Yuan Y, Yan SC, Hao JX, Terenius L: Effect of low- and high-frequency TENS on met-enkephalin-arg-phe and dynorphin a immunoreactivity in human lumbar CSF. Pain 1991;47:295–298.

56 Salar G, Job I, Mingrino S, Bosio A, Trabucchi M: Effect of transcutaneous electrotherapy on CSF beta-endorphin content in patients without pain problems. Pain 1981;10:169–172.

57 Sabino GS, Santos CM, Francischi JN, de Resende MA: Release of endogenous opioids following transcutaneous electric nerve stimulation in an experimental model of acute inflammatory pain. J Pain 2008;9:157–163.

58 Sluka KA, Deacon M, Stibal A, Strissel S, Terpstra A: Spinal blockade of opioid receptors prevents the analgesia produced by TENS in arthritic rats. J Pharmacol Exp Ther 1999;289:840–846.

59 Chandran P, Sluka KA: Development of opioid tolerance with repeated transcutaneous electrical nerve stimulation administration. Pain 2003;102: 195–201.

60 Desantana JM, da Silva LF, Sluka KA: Cholecystokinin receptors mediate tolerance to the analgesic effect of TENS in arthritic rats. Pain 2010; 148:84–93

61 Hingne PM, Sluka KA: Blockade of NMDA receptors prevents analgesic tolerance to repeated transcutaneous electrical nerve stimulation (TENS) in rats. J Pain 2008;9:217–225.

62 Chen XH, Geller EB, Adler MW: CCK(b) receptors in the periaqueductal grey are involved in electroacupuncture antinociception in the rat cold water tail-flick test. Neuropharmacology 1998;37:751–757.

63 Tortorici V, Robbins CS, Morgan MM: Tolerance to the antinociceptive effect of morphine microinjections into the ventral but not lateral-dorsal periaqueductal gray of the rat. Behavioral Neurosci 1999; 113:833–839.

64 Simpson B: Spinal cord and brain stimulation; in Melzack R, Wall PD (eds): Textbook of Pain. New York, Churchill-Livingstone, 1999, pp 1353–1381.

65 Goadsby PJ, Bartsch T, Dodick DW: Occipital nerve stimulation for headache: mechanisms and efficacy. Headache 2008;48:313–318.

66 Ignelzi RJ, Nyquist JK: Excitability changes in peripheral nerve fibers after repetitive electrical stimulation. Implications in pain modulation. J Neurosurg 1979;51:824–833.

67 Magis D, Allena M, Bolla M, De Pasqua V, Remacle JM, Schoenen J: Occipital nerve stimulation for drug-resistant chronic cluster headache: a prospective pilot study. Lancet Neurol 2007;6:314–321.
68 Chung JM, Lee KH, Hori Y, Endo K, Willis WD: Factors influencing peripheral nerve stimulation produced inhibition of primate spinothalamic tract cells. Pain 1984;19:277–293.
69 Doubell T, Mannion, RJ, Woolf, CJ: The dorsal horn: state dependent sensory processing, plasticity and the generation of pain; in Melzack R, Wall PD (eds): Textbook of Pain. New York, Churchill-Livingstone, 1999, pp 165–180.
70 Kolmodin GM, Skoglund CR: Analysis of spinal interneurons activated by tactile and nociceptive stimulation. Acta Physiol Scand 1960;50:337–355.
71 Woolf CJ: Transcutaneous electrical nerve stimulation and the reaction to experimental pain in human subjects. Pain 1979;7:115–127.
72 Burns B, Watkins L, Goadsby PJ: Treatment of medically intractable cluster headache by occipital nerve stimulation: long-term follow-up of eight patients. Lancet 2007;369:1099–1106.
73 Burns B, Watkins L, Goadsby PJ: Treatment of intractable chronic cluster headache by occipital nerve stimulation in 14 patients. Neurology 2009;72: 341–345.
74 Goadsby PJ, Dodick DW, Saper JR, Silberstein SD: Occipital nerve stimulation (ONS) for the treatment of intractable chronic migraine (ONSTIM). Cephalalgia 2009;29:133.
75 Radhakrishnan R, Sluka KA: Deep tissue afferents, but not cutaneous afferents, mediate transcutaneous electrical nerve stimulation-induced antihyperalgesia. J Pain 2005;6:673–680.
76 Matharu M, Bartsch T, Ward N, Frackowiak R, Weiner R, Goadsby P: Central neuromodulation in chronic migraine patients with suboccipital stimulators: a PET study. Brain 2004;127:220–230.
77 Weiller C, May A, Limmroth V, Juptner M, Kaube H, Schayck RV, Coenen HH, Diener HC: Brain stem activation in spontaneous human migraine attacks. Nat Med 1995;1:658–660.
78 Bahra A, Matharu MS, Buchel C, Frackowiak RS, Goadsby PJ: Brainstem activation specific to migraine headache. Lancet 2001;357:1016–1017.
79 Mayanagi Y, Bouchard G: Evaluation of stereotactic thalamotomies for pain relief with reference to pulvinar intervention. Appl Neurophysiol 1976;39: 154–157.
80 Choi CR, Umbach W: Combined stereotaxic surgery for relief of intractable pain. Neurochirurgia (Stuttg) 1977;20:84–87.
81 Magis D, Schoenen J: Neurostimulation in chronic cluster headache. Curr Pain Headache Rep 2008;12: 145–153.
82 Hansson P, Lundeberg T: Transcutaneous electrical nerve stimulation, vibration and acupuncture as pain-relieving measures; in Melzack R, Wall PD (eds): Textbook of Pain. New York, Churchill-Livingstone, 1999, pp 1341–1351.

Professor Peter J. Goadsby
Headache Group, Department of Neurology
University of California, San Francisco
1701 Divisadero St, Suite 480, San Francisco, CA 94115 (USA)
E-Mail pgoadsby@headacheucsf.edu

Slavin KV (ed): Peripheral Nerve Stimulation.
Prog Neurol Surg. Basel, Karger, 2011, vol 24, pp 27–40

Peripheral Nerve Stimulation for Chronic Neurogenic Pain

Hosam Al-Jehani · Line Jacques

Department of Neurology and Neurosurgery, Montreal Neurological Institute/Hospital, McGill University, Montreal, Canada

Abstract

Peripheral nerve stimulation (PNS) has been used for the treatment of neuropathic pain for more than 40 years. Recent interest in the utilization of this technique stems from the many modifications of the original procedure and the refinement of the available hardware. This rendered the procedure less traumatic and more effective, and thus more widely accepted as a neuromodulation technique for the treatment of various chronic pain syndromes including post-traumatic and postsurgical neuropathy, occipital neuralgia, and complex regional pain syndromes, and in relatively new indications for neuromodulation, such as migraines and daily headaches, cluster headaches. We present a review of the principle and indications for the use of PNS, and review our single institution experience that comprises 24 peripheral nerve stimulators as well as 8 occipital nerve stimulators over 13 years. We review the protocol of our approach including the surgical nuances for our implantation technique. Collaborative efforts in future research will lead to a growth in our clinical experience with the utilization of PNS and will help in identifying the best candidates for it. This, along with the development and refinement of the available hardware would lead to a more specific patient selection for each modality of treatment, increasing the efficacy and success of the intended treatment.

Peripheral neuropathic pain refers to a primary lesion or dysfunction in the peripheral nervous system (PNS). The most common problems include neuralgia and complex regional pain syndromes (CRPS) type 1 (previously known as reflex sympathetic dystrophy – RSD) and type 2 (previously known as causlagia), and both neuralgia and CRPS type 2 involve malfunction of a named nerve that may become a target of neurosurgical interventions. According to the International Association for the Study of Pain (IASP), neuralgia refers to pain in the distribution of a nerve. Causalgia is a 'syndrome of sustained burning pain after a traumatic nerve lesion combined with vasomotor and sudomotor dysfunction and later trophic changes' [1]. Injuries to select nerves such as the median, tibial, brachial, and lumbar plexuses can cause this syndrome. The term RSD is used to describe a syndrome of pain, sensory changes and swelling in an extremity, where the responsible nerve is not identifiable but the function of the limb is often considerably impaired, and osteoporosis is commonly observed in the affected limb [1].

Nerve lesions such as neuromas have long been suspected to cause neuropathic pain. Damaged nerves often have a regenerative response following a wide variety of nerve injuries [2]. Severed nerves, which lack of continuity, can also be painful secondary to the internal changes of that nerve itself [3]. This is often the result of activated nociceptive fibers or of external influences, such as tethering or compression of the nerve. The origin of pain in some cases is centralized, particularly in phantom limb pain. Direct reconstructive surgical procedures might contribute to reducing nerve pain, but occasionally fail to achieve full pain remission or complete return of the limb's function. When this occurs, the patient is left with an extremity which has poor or virtually no useable function.

Tricyclic antidepressants, anticonvulsants, cannabinoids and narcotics can be used alone or in combination to provide a degree of pain management.

Physiotherapy, occupational therapy and psychological techniques can be employed to help these patients develop better coping skills and manage their symptoms more appropriately.

Neuromodulation has been found to be efficacious in treating patients suffering from chronic pain as a result of nerve injuries. Peripheral nerve stimulation may be applied proximally to the lesion allowing direct stimulation of the injured nerve. Some nerve injuries may not respond well to PNS and therefore may be more effectively treated with spinal cord stimulation (SCS). This is especially the case when more than one nerve group is affected or the lesion is very proximal. Peripheral nerve field stimulation (PNFS) or sub-cutaneous stimulation is a novel approach used to stimulate painful areas of the skin, which are difficult to treat using conventional spinal cord stimulation techniques.

The first permanent implantation of a peripheral nerve electrode in an attempt to obtain long-term pain relief was done by Wall et al. [4] in 1967 and one of the first clinical reports was published by Nashold and Goldner [2] in 1982. Racz et al. [3] reported the largest experience with 125 patients treated with this treatment modality.

There has been significant interest in PNS for the treatment of craniofacial neuropathic pain, occipital neuralgia, cervical headaches and more recently the treatment of chronic refractory migraine headaches. Weiner and his group in Dallas led this work in the 1990s [5, 6]. There is currently a significant amount of research into the treatment of these conditions, which are severely debilitating for patients who suffer from them. The application of PNS continues to expand including new and modified techniques to treat other types of facial and headache syndromes such as intractable and transformed migraine, cervicogenic headache, cluster headache and neuropathic facial pain.

The impact of intractable migraine, cervicogenic and secondary headache syndromes such as occipital neuralgia are profound. It is estimated that 40 million Americans are affected by these conditions [7], a further 5% experience chronic daily headaches and 2% of these patients are refractory to conventional medical management (CMM). With such a large volume of patients needing some form of effective treatment, this translates into a treatment cost of a billion dollars annually in the USA. Of this cost, less than 1% is attributed to ER visits. The cost of lost wages due to absence and impaired performance are estimated to be 18 billion dollars annually [6].

Mechanism of Action

The mechanisms of action for peripheral neuromodulation techniques cannot be discerned well without a proper understanding of the mechanisms by which the chronic pain is produced. The most widely accepted mechanisms of action for the generation of chronic neuropathic pain are as follows: cross-talk between A-fibers and C-fibers, purinergic signaling pain pathway activation [8] and excitability-dependent calcium transients. Excitability-dependent calcium transients are thought to be produced by changes in the distribution and expression of sodium channels along the axon of the injured nerve in response to nerve growth factor.

The gate control theory of pain devised by Melzack and Wall [9] was known as the basis for the analgesic effect of electrical stimulation. Subsequent investigations and basic science research in this area have revealed that this model is too simplistic in identifying all of the complex changes that have been observed in chronic pain patients. The proposed mechanisms of action of PNS are firstly by a central inhibitory mechanism. In 1984, Chung et al. [10, 11] demonstrated a profound inhibition of primate spinothalamic tract cells after noxious and thermal stimuli, which were dependant on spinal cord circuitry. To activate the A-fibers, an electrical stimulation with high frequency and significant intensity was required.

Experimental work by Ignelzi and Nyquist [12], recorded transient excitability changes in both large and small diameter fibers, which resulted in slowing of single fiber conduction velocities and an increasing electrical threshold. Racz et al. [3] recorded 9 patients during 3-day trials with implanted electrodes and observed unexpected spontaneous activity that can reflect pain status conditions.

Electrical stimulation should not be viewed as a simple electrical phenomenon. There are several other elements that are involved in the stimulation process. These include subcutaneous electrical conductance, dermatomal and myotomal stimulation, sympathetic stimulation, local blood flow alteration, peripheral and central neurochemical mechanisms, and the trigeminovascular system.

The most important of these elements appears to be the effect on the trigeminovascular system [13]. This phenomenon was demonstrated by an animal study. When the greater occipital nerve was electrically stimulated, it led to a 2-fold increase in the metabolic activity of the ipsilateral trigeminal nucleus and cervical dorsal horn. PET studies were used to show that activation of the dorsal pontine regions in migraine patients after PNS, directly correlate to a significant reduction of pain symptoms experienced by the patients [14].

Indications and Patient Selection

Having a clear-cut etiology for the pain is one of the most important criteria for patient selection. The pain has to be in the distribution of a single nerve. Otherwise, SCS would be a more appropriate choice of therapy. Detailed imaging of the nerve might exclude the presence of a tumor, neuroma or a correctable pathology. MRI with gadolinium, MRN (neuronography), high-frequency ultrasound and electrodiagnostic study will help define the nerve pathology. It is prudent for clinicians to exhaust less-invasive interventions first, and confirm that the patient is refractory to all conventional medical treatments. The patients that we typically treat in our center at the Montreal Neurological Institute (MNI) have VAS scores of 5 or more and tend to have other disability ratings consistent with major reduction in quality of life and function.

In our experience, sciatic nerve injuries tend to respond more effectively to SCS therapy. PNS tends to be unsuccessful in this patient group as a result of the size of the nerve and the amount of movement within the nerve. This creates a poor electrode-to-nerve contact ratio and yields inconsistent conduction characteristics. Proximal nerve root injuries, such as in brachial plexus injuries (mixed spinal cord and root injuries with or without avulsion) will also be poor responders to PNS, and therefore it is not recommended as a treatment option.

PNS is specifically used for patients with neuropathic pain of various etiologies as long as there is some sensory response in the area of their pain [15]. An interdisciplinary team approach to patient assessment will provide a vital tool for evaluating patient susceptibility. It is common for patients to be seen by the following specialists during the patient selection process: neurosurgeons, neurologists, anesthesiologists, psychologists, specialized pain physicians, nurses, occupational therapists, and physiotherapists. It is necessary and beneficial for all patients to have a psychological and behavioral assessment prior to implantation to detect somatization, untreated depression, as well as identifying and treating any secondary gain issues. The patients should be motivated to have this procedure and have adequate comprehension to become 'partners' in their own treatment and take ownership for their long-term treatment goals, which may include dramatic lifestyle changes. The patient's goals and expectations must be clear and realistic, as the neuromodulation techniques are not 'curative' procedures. Instead, these therapies are often adjunctive treatments, which will provide the patient additional tools to assist them in the management of their pain syndromes.

Contraindications to PNS include major medical comorbidities, infection at the site of the target nerve, failed stimulation trial, and pregnancy.

A diagnostic local anesthetic block is used to confirm the involvement of the target nerve if this region is the major component in the generation of the patient's pain syndrome [16]. The result of the diagnostic block is not predictive of the response to the PNS itself. In a select group of patients, transcutaneous electrical nerve stimulation (TENS) was used as a trial modality [17]. The only way to truly verify a patient's candidacy for PNS therapy is by placing a temporary or permanent lead into the patient that is connected to an external pulse generator that directly mimics the sensations produced by the permanent implantable system. Directly stimulating the target nerve and having the patients maintain a detailed log of their pain symptoms and drug usage achieves this. The goal of the trial is to demonstrate at least a 50% improvement in pain symptoms, and assess the overall satisfaction with the treatment. These early observations are often useful in managing the patients' expectations and keeping them focused on their expected outcomes with the therapy. Rarely if ever, do patients who had an unsatisfactory trial ever achieve satisfaction with a permanent implanted device. Therefore, a careful review of the patients' logs and an extensive debriefing are useful in making the decision to partner with the patient in this treatment modality. This is often most successful when discussed and agreed to by an interdisciplinary pain team, who will be involved in the patient's long-term partnered care. Red flags by any of the team members should be seriously considered prior to making the decision to proceed with PNS or any neuromodulation therapy.

Surgical Insertion Technique

The procedure is performed in 2 stages, the first one being the trial. In our center, this is performed under local anesthesia and heavy sedation. The second is performed under general anesthesia and involves placement of the pulse generator. The lead is placed proximal to the nerve injury. A longitudinal incision along the nerve is performed and a flap is created adjacent to that nerve to prevent direct contact with the lead. The flap is sutured in place to prevent migration and allow the nerve to slide freely (fig. 1). One has to be cautious not to aggressively denude the nerve in order to not jeopardize its structural integrity and future healing. It is important that the limb remains in motion to minimize the formation of scar tissue.

The electrical stimulation parameters include a rate of 65–80 Hz, voltage of 0.8–1.2 V and pulse width between 400 and 500 µs. A bipolar electrode combination 0– and 3+ or 0+ and 3– tends to provide the best results, and a trial duration of 3–10 days with broad-spectrum prophylactic antibiotics to minimize the patient's risk of infection.

The second phase of the procedure involves removal of the extension wires and insertion of a permanent extension wire to connect to the implantable pulse generator (IPG). The placement of that pulse generator takes into account the proximity to the lead, the anatomy of the patient and the potential motion of the affected limb. The infraclavicular area is often used for IPG placement for the upper extremities and

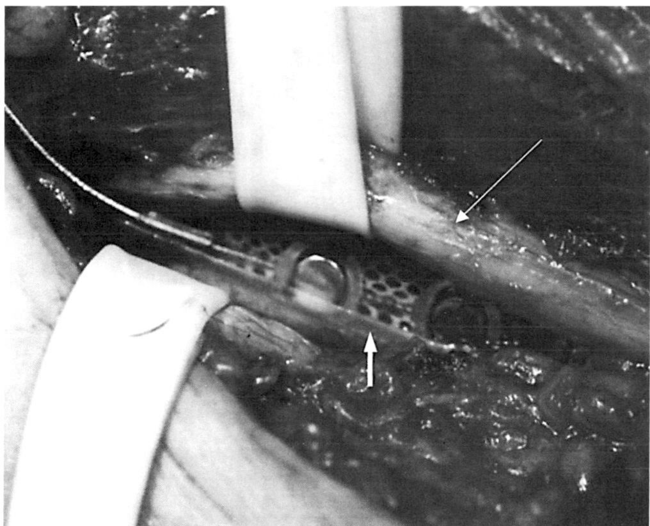

Fig. 1. Peripheral nerve stimulator insertion. This demonstrates the open exposure for peripheral nerve stimulation electrode insertion on the median nerve at the forearm level. Note that the lead inserted in a sub-fascial plane deeper to the target nerve. Long arrow = Median nerve at the level of the forearm in a patient with multiple carpal tunnel release operations, which is retracted to reveal the underlying paddle lead. Short arrow = Edge of the fascia under the nerve which is going to be tacked over the electrode to prevent excessive scarring around the nerve but allowing the nerve to slide in an intact fascial plane.

the lower abdomen or the thigh for the lower extremities. It is vitally important to avoid the patient's ribs or superior iliac crest and areas such as the iliohypogastric or genitofemoral nerves [5].

The PNS insertion technique includes the open nerve dissection technique, which requires a comprehensive knowledge of peripheral nerve anatomy, and percutaneous insertion of the stimulating lead. There are many technical variables, which may result in the need to use different lead types, extension wires or electrical stimulators. Different leads may include surgical or flat paddle leads, cylindrical leads with variable contact numbers or spacing, single or bifurcated extensions and IPGs with 4, 8 or 16 contacts programmability to target unilateral or bilateral nerve regions.

In cases of craniofacial pain, a unifying system is lacking, but several anatomic patterns have been described [6]. In the C2 pattern, the pain radiates from the occiput to the vertex or the frontal region and vice versa. The other patterns include the frontal and the holocranial patterns. These patterns can be unilateral or bilateral. Knowledge of these patterns can influence the type of lead or combinations of leads to be used to provide maximal coverage for the painful area.

These implantations are performed with the patient in the prone (or lateral) position for occipital targets and in the supine position for trigeminal distribution targets

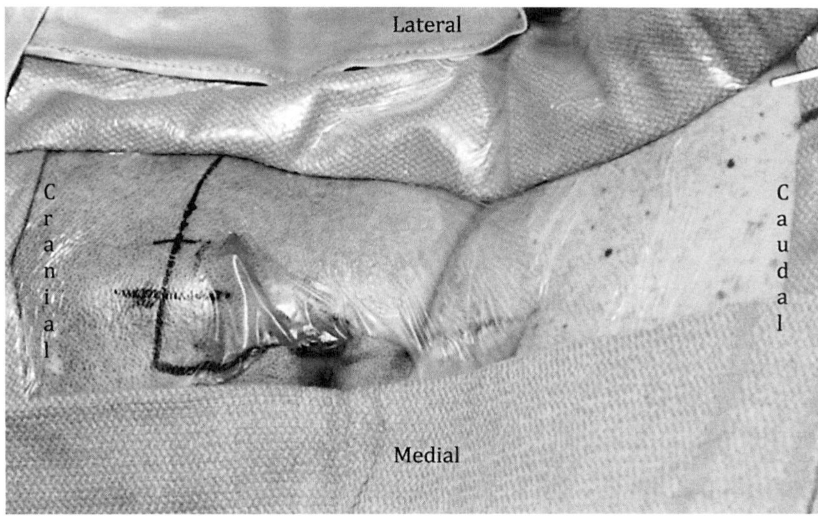

Fig. 2. Landmarks for insertion of occipital lead. The patient is in the prone position with the vertical line representing the midline and the horizontal line representing the lead trajectory. The entry site is 1.5–2 cm lateral to the midline.

as well as peripheral nerve exposures. The procedures are well tolerated using light sedation and local anesthesia, which should be used with caution to not interfere with nerve stimulation. Fluoroscopy [18] or ultrasonography [19, 20] are useful adjuncts in the placement process, depending on anatomical localization and the anticipated difficulty of finding the target nerve.

After the lead is inserted in to the target region, several anchoring devices are used to prevent lead migration, which is reported to occur in 20–50% of stimulation trials.

The exposure for occipital neuralgia patients starts with a 2-cm incision medial to the posterior margin of the mastoid process and 2-cm inferior to the superior nuchal line to ensure contact with the occipital nerve as they pierce the fascial attachment of the axial muscles along the superior nuchal line. This incision in carried down to the subcutaneous fat after which, using a curved hemostat, a tract is created to accommodate the paddle lead from lateral to medial up to the midline. Keeping the tract narrow is an important surgical detail to prevent lead movement or migration. Anchoring the paddle lead to the underlying fascial layer also reduces the chances of lead migration (fig. 2–4). Another technical nuance during this procedure is to provide a strain-reducing loop prior to externalizing the wires out of the incision to avoid lead migration. For cases of transformed migraine, a 1.5-cm vertical incision is placed over C1 at the level of the skull base. The paddle leads are passed from medial to lateral [21].

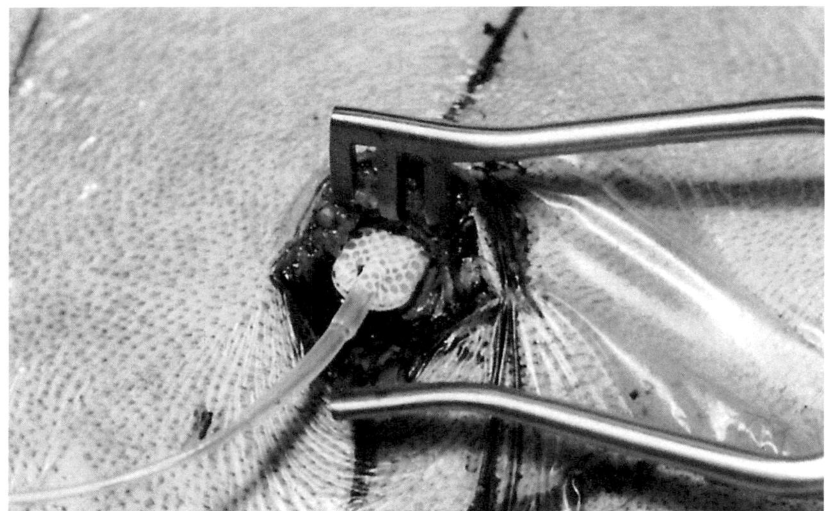

Fig. 3. Insertion of subcutaneous occipital lead. The lead is inserted in the subcutaneous fatty access plane. Entry into this plane lowers the risk of damaging the occipital nerve during the insertion process.

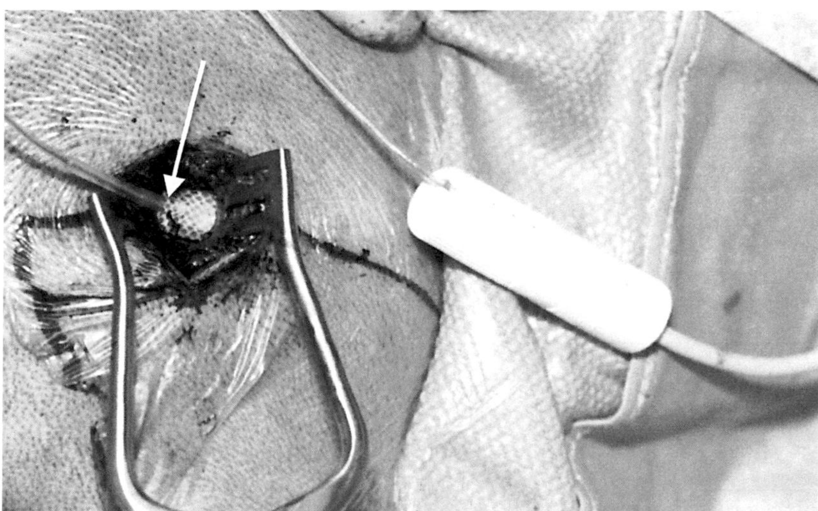

Fig. 4. Anchoring of the lead. The surgical paddle lead (Resume 2, Medtronic) is anchored to the underlying fascial layer to prevent lead migration (arrow). Other paddle lead designs (e.g. On-Point and Specify from Medtronic) have pitted edges to facilitate the anchoring process and avoid injuring the contacts.

Trial of Stimulation

The general consensus for a successful trial is a reduction in pain of at least 50%, although some centers may use additional criteria as well. In the specific indication of transformed migraine, the MIDAS scale [22] can be used to objectively assess the patient's response. Similar scales do not exist for many other pathologies, so one has to rely on other patient observations to better decide on the success of the trial. Some implanters recommend a soft collar during the trial period as a reminder for the patients not to vigorously move their head and promote scarring of the lead body without disruption. The duration of the trial is variable depending on different centers.

Permanent Implantation

Replacing the lead over the target region with a new lead is debatable, as identical lead placement cannot be guaranteed. The location of the IPG pocket is dependent on the location of the target area, body habitus and, if feasible, patient preference to avoid disfiguring scars and conspicuous hardware.

Patients are provided with antibiotics for 24 h after the permanent implantation. Some recommend physiotherapy to extend the extension wire loops to reduce the stress on the lead and prevent loss of efficacy due to traction on the target lead.

Results

Review of the literature consistently shows 75% good-to-excellent long-term pain relief with 15% fair response and 10% poor response. This is a reflection of the variability of responses based on original diagnoses for which the PNS is implanted (tables 1, 2). Occipital neuralgia and transformed migraine shows a pain reduction of 80–90% while pain syndromes of trigeminal distribution and peripheral nerve distribution show lower improvement rates of between 60 and 80% (tables 1, 2).

Authors' Experience

Between 1997 and 2010, 24 PNS implants have been inserted, and 8 ONS devices have been placed between 2007 and 2010. The male:female ratio was 1:1.4 for PNS average age 48 years (range 28–62) and 6:2 for ONS average age of 52 years (range 35–60). The mechanism of nerve injuries for PNS patients includes repaired lacerations, previous nerve entrapment (after carpal tunnel release), repaired crush injury, and previous nerve tumor resection. All ONS patients were diagnosed with occipital neuralgia following whiplash injuries. None of them were involved in litigation.

Table 1. Summary of studies on peripheral nerve stimulation for nerve pain

Patient no.	First author	Year	Number of patients	Duration of follow-up	Outcome	Complications
1	Wall [4]	1967	8	N/A	50% reduction	
2	Picaza [17]	1975	32	6–20 months	20/32 >50% reduction	
3	Cauthen [26]	1975	120	N/A	58/120 good relief	
4	Sweet [16]	1976	69	10 years	25% reduction	
5	Campbell [27]	1976	33	12 months	8/33 excellent 7/33 intermediate 17 failures (12 sciatic and metastatic)	
6	Picaza [28]	1977	12	12–46 months	N/A	
7	Long [29]	1977	34	6–12 months	UE excellent to good 12/14 LE satisfactory 5/20	
8	Law [30]	1980	22	9–88 months 25 months	62% reduction	1 infection 5 no effect
9	Nashold [2]	1982	38 19 U 16 L	4–9 years	UE 52% reduction LE 31% reduction	
10	Waisbrod [31]	1985	19	11.5 months	58% complete relief 21% good relief	
11	Strege [32]	1994	24	12–120 months, mean 32 months	18/24 good to excellent relief	
12	Eisenberg [33]	2004	46	3–16 years	78% patients >50% reduction	
13	Mobbs [34]	2007	38	31 months	61% patients >50% reduction 39% poor result	
14	Van Calenbergh [35]	2009	5	20 years	80% excellent pain relief of 11, 4 removed, 2 not reviewed (1 died, 1 lost)	

Table 2. Summary of studies on occipital nerve stimulators for headache syndromes

Patient no.	First author	Year	Number of patients	Duration of follow-up	Outcome	Complications
1	Picaza[1] [28]	1977	6	12–46 months	3/6 good to excellent	
2	Weiner [36]	1999	13, 17 implants	1.5–6 years	12/13 >50% reduction	1 migration 1 infection
3	Hammer [37]	2001	1	9 months	90% reduction	none
4	Jones [38]	2003	3	N/A	excellent outcome 3/3	
5	Popeney [39]	2003	25	18 months	89% improvement	9 migrations 1 infection
6	Oh [21]	2004	10 ON 10 TM	6 months (1 patient 4 years)	15/20 excellent 4/20 good to fair 1/20 poor	7 migrations 2 infections 2 IPG site complication
7	Matharu [14]	2004	8	7 months to 3 years mean 1.5	4/8 complete relief 2/8 very good 2/8 50% reduction	
8	Kapural [18]	2005	6	3 months	VAS 8–2 PDI 48–14 in all 6	none
9	Rodrigo-Royo [40]	2005	4	4–16 months	good response in all	none
10	Johnstone [41]	2006	7	6–47 months mean 25	7/7 improvement in QoL	2 infection
11	Slavin [42]	2006	10	5–32 months mean 22	70% adequate pain control	1 infection 1 loss of stimulation 1 no stimulation
12	Magis[2] [43]	2007	8	3–22 months mean 15	2/8 pain free 3/8 >90% reduction	1 migration 1 loss of stimulation
13	Burns[2] [44]	2007	8	8–27 months mean 20	2/8 >90% reduction 3/8 40–80% reduction 1/8 25% reduction	1 muscle stimulation 2 wire kink
14	Schwedt[2] [23]	2007	15	5–42 months mean 19	50% reduction of pain 60% revision in 1 year	8 migrations
15	Melvin [45]	2007	11	12 weeks	67% pain reduction	1 migration 1 loss of stimulation

[1]Mixed occipital headache and hemicrania.
[2]Included cluster headache.

All patients underwent psychological evaluation and were seen by a neurologist, anesthesiologist, physiotherapist and/or occupational therapist for conservative measures. They all underwent nerve blocks that produced temporary relief.

The location of PNS implants for the upper extremities (n = 16) included ulnar (n = 9), median (n = 6) and radial (n = 1), and for the lower extremities (n = 8) included common peroneal (n = 4), posterior tibial (n = 2), sural (n = 1) and saphenous (n = 1). Follow-up was 10–90 months with a mean of 24 months.

Five of 8 ONS implants were unilateral. Follow-up was 8–30 months with a mean of 12 months.

In the PNS group, 72% of patients reported good-to-excellent pain relief, 10% had minimal pain relief but increased function in the affected limb, and 78% were satisfied with their outcome. Two patients had their lead repositioned more proximally after 5 and 6 years of good relief. Two patients (one with upper and the other with lower extremity PNS) were converted to SCS. One patient lost coverage after a difficult delivery and was explanted after a trial of SCS. We did not experience compressive neuropathy secondary to the paddle use.

Of 8 ONS patients, 6 reported good-to-excellent pain relief (50–75%) and the remaining 2 reported poor (<50%) pain relief.

One patient had to be re-operated twice due to connector pulling sensation and had to be repositioned. One patient required antibiotic therapy for another 7 days after permanent implant for incision site infection.

Complications

Most complications of PNS are related to hardware malfunction. These include migration of leads and lead breakage [23, 24]. Paying attention to the length of the strain-reducing loop and the use of silicone medical adhesive to the hardware elements prior to suturing them to the fascial planes can minimize these events. Compressive neuropathy due to the pressure of the paddle lead has been reported [2, 17]. Properly placing the anchoring device and not applying too much torque on the target nerve could minimize this. The typical infection rates are low at around 3%. Wound dehiscence and erosion of the wire through the skin occur infrequently [25].

Conclusion

PNS for chronic neuropathic pain syndromes is an exciting field of neuromodulation. Improving our understanding of the pain syndromes treated as well as that of the modulators of the pain pathway must parallel the development of the available technology. That, along with the growing acceptance of these techniques among the neuromodulation clinicians, will result in better surgical selection and a refined implantation technique to improve the outcome of these patients. These therapies would achieve greater acceptance and result in better efficacy from the use of well-designed and well-conducted multicenter prospective trials.

References

1 Merskey H, Bogduk N: Pain terms, a current list with definitions and notes on usage; in Merskey H, Bogduk N (eds): Classification of Chronic Pain, ed 2. Seattle, IASP Press, 1994, pp 209–214.

2 Nashold BS Jr, Goldner JL, Mullen JB, Bright DS: Long-term pain control by direct peripheral-nerve stimulation. J Bone Joint Surg Am 1982;64:1–10.

3 Racz GB, Lewis R Jr, Heavner JE, Scott J: Peripheral nerve stimulator implant for treatment of causalgia; in Stanton-Hicks M (ed): Pain and the Sympathetic Nervous System. Boston, Kluwer Academic Publishers, 1990, pp 225–239.

4 Wall PD, Sweet WH: Temporary abolition of pain in man. Science 1967;155:108–109.

5 Weiner RL: Peripheral nerve neurostimulation. Neurosurg Clin N Am 2003;14:401–408.

6 Rogers LL, Swidan S: Stimulation of the occipital nerve for the treatment of migraine: current state and future prospects. Acta Neurochir Suppl 2007;97:121–128.

7 Weiner RL: Occipital neurostimulation for treatment of intractable headache syndromes. Acta Neurochir Suppl 2007;97:129–133.

8 Burnstock G: Purinergic receptors and pain. Curr Pharm Des 2009;15:1717–1735.

9 Melzack RA, Wall PD: Pain mechanisms: a new theory. Science 1965;150:971–979.

10 Chung JM, Fang ZR, Hori Y, Lee KH, Willis WD: Prolonged inhibition of primate spinothalamic tract cells by peripheral nerve stimulation. Pain 1984;19:259–275.

11 Chung JM, Lee KH, Hori Y, Endo K, Willis WD: Factors influencing peripheral nerve stimulation produced inhibition of primate spinothalamic tract cells. Pain 1984;19:277–293.

12 Ignelzi RJ, Nyquist JK: Excitability changes in peripheral nerve fibers after repetitive electrical stimulation: implications in pain modulation. J Neurosurg 1979;51:824–833.

13 Moskowitz MA: Defining a pathway to discovery from bench to bedside: the trigeminovascular system and sensitization. Headache 2008;48:688–690.

14 Matharu MS, Bartsch T, Ward N, Frackowiak RS, Weiner R, Goadsby PJ: Central neuromodulation in chronic migraine patients with suboccipital stimulators: a PET study. Brain 2004;127:220–230.

15 Slavin KV, Colpan ME, Munawar N, Wess C, Nersesyan H: Trigeminal and occipital peripheral nerve stimulation for craniofacial pain: a single-institution experience and review of the literature. Neurosurg Focus 2006;21:E5.

16 Sweet WH: Control of pain by direct electrical stimulation of peripheral nerves. Clin Neurosurg 1976;23:103–111.

17 Picaza JA, Cannon BW, Hunter SE, Boyd AS, Guma J, Maurer D: Pain suppression by peripheral nerve stimulation. II. Observations with implanted devices. Surg Neurol 1975;4:115–126.

18 Kapural L, Mekhail N, Hayek SM, Stanton-Hicks M, Malak O: Occipital nerve electrical stimulation via the midline approach and subcutaneous surgical leads for treatment of severe occipital neuralgia: a pilot study. Anesth Analg 2005;101:171–174.

19 Eldrige JS, Obray JB, Pingree MJ, Hoelzer BC: Occipital neuromodulation: ultrasound guidance for peripheral nerve stimulator implantation. Pain Pract 2010;10:580–585.

20 Huntoon MA, Burgher AH: Ultrasound-guided permanent implantation of peripheral nerve stimulation (PNS) system for neuropathic pain of the extremities: original cases and outcomes. Pain Med 2009;10:1369–1377.

21 Oh MY, Ortega J, Bellotte JB, Whiting DM, Aló K: Peripheral nerve stimulation for the treatment of occipital neuralgia and transformed migraine using a C1-2-3 subcutaneous paddle style electrode: a technical report. Neuromodulation 2004;7:103–112.

22 Stewart WF, Lipton RB, Whyte J, Dowson A, Kolodner K, Liberman JN, Sawyer J: An international study to assess reliability of the Migraine Disability Assessment (MIDAS) score. Neurology 1999;53:988–994.

23 Schwedt TJ, Dodick DW, Hentz J, Trentman TL, Zimmerman RS: Occipital nerve stimulation for chronic headache: long-term safety and efficacy. Cephalalgia 2007;27:153–157.

24 Trentman TL, Zimmerman RS: Occipital nerve stimulation: technical and surgical aspects of implantation. Headache 2008;48:319–327.

25 Slavin KV: Peripheral nerve stimulation for neuropathic pain. Neurotherapeutics 2008;5:100–106.

26 Cauthen JC, Renner EJ: Transcutaneous and peripheral nerve stimulation for chronic pain states. Surg Neurol 1975;4:102–104.
27 Campbell JN, Long DM: Peripheral nerve stimulation in the treatment of intractable pain. J Neurosurg 1976;45:692–699.
28 Picaza JA, Hunter SE, Cannon BW: Pain suppression by peripheral nerve stimulation: chronic effects of implanted devices. Appl Neurophysiol 1977–1978;40:223–234.
29 Long DM: Electrical stimulation for the control of pain. Arch Surg 1977;112:884–888.
30 Law JD, Sweet J, Kirsch WM: Retrospective analysis of 22 patients with chronic pain treated by peripheral nerve stimulation. J Neurosurg 1980;52:482–485.
31 Waisbrod H, Panhans C, Hansen D, Gerbeshagen HU: Direct nerve stimulation for painful peripheral neuropathies. J Bone Joint Surg (Br) 1985; 67:470–472.
32 Strege DW, Cooney WP, Wood MB, Johnson SJ, Metcalf BJ: Chronic peripheral nerve pain treated with direct electrical nerve stimulation. J Hand Surg Am 1994;19:931–939.
33 Eisenberg E, Waisbrod H, Gerbershagen HU: Long-term peripheral nerve stimulation for painful nerve injuries. Clin J Pain 2004;20:143–146.
34 Mobbs RJ, Nair S, Blum P: Peripheral nerve stimulation for the treatment of chronic pain. J Clin Neurosci 2007;14:216–223.
35 Van Calenbergh F, Gybels J, Van Laere K, Dupont P, Plaghki L, Depreitere B, Kupers R: Long term clinical outcome of peripheral nerve stimulation in patients with chronic peripheral neuropathic pain. Surg Neurol 2009;72:330–335.
36 Weiner RL, Reed KL: Peripheral neurostimulation for control of intractable occipital neuralgia. Neuromodulation 1999;2:217–221.
37 Hammer M, Doleys DM: Perineuromal stimulation in the treatment of occipital neuralgia: a case study. Neuromodulation 2001;4:47–51.
38 Jones RL: Occipital nerve stimulation using a Medtronic Resume II® electrode array. Pain Physician 2003;6:507–508.
39 Popeney CA, Aló KM: Peripheral neurostimulation for the treatment of chronic, disabling transformed migraine. Headache 2003;43:369–375.
40 Rodrigo-Royo MD, Azcona JM, Quero J, Lorente MC, Acín P, Azcona J: Peripheral neurostimulation in the management of cervicogenic headaches: four case reports. Neuromodulation 2005;4:241–248.
41 Johnstone CS, Sundaraj R: Occipital nerve stimulation for the treatment of occipital neuralgia: eight case studies. Neuromodulation 2006;9:41–47.
42 Slavin KV, Nersesyan H, Wess C: Peripheral neurostimulation for treatment of intractable occipital neuralgia. Neurosurgery 2006;58:128–132.
43 Magis D, Allena M, Bolla M, De Pasqua V, Remacle JM, Schoenen J: Occipital nerve stimulation for drug-resistant chronic cluster headache: a prospective pilot study. Lancet Neurol 2007;6:314–321.
44 Burns B, Watkins L, Goadsby PJ: Treatment of medically intractable cluster headache by occipital nerve stimulation: long-term follow-up of eight patients. Lancet 2007;369:1099–1106.
45 Melvin EA Jr, Jordan FR, Weiner RL, Primm D: Using peripheral stimulation to reduce the pain of C2-mediated occipital headaches: a preliminary report. Pain Physician 2007;10:453–460.

Dr. Line Jacques
Montreal Neurological Institute & Hospital
3801 University Street, Room 109
Montreal, QC H3A 2B4 (Canada)
Tel. +1 514 398 6644, E-Mail ljacques2@yahoo.com

Slavin KV (ed): Peripheral Nerve Stimulation.
Prog Neurol Surg. Basel, Karger, 2011, vol 24, pp 41–57

Percutaneous Peripheral Nerve Stimulation

Kenneth M. Aló[a,b] · Marina V. Abramova[c] · Erich O. Richter[c]

[a]Pain Management, The Methodist Hospital, The Methodist Hospital Research Institute, The Texas Medical Center Houston, Houston, Tex., [b]Section of Neurocardiology, Monterrey, Technical University Monterrey, Monterrey, Mexico and [c]LSU Health Sciences Center, New Orleans, La., USA

Abstract

Since its inception in the 1970s, peripheral neuromodulation has become an increasingly common procedure to treat chronic neuropathic disorders. Historically, peripheral nerve stimulation (PNS) originated with the placement of large surface cuff electrodes, which was refined by the introduction of functional nerve mapping with circumferential electrical stimulation. This substantially improved the targeting of sensory fascicles. Surgical placement of spinal cord stimulation (SCS) 'button type' paddle electrodes was replaced when the introduction of percutaneous cylindrical SCS electrodes expanded the spectrum of PNS applications and improved the ability to target afferent sensory fibers as well as reducing the complication rate. To further refine functional mapping for the placement of these percutaneous electrodes, radiofrequency needle probes have more recently been employed to elicit paresthesias in awake patients to map the pain generators and guide treatment. In this chapter, we provide a description of the development and basic mechanisms of peripheral nerve stimulation, as well as a more detailed description of the two most commonly employed forms of peripheral nerve stimulation: occipital nerve stimulation for occipital neuralgia, and subcutaneous peripheral nerve field stimulation to stimulate free nerve endings within the subcutaneous tissue when the pain is limited to a small, well-localized area. The closely related ideas of internal and external targeted subcutaneous stimulation are also discussed.

The basic science of neurostimulation was advanced into clinical practice by the gate control theory of pain [1]. Following the seminal publication of stimulation-produced analgesia (SPA) by Reynolds [2], clinicians and basic scientists – working both independently and in collaboration – tested the gate theory in both animals and humans in a variety of experiments. These experiments led to the introduction of spinal cord stimulation (SCS) by Shealy and coworkers and cutaneous electrical nerve stimulators by Long and Shealy, later named transcutaneous electrical nerve stimulation (TENS) by Burton [3–8]. Both transcutaneous and spinal cord neurostimulators were subsequently applied clinically [9, 10]. SCS initially focused on the central nervous system (CNS), but neuropathic pain localized to a specific nerve territory – cranial, peripheral, or visceral nerve complex – frequently did not respond to SCS. Thus, the combination of SCS and peripheral neuromodulation or peripheral nerve nerve stimulation (PNS) was investigated during the 1970s. In many of those early cases, PNS failed to achieve consistent analgesia due to inadequate scientific research, poor patient selection, and limitations related to existent hardware. As a result, PNS was seldom performed in the 1970s due to high morbidity and poor surgical outcomes. Still, some surgeons recognized its potential and persisted with its development for refractory neuropathic pain.

Initial Surgical Electrode Placements

Even though selective fascicular stimulation was the recognized means by which an optimal peripheral clinical response was to be achieved, the initial peripheral nerve stimulators were surgical placements with large surface cuff electrodes. To test the viability and location of these initial surgical PNS placements, percutaneous electrodes were commonly trialed [11, 12]. After implantation of percutaneous electrodes on the target nerve, a trial of PNS was undertaken by attaching the lead cable to an externalized pulse generator and later removed. Prior to surgical placement, electrophysiological studies, at least two nerve blocks that gave relief from pain during the anesthetic phase (first 2–3 days), and a percutaneous trial stimulation proximal to the nerve pathology that provided at least 50% pain relief was desired. Functional improvement, reduced disability, a reduction of allodynia and hyperalgesia, and improvement in blood flow and motor function were also commonly measured.

In an effort to further define the best surgical placement, functional nerve mapping by circumferential electrical stimulation to localize sensory fascicles was also introduced [13, 14]. Sunderland [15, 16] demonstrated that motor and sensory components are more randomly arranged in the proximal segments of large nerve trunks, and more discretely localized in the distal extremities. Law et al. [17] were able to develop a success rate of 60% after mapping patients with upper extremity postherpetic or traumatic neuropathies, but lower extremity reports [11, 18–22] generally continued to show poor outcomes with initial surgical cuff PNS surgeries. An example case of such failure for lower extremity pain is a saddle electrode with eight contacts placed subepineurally on the sciatic nerve [23]. This arrangement failed to produce meaningful sensory stimulation. The failure was part anatomic, part technical, and part scar based as the cuff surface electrodes became adherent over time. These electrodes have since undergone extensive development for use in functional efferent motor electrical stimulation [24–26]. As the efficiency of the surgical electrode surface interface was influenced by epineural tissue and the deep location of sensory fascicles, the stimulation amplitude required to achieve threshold for afferent fascicular sensory stimulation was quite close to the threshold for motor stimulation [14].

In the 1980s, cuff electrodes gave way to direct surgical placement of SCS paddle 'button type' electrodes for PNS. When compared with cuffs, a thin layer of fascia or tendon had to be interposed between the SCS paddle electrode and the nerve to improve the activation threshold and reduce direct scarring to the fascicles [27, 28]. Several reports acknowledge the success of this modification, but widespread application of SCS paddles for PNS remained limited due to a variety of problems [29–32], such as the inability to provide uniform, stable stimulation to a nerve trunk due to their rigid rectangular shape. Subsequent rotation, torsion, translation, direct adhesion, and/or distraction away from the PNS target produced a loss of nerve fiber recruitment and analgesic effect. Despite an overall improvement compared to cuff electrodes, surgical paddle approaches still did not achieve the ultimate goal of selective fascicular sensory stimulation. With the subsequent lack of more selective surgical electrode systems, PNS as a field was stagnant until the late 1990s when percutaneous cylindrical SCS-type PNS techniques where introduced for C1–2-3 neuralgia, occipital neuralgia, and transformed migraine [33–36, 45].

Peripheral Neurostimulation: Pertinent Anatomy and Physiology

In the past decade, the scope of PNS has increased markedly for upper and lower extremity, cranial, occipital, lumbar, sacral, genitofemoral, ilioinguinal, axial, segmental and ilio-hypogastric nerves. The primary reason for this dynamic recent expansion, compared with the previous static 3 decades, has been the introduction of percutaneous cylindrical SCS-type electrodes for use in PNS [33–36, 45]. The ability to place the electrical field near the neural fascicles without open dissection has not only reduced the morbidity of scarring and the mechanical challenges of the previous surgical systems, but also improved the ability to differentially stimulate the afferent sensory fascicles. To better appreciate this, a general review of neural microanatomy and physiology follows. The mammalian nerve is comprised of an axon bounded by an axolemma and contained within a complex sheath. In myelinated fibers, the single axon is surrounded by many laminae, and interrupted at variable distance by internodes. The myelin sheath is surrounded by the endothelial tube. For unmyelinated fibers, these tubes may contain several axons. Throughout its length the diameter of an axon may vary [37].

Nerve fibers undergo extensive branching; therefore, the total number of nerve fibers is greater in distal sections than in proximal sections of the nerve trunk [38]. Because this configuration enables a single neuron to influence a comparatively large mass of tissue, nociception from an injured branch may be referred to undisturbed tissue. In addition, by way of the axon reflex in branching axons, algesic substances are released in noninjured tissue. Axon reflexes also occur in unmyelinated cutaneous nociceptive fibers; when stimulated, they generate both orthodromic impulses, and antidromic impulses in efferent collateral fibers to blood vessels and skin. These physiologic actions have a significant bearing not only on the effects of central neurostimulation but also on PNS. Skin, subcutaneous tissue, and fascia are supplied with free nerve endings (sensory fibers, nodal fibers, and postganglionic sympathetic fibers), and a range of nociceptors [39]. The function of peripheral afferent end terminals, or nociceptors, in neuropathic and other pain syndromes is severely compromised; particularly in terms of alteration of local conductance activity and changed terminal chemistry [39]. The delivery of neurostimulation to an affected painful area close to free nerve endings can act as a catalyst that reduces this abnormal electrical activity, subsequently returning neuronal conductance to normal sodium-channel transmission [40, 41]. Mechanoreceptors and sympathetic efferent fibers also have a role in the development of pain and the subsequent response to peripheral neuromodulation [42]; the local release of neurotransmitters and neuromodulators may also play a role following neurostimulation [43].

Nerve Trunks

Nerve trunks consist of fascicles which are invested with a thin, laminated sheath of perineural cells and collagen with endoneural tubes investing each nerve fiber. The fascicles within a nerve trunk are surrounded by loose areolar tissue, the epineurium.

Fascicular Anatomy

Fascicles do not run in strictly parallel groups, but repeatedly divide, unite, and re-divide to form an extensive plexus throughout the length of a nerve to its terminal branches. The number of fascicles varies along the course of the nerve. For example, where a nerve crosses a joint, the fascicles are more numerous [44]. The localization of specific fascicles, while random in the proximal portion of their nerve trunks, begins to orient in functional terms as they approach their terminal branches. The nerve fascicles are supported by and receive their nutrition from the epineurium. The amount of epineural tissue, which varies among nerves, influences the amount of electrical energy necessary to achieve a clinical effect during neurostimulation. The epineural tissue acts as a diffusion barrier that effects local anesthetic action; nerves with fewer fascicles and a thicker perineurium are more difficult to block.

Blood Supply of Peripheral Nerves

The vasa nervorum are an irregular source of nutrition that supplies each peripheral nerve from adjacent blood vessels. After entering a nerve, a nutrient artery branches

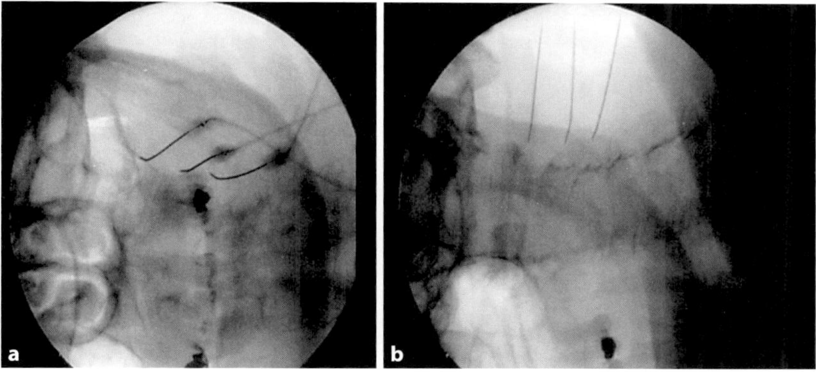

Fig. 1. Anteroposterior (**a**) and lateral (**b**) radiographic images of an awake patient with intra-operative right C1–C2–C3 stimulating needles 'mapping' dermatomal paresthesia into the distal right C2, C3 (lesser C1) dermatomes (50 Hz at 2.0 V).

into plexuses. Some of the early morbidity associated with PNS during the 1970s was undoubtedly due to intra-epineural sclerosis and extraneural constriction interfering with the nutritional blood supply. Disturbance to adjacent anastomotic vessels should be minimized during any surgical procedure on a nerve. This is much less concerning with newer percutaneous PNS approaches.

Percutaneous Surgical Techniques

Percutaneous Needle Stimulation: Mapping the Painful Neural Structure

Percutaneous PNS electrodes will only be effective if they are placed in the vicinity of the painful peripheral nerve(s) close enough to elicit appropriate sensory paresthesia into the affected pain distribution [33–35]. In fact, Weiner described very poor success using a deep fascial dissection with the first 6 occipital PNS systems placed. This was due to an inability to map paresthesia into the correct distal C2 or C3 painful nerve branches [Weiner, pers. commun., 1996]. As a result, we suggested first eliciting paresthesia in the awake patient via a radiofrequency (RF) needle (Radionics, Boston, Mass., USA) at the extraspinal respective C2, or C3 rami (to lesser extent C1), or via an epidural Racz catheter (Epimed International, Lubbock, Tex., USA) at the same levels [Alo, 1996, unpubl. results]. This allowed the patient to precisely confirm that the paresthesia was reproduced into the specific painful dermatome(s) to guide the subsequent local anesthetic blockade and/or subcutaneous (not deep fascial) percutaneous PNS electrode placement (fig. 1a, b).

If as in figure 1, the awake patient is able to confirm concordant dermatomal needle stimulation paresthesia into their painful distribution prior to placement of local anesthetic blockade, then a 'dermatomal map' is recorded and local anesthetic and

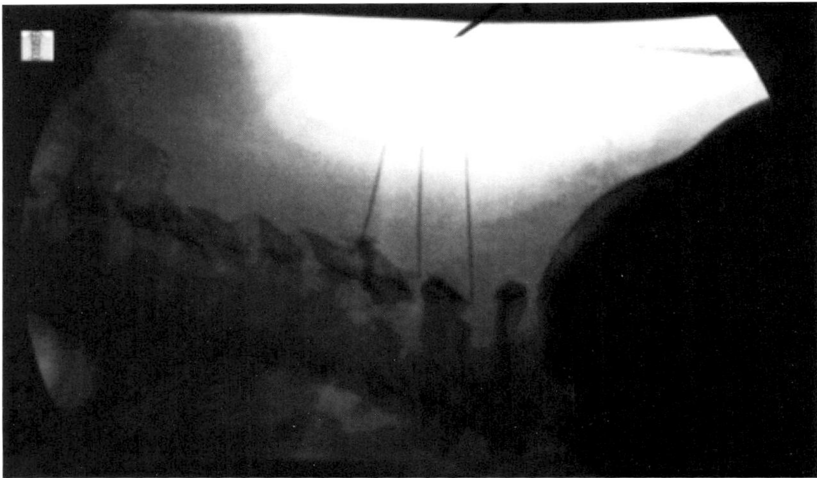

Fig. 2. Intra-operative, pre-injection, percutaneous needle stimulation in the awake patient of the right intra-articular C1/C2, C2/C3, C3/C4 facet joints (50 Hz at 3.5 V) reproducing nondermatomal aching into the right neck.

corticosteroid injected. Thereafter, their postoperative anesthetic (days 1–3) and corticosteroid (days 3+) responses are documented in diary fashion.

However, if the dermatomal mapping is nonconcordant, or only partially concordant, then other non-nervous structures need to be assessed in the same fashion to further refine the pain source(s). For example, the upper interarticular facet joints may be stimulated with the RF needle (50 Hz and 3.5 V) to produce a 'sclerotomal map'. They may also then be blocked with local anesthetic and corticosteroid to identify if a potentially confounding non-dermatomal cervicocranial pain trigger is present (fig. 2). Likewise, the same process could be applied systematically in other cervical structures (uncovertebral joint, muscles, discs, etc.) This is especially important in complex presentations with overlapping pain sources to exclude sources that may be less responsive to PNS. If, in the patient depicted in figure 2, for example, a nondermatomal, painful, aching into the upper neck is concordantly produced with stimulation, and then resolves in the postoperative anesthetic and/or corticosteroid phases, an upper cervical neurotomy, rather than a percutaneous PNS trial would be performed.

Since the authors have adopted this technique (differentiation/clarification of neural vs. non-neural painful structures), outcomes of Weiner's original percutaneous C1–C2–C3 PNS approach immediately improved while indications expanded. As a result, the extension of this strategy to many other dermatomal, sclerotomal, and discogenic pain generators (see illustrative cases below) also ensued. While this technique is not our primary focus here, and a complete discussion of these techniques is beyond the scope of this chapter, we have included this brief description to clarify how percutaneous needle stimulation can help identify pain sources that may be more responsive to longer-term percutaneous PNS catheter placement.

Occipital Nerve Stimulation

The original description for percutaneous PNS was that of occipital lead placement into the subcutaneous tissues innervated by the distal C1, C2, and C3 posterior primary rami for occipital neuralgia. The first reported cases [33] described a percutaneous wire electrode lead placement. Since then, numerous uses of neuromodulation for occipital neuralgia and headache, including transformed migraine, have been reported [34–36, 45–47]. In an effort to reduce electrode migration and improve tissue contact and conduction, percutaneous paddle electrode placement has also been developed [45].

To demonstrate initial efficacy and pain control, almost all potential candidates for occipital nerve stimulation (ONS) implant undergo a percutaneous trial electrode placement of up to 1 week or more. Percutaneous needle stimulation mapping (as described above), applied at the time of occipital nerve or C1, C2, or C3 blockade can further focus trial placement. This procedure can be done in an office or other outpatient setting with minimal or no sedation. The general electrode implant steps are identical to those applied for the permanent device (outlined below). After placement, the electrodes are sutured to the skin, covered with generous dressings, and connected to the supplied transmitter. During the trial, patients measure the percentage of pain relief and symptom control obtained, as well as any functional or medication improvements. Following the trial period the electrodes are removed, the patient is interviewed, and a decision is made regarding permanent implantation. Pain and/or associated symptom relief of 50% is generally acceptable to proceed. For the wounds to heal and to minimize risks of infection, at least 1–2 weeks are required before a new incision is made for permanent implantation. Alternatively, permanent electrodes can be placed at the initial procedure, tunneled with extension wires during the trial period, and then connected to a pulse generator with removal of the extensions if the trial is successful.

Implant – Percutaneous Wire Electrodes

Most implants are bilateral lead placements at or near the level of C1, with trajectories ranging from zero to almost 90° from the vertex of the occipital scalp. Implants of percutaneous electrodes for ONS (and most other percutaneous applications) include the following considerations:

1 Obtain informed consent. Describe to the patient if the application is on or off label.
2 Clip the suboccipital scalp as necessary.
3 Place a nasal cannula for O_2 and an IV.
4 Position the patient awake, lateral or prone, with the arms tucked at the sides.
5 Prep all involved skin areas sterilely, cover with antibacterial adhesive film, drape widely.

6 Mark incision sites.
7 Administer a small dose of propofol, midazolam, or other short-acting anesthetic agent prior to a local anesthetic (with epinephrine for hemostasis) injection of the incision site.
8 Make an incision through the skin and subcutaneous tissue to the level of the cervical fascia, obtain hemostasis with electrocautery.
9 Create small subcutaneous pockets on either side of the incision with Metz scissors to allow seating of the electrode loops created at the end of the case. These loops help avoid migration of the electrodes.
10 Bend the supplied Tuohy needle gently.
11 Place the needle subcutaneously from the midline incision laterally, or angled somewhat superiorly staying superficial to the fascia at all times. Extend the needle beyond the point of maximal occipital tenderness or pain as reported by the patient to allow for some repositioning of the electrode more proximally if necessary during 'on-the-table' test stimulation with C-arm fluoroscopic guidance.
12 Remove the stylet and place the multicontact electrode through the needle to its tip, then gently pull the needle out while keeping mild forward pressure on the electrode.
13 Once the needle has been completely removed, connect the distal end of the electrode to a lead extension wire for intraoperative stimulation testing, with the patient awake to report and record the paresthesia perception and maximum tolerable threshold(s) and location.
14 Once acceptable coverage has been attained, affix the electrode to the underlying fascia with the supplied anchors.
15 Repeat this procedure on the other side.
16 Sedate patient with short-acting anesthetic agents in preparation for tunneling and generator pocket dissection and placement if an entire permanent implantation is to be performed.
17 Create tension-relieving loops in the electrode within the cervical incision and secure the electrode gently to the fascia with absorbable suture prior to wound closure to maintain the loop and reduce migration as well as to avoid electrode twisting.

Permanent Implant Paddle

Permanent implant with a paddle requires additionally the following:

1 Settle patient in lateral or prone position, and mark the pain site.
2 Make the incision medial to the pain site.
3 Perform a sharp subcutaneous dissection to accommodate the paddle electrode face down with contacts toward the fascia in the fat layer.
4 Create a pocket with a plastic or metal dissector to accept the paddle.
5 Attend to hemostasis meticulously with cautery.

6 Test, anchor, tunnel, and connect the pulse generator and verify the connection as usual.

We expect that these techniques will continue to be improved, with fewer complications, to more refined total local implants and wireless products as microcircuitry evolves.

Subcutaneous Peripheral Nerve Field Stimulation

Subcutaneous peripheral nerve field (PNfS) stimulation is a technique in which the lead or leads stimulate not a main nerve trunk but rather the small endings of the distribution of the nerve within the subcutaneous tissue directly beneath the dermis. It has been described by many authors [48, 49].

Entry in the subcutaneous tissue is usually characterized by a 'pop' feeling from the loss of resistance once the needle has penetrated the epidermis and dermis. This technique, a revolutionary change in the paradigm of classical neurostimulation, was developed to direct stimulation to areas that are difficult to reach from the spinal cord or major nerve trunk level. In the classical stimulation, the goal is to stimulate some major nervous sensory structures upstream from the painful area to convey paresthesiae in that area. In contrast, with PNfS the lead is actually placed in or near the area of the pain or the area of the projection of the pain. If the pain is limited to a relatively small and well-defined area, PNfS is now sometimes utilized as a first, minimally invasive, neurostimulation procedure.

PNfS is best accomplished with percutaneous cylindrical leads and not with paddle leads. When performing dorsal column, nerve root, or large peripheral nerve stimulation, the target is well defined and the lead is placed on top of it; the current is therefore unidirectional and best delivered by a paddle lead. With PNfS, however, the lead is placed within the target, which is made of all the small sensory nerve endings within the subcutaneous tissues. The best electrical field is therefore circumferential, like that delivered by a percutaneously placed cylindrical lead.

With PNfS, the lead should be placed within or as near as possible to the painful area. The number, spacing, and distribution of the electrical contacts should be carefully planned according to the size and shape of the painful area.

If mild allodynia exists, the lead or leads may still be placed within the painful area. In the case of severe allodynia, however, the best strategy is to insert the leads on each side of the allodynic area to 'bracket' it. It is crucial to carefully map the transition zone between the allodynic area and the nonallodynic area and place the lead exactly in that zone; the difference of only a centimeter could substantially impact the success or failure of the modality.

Almost any area of the body can be reached with this technique. Most commonly addressed are the lumbar area, the posterior thoracic area, the scapular area, the inguinal area, and various regions of the head and face.

The trial is performed without an incision, by inserting the leads in the subcutaneous tissue through the needle provided in the kit or some other inserting device.

Although the procedure is simple, it must be done with short intravenous sedation. Once the leads are inserted, the trial is undertaken similar to a regular spinal cord stimulation trial. If the pain is reduced, the whole system is implanted at a second sitting. Although more experience is needed with this technique, a positive response to transcutaneous stimulation may be an indicator of success with PNfS.

PNfS can also be utilized in conjunction with intraspinal stimulation or large peripheral nerve stimulation. Although the technique is not particularly invasive, great care must be taken in surgical planning and execution. The leads must be placed exactly in the painful area or areas, which requires careful assessment of the topography of the pain. The most common indications include intractable axial lumbar pain, posterior thoracic pain, and scapular pain; inguinal pain; thoracic wall pain; and shoulder pain.

Subcutaneous Targeted Peripheral Stimulation

The original percutaneous PNS [33] and then PNfS techniques soon evolved to include other mononeural neuralgias [50–55]. In addition, a multiple needle stimulation technique using alternating frequencies of 15 and 30 Hz, for diabetic neuropathic pain and for low back pain was described, called percutaneous electrical nerve stimulation (PENS). This involved percutaneous implantation at multiple locations using a stimulating needle as taught initially by Racz (Racz-stimulating epidural catheter, circa 1983) and refined at various pain structures by Aló in 1996 with the stimulation mapping techniques described above. This improved the precision of the therapy, expanding applications for PNS to neural structures such as the brachial plexus [56], the lumbar plexus [57], single peripheral nerves [58], the paravertebral space [59], and the sympathetic chain [60].

Here, the concept of applying percutaneous PNS to pain in a non-dermatomal distribution by targeting the stimulation via a stimulating needle or subcutaneous placement of a stimulating electrode array to the nerve distribution for that area, led to the term targeted stimulation (TS). Subsequent introductions of nerve localization approach (percutaneous electrode guidance – PEG) into clinical practice by Urmey and Grossi [61] led to the application of this device for the treatment of neuropathic pain and resulted in the development of external neuromodulation (EN) [56, 62, 63]; EN involves application of electrical stimulation via an external nerve mapping probe connected to an impulse generator. Albeit noninvasive, the adoption of a nerve mapping probe similar to previous applications of single episode needle stimulation or stimulating catheter placement proved to be as effective as direct needle or stimulating catheter application [58, 64]. These preliminary reports provide anecdotal evidence for the effectiveness of EN [62, 63]. Khan et al. [65] introduced a concept similar to EN, subcutaneous electrical nerve stimulation (SENS). They employed SENS in the treatment of chronic neuropathic pain in 2 patients who were unsuitable for conventional therapy. Buchser et al. [66] used this principle of targeted stimulation, which they called subcutaneous peripheral nerve stimulation (SPNS), for application in patients with failed back surgery syndrome (FBSS). Krutsch et al. [67] reported successful application of SENS in a patient with FBSS who remained nearly pain-free at 1-year follow up. The beneficial effects of peripheral stimulation, percutaneous stimulation, and TS, using low-frequency modulation, can be partially explained by the interruption of the input of nociceptive afferents [68].

Local suppression of Aβ-fiber activity by TS is another attractive mechanistic hypothesis, but central mechanisms have also been suggested for the effects seen from peripheral neuromodulation [69, 70].

Indications and Rationale for Patient Selection
When conservative medical management, nerve blocks, or neuroablation have failed to provide adequate relief in patients with chronic pain in a localized nondermatomal area, subcutaneous neuromodulation may be considered. When selecting a patient for PNfS, it is important to consider the level of invasiveness, efficacy, and cost of the procedure compared with other remaining options. The neurostimulation coverage of a painful target area with an electrical field applied subcutaneously, or oriented to deeper structures permits for effective direct stimulation and therefore neuromodulation of peripheral receptors in the affected area without specific direct application to either nerves or plexuses. In general, for PNfS to be effective, stimulation must be localized within the topographical area of pain; however, outcomes may still be positive even if the stimulation does not cover the marginal areas of the pain complaint, as noted in the concepts of PNfS and TS above. The application of stimulation via multicontact leads which are situated directly at the epicenter of the painful area and targeted to the site of pain as directed by the patients is a safe, simple, and effective mode of treatment.

Discussion and Conclusion

We have reviewed the basic principles and historical development of PNS, including the two most prominent forms in current usage, ONS and PNfS. These technologies and techniques will continue to evolve and improve over the years to come. We expect that the percutaneous RF needle stimulation mapping techniques will further refine dermatomal vs. sclerotomal stimulation, and help with other less responsive neurostimulation targets. In distinction to epidural SCS, in which the trend is toward refined steering of lateral and cephalocaudal current to improve neural targeting, PNS will move toward smaller devices capable of direct regional current targeting. On the other hand, newer systems may also allow a more diffuse stimulation grid to be implanted over larger surface areas with less invasiveness, increasing the prominence of subcutaneous field stimulation. Regardless, the coming years promise to be an era of clinical innovation and advance in the treatment of chronic neuropathic pain with percutaneous PNS neuromodulatory techniques.

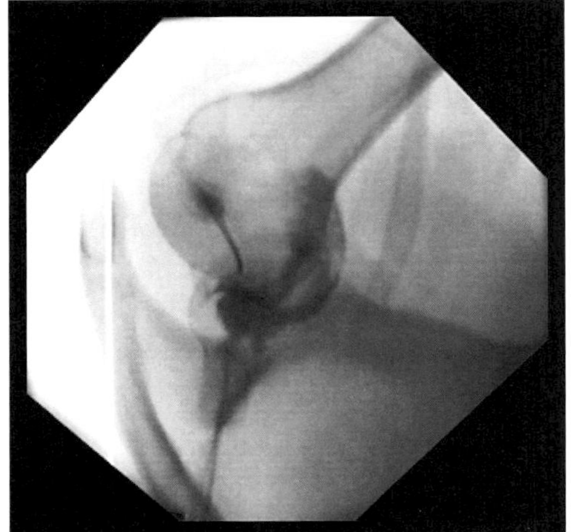

Fig. 3. Radiograph showing radiofrequency needle positioned in the interarticular aspect of the shoulder joint.

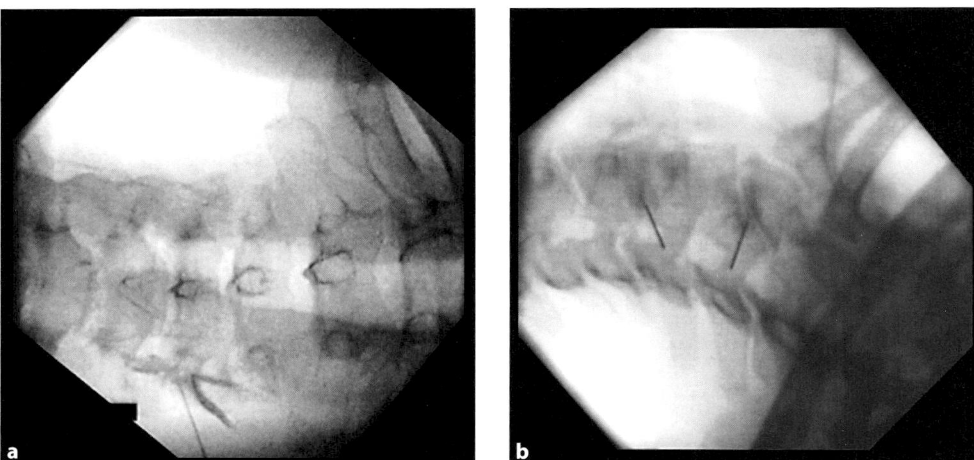

Fig. 4. Radiographic images (**a** – anteroposterior view; **b** – lateral view) of radiofrequency needle positioned at the C7 foraminal level.

Illustrative Cases

The first patient we discuss presents with neck and shoulder pain into the right upper extremity with mechanical and neuropathic elements suspected. Figure 3 shows intraoperative RF needle stimulation (50 Hz at 5 V) of the interarticular aspect of right shoulder joint in the awake patient, with referred aching confirmed (reproduced) in the subdeltoid, subacromial region. The aching pain was reduced after local anesthetic and corticosteroid injection during the anesthetic and corticosteroid phases without reduction in the radicular element. Figures 4a and b show the anteroposterior and lateral image of intraoperative RF awake needle stimulation (50 Hz at 2 V) mapping

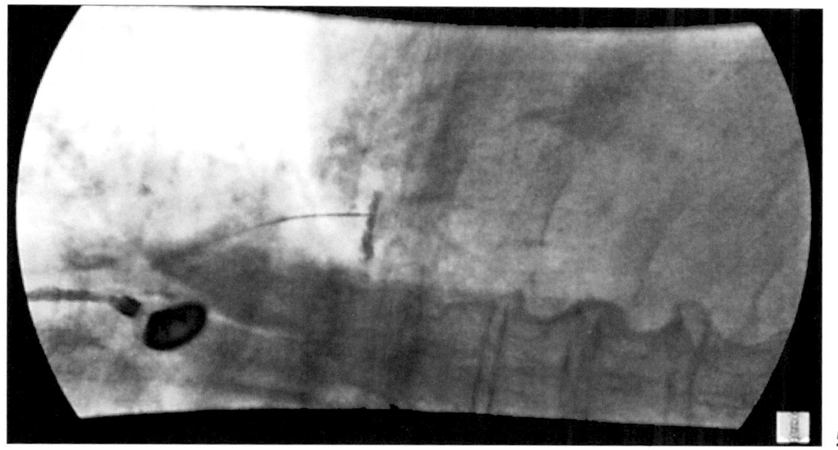

5

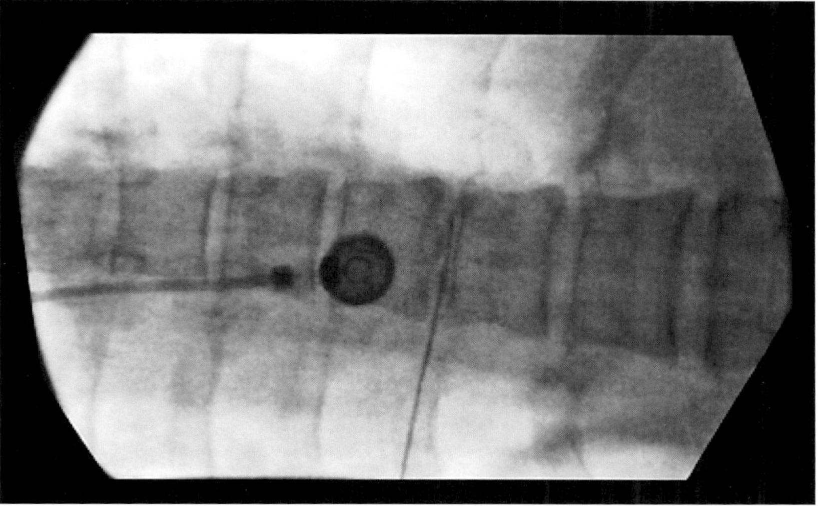

6

Fig. 5. Radiograph of radiofrequency needle positioned in the vicinity of the right T6 intercostal nerve.
Fig. 6. Radiograph of radiofrequency needle positioned in the T6-T7 disc space.

the residual right radicular C7 pain separate from the shoulder symptoms. Note the placement of the selective cervical 'foraminal needle' at the extraforaminal, extraspinal, posterior inferior laminar bone position for performance of the selective nerve root block and dermatomal mapping. This minimizes pressure and absorption within the foramen during the injection of short acting local anesthetic and nonparticulate steroid.

Another patient presented with a complex combination of right mid (T6-L7) and left and right low back (L3-L4) region pain with radiation to the left sacroiliac joint (SIJ) and right lower extremity, in the face of previous lumbar fusion and thoracic disc herniation. Figure 5 shows awake 'dermatomal mapping' (50 Hz at 2 V) of the right T6 intercostal nerve for a potential element of

7 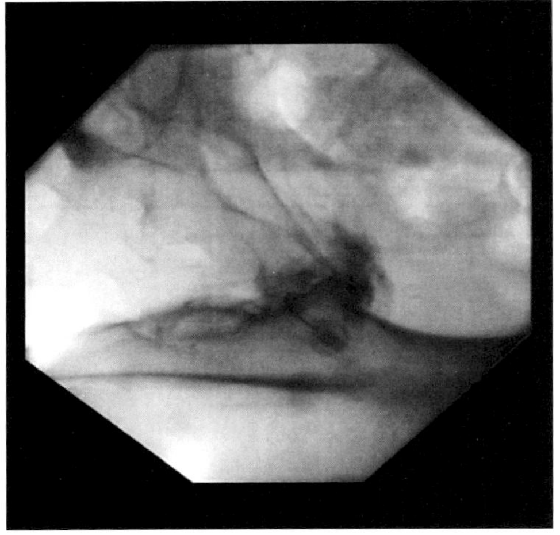

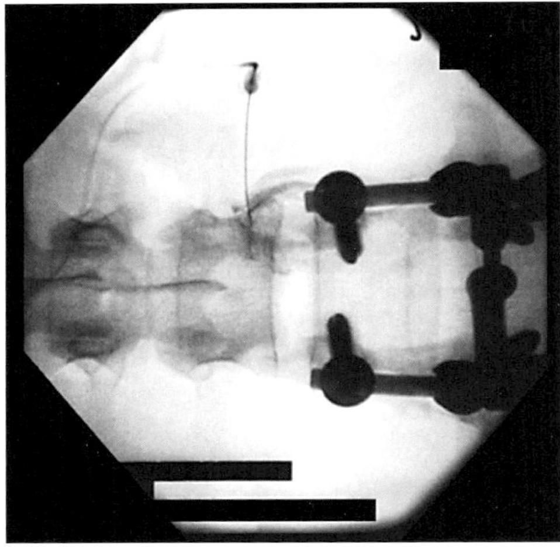 8

Fig. 7. Radiographic image of radiofrequency needle positioned in the left sacroiliac joint.
Fig. 8. Radiographic image of radiofrequency needle positioned in the vicinity of the right L3 nerve root.

radicular pain; figure 6 shows awake intradiscal 'discogenic mapping' (50 Hz at 8 V) of the T6-T7 disc for a potential element of discogenic pain; figure 7 shows awake 'sclerotomal mapping' (50 Hz at 5 V) of a posteriorly provocative left SIJ (as opposed to lateral transverse branch innervations at the L5-S1-S2-S3 foramina), and figure 8 shows awake 'dermatomal mapping' (50 Hz at 2 V) of the right L3 root at the potentially 'transitionally stressed' L3-L4 disc level. All intraoperative responses were recorded and documented in conjunction with postoperative anesthetic (days 1–3) and corticosteroid phases (days 3–7+) diaries.

References

1 Melzack R, Wall PD: Pain mechanisms: a new theory. Science 1965;150:971–979.
2 Reynolds DV: Surgery in the rat during electrical analgesia induced by focal brain stimulation. Science 1969;164:444–445.
3 Burton C: Pain suppression through peripheral nerve stimulation. Annual Houston Neurological Symposium, Houston, 1973.
4 Long DM, Hagfors N: Electrical stimulation in the nervous system: the current status of electrical stimulation of the nervous system for relief of pain. Pain 1975;1:109–123.
5 Shealy CN: Dorsal column stimulation: optimization of application. Surg Neurol 1975;4:142–145.
6 Shealy CN, Mortimer JT, Hagfors NR: Dorsal column electroanalgesia. J Neurosurg 1970;32: 560–564.
7 Shealy CN, Mortimer JT, Reswick JB: Electrical inhibition of pain by stimulation of the dorsal columns: preliminary clinical report. Anesth Analg 1967;46:489–491.
8 Long DM, Carolan MT: Cutaneous afferent stimulation in the treatment of chronic pain; in Bonica JJ (ed): International Symposium on Pain. Adv Neurol. New York, Raven Press, 1974, vol 4, pp 755–759.
9 Sweet WH: Lessons on pain control from electrical stimulation. Trans Stud Coll Physicians Phila 1968; 35:171–184.

10 Wall PD, Sweet WH: Temporary abolition of pain in man. Science 1967;155:108–109.
11 Campbell JN, Long DM: Peripheral nerve stimulation in the treatment of intractable pain. J Neurosurg 1976;45:692–699.
12 Nashold BS Jr, Mullen JB, Avery R: Peripheral nerve stimulation for pain relief using a multicontact electrode system: technical note. J Neurosurg 1979;51: 872–873.
13 Nashold BS Jr, Goldner JL: Electrical stimulation of peripheral nerves for relief of intractable chronic pain. Med Instrum 1975;9:224–225.
14 Goldner JL, Nashold BS Jr, Hendrix PC: Peripheral nerve electrical stimulation. Clin Orthop Relat Res 1982;163:33–41.
15 Sunderland S: The intraneural topography of the radial, median and ulnar nerves. Brain 1945;64:242–299.
16 Sunderland, S: Nerves and Nerve Injuries, ed 2. Edinburgh, Churchill-Livingstone, 1978.
17 Law, JT, Swett J, Kirsch W: Retrospective analysis of 22 patients with chronic pain treated by peripheral nerve stimulation. J Neurosurg 1981;52:482–485.
18 Kirsch WM, Lewis JA, Simon RH: Experience with electrical stimulation devices for the control of chronic pain. Med Instr 1975;9:217–220.
19 Picaza JA, Cannon BW, Hunter SE, Boyd AS, Guma J, Maurer D: Pain suppression by peripheral nerve stimulation. II. Observations with implanted devices. Surg Neurol 1975;4:115–126.
20 Sweet WH: Control of pain by direct electrical stimulation of peripheral nerves. Clin Neurosurg 1976; 23:103–111.
21 Waisbrod H, Panhan C, Hansen D, Gerbershagen HU: Direct nerve stimulation for painful peripheral neuropathies. J Bone Joint Surg 1985;67B: 470–472.
22 Gybels J, Kupers R: Central and peripheral electrical stimulation of the nervous system in the treatment of chronic pain. Acta Neurochir Suppl 1987; 38:64–75.
23 Buschman DN, Oppel F: Peripheral nerve stimulation for pain relief in CRPS II and phantom-limb pain (in German). Schmerz 1999;13:113–120.
24 Brummer SB, Turner MJ: Electrochemical considerations for safe electrical stimulation of the nervous system with platinum electrodes. IEEE Trans Biomed Eng 1977;24:59–63.
25 Brummer SB, Turner MJ: Electrical stimulation with Pt electrodes. I. A method for determination of 'real' electrode areas. IEEE Trans Biomed Eng 1977; 24:436–439.
26 Brummer SB, Turner MJ: Electrical stimulation with Pt electrodes. II. Estimation of maximum surface redox (theoretical non-gassing) limits. IEEE Trans Biomed Eng 1977;24:440–443.
27 Racz GB, Brown NT, Lewis R: Peripheral stimulator implant for treatment of causalgia caused by electrical burns. Tex Med 1988;84:45–50.
28 Racz GB, Lewis R, Heavner JE, Scott J: Peripheral nerve stimulator implant for treatment of causalgia; in Stanton-Hicks M (ed): Pain and the Sympathetic Nervous System. Boston, Kluwer Academic Publishers, 1990, pp 225–239.
29 Strege W, Cooney WG, Wood MB, Johnson SJ, Metcalf BJ: Chronic peripheral nerve pain treated with direct electrical nerve stimulation. J Hand Surg Am 1994;19:931–939.
30 Hassenbusch SJ, Stanton-Hicks M, Schoppa D, Walsh JG, Covington EC: Long-term peripheral nerve stimulation for reflex sympathetic dystrophy. J Neurosurg 1996;84:415–423.
31 Cooney WP: Electrical stimulation in the treatment of complex regional pain syndrome of the upper extremities. Hand Clin 1997;13:519–26.
32 Novak CV, Mackinnon SD: Outcome following implantation of peripheral nerve stimulator in patients with chronic pain. Plast Reconstr Surg 2000;105:1967–1972.
33 Weiner RL, Reed KL: Peripheral neurostimulation for the control of intractable occipital neuralgia. Neuromodulation 1999;2:217–221.
34 Weiner RL, Aló KM, Reed K: Peripheral neurostimulation for control of intractable occipital headaches. Abstr World Pain Meet, San Francisco, 2000.
35 Weiner RL, Aló KM, Reed KL, Fuller ML: Subcutaneous neurostimulation for intractable C_2 mediated headaches. J Neurosurg 2001;94:398A.
36 Popeney CA, Aló KM: C1–2–3 peripheral nerve stimulation (PNS) for the treatment of disability associated with transformed migraine. Headache 2003;43:369–373.
37 Peters A, Palay SL, Webster HF: the Fine Defined Structure of the Nervous System: The Neuron and Supporting Cells. Philadelphia, Saunders, 1976
38 Sunderland S: Nerve Injuries and Their Repair: a Critical Appraisal. Edinburgh, Churchill-Livingstone, 1991, pp 31–45.
39 Byers MR, Bonica JJ: Peripheral pain mechanisms and nociceptor plasticity; in Loeser JD (ed): Bonica's Management of Pain, ed 3. Philadelphia, Lippincott Williams & Wilkins, 2001, pp 26–72.
40 Priestley T: Voltage-gated sodium channels and pain. Curr Drug Targets CNS Neurol Disord 2004;3: 441–456.

41 Devor M: Sodium channels and mechanisms of neuropathic pain. J Pain 2006;7(suppl 1):S3–S12.
42 Na HS, Leem JW, Chung JM: Abnormalities of mechanoreceptors in a rat model of neuropathic pain: possible involvement in mediating mechanical allodynia. J Neurophysiol 1993;70:522–528.
43 Linderoth B, Stiller CO, Gunasekera L, O'Connor WT, Franck J, Gazelius B, Brodin E: Release of neurotransmitters in the CNS by spinal cord stimulation: survey of present state of knowledge and recent experimental studies. Stereotact Funct Neurosurg 1993;61:157–170.
44 DiRosa F, Giuzzi P, Battiston B: Radial nerve anatomy and fascicular arrangement; in Brunelli G (ed): Textbook of Microsurgery. Milan, Masson, 1988, p 571.
45 Oh MY, Ortega J, Bellotte JB, Whiting DM, Aló KM: Peripheral nerve stimulation for the treatment of occipital neuralgia and transformed migraine using a C1–2–3 subcutaneous paddle style electrode: a technical report. Neuromodulation 2004;7:-103–112.
46 Weiner RL: The future of peripheral nerve neurostimulation. Neurol Res 2000;22:299–304.
47 Aló KM, Holsheimer J: New trends in neuromodulation for the management of neuropathic pain. Neurosurgery 2002;50:690–704.
48 Paicius RM, Bernstein CA, Lempert-Cohen C: Peripheral nerve field stimulation in chronic abdominal pain. Pain Physician 2006;9:261–266.
49 Bernstein CA, Paicius, RM, Barkow, SH, Lempert-Cohen C: Spinal cord stimulation in conjunction with peripheral nerve field stimulation for the treatment of low back and leg pain: a case series. Neuromodulation 2008;11:116–123.
50 Hammer M, Doleys DM: Perineuromal stimulation in the treatment of occipital neuralgia: a case study. Neuromodulation 2001;4:47–51.
51 Stinson LW, Roderer GT, Cross NE, Davis BE: Peripheral subcutaneous. electrostimulation for control of intractable post-operative inguinal pain; a case report series. Neuromodulation 2001;4: 99–104.
52 Dunteman E: Peripheral nerve stimulation for unremitting ophthalmic post-herpetic neuralgia. Neuromodulation 2002;5:32–37.
53 Monti E: Peripheral nerve stimulation: a percutaneous minimally invasive approach. Neuromodulation 2004;7:193–196.
54 Ghoname EA, Craig WF, White PF, Ahmed HE, Hamza MA, Henderson BN, Gajraj NM, Huber PJ, Gatchel RJ: Percutaneous electrical nerve stimulation for low back pain: a randomized crossover study. JAMA 1999;282:941–942.
55 Hamza MA, White PF, Craig WF, Ghoname ES, Ahmed HE, Proctor TJ, Noe CE, Vakharia AS, Gajraj N: Percutaneous electrical nerve stimulation: a novel analgesic therapy for diabetic neuropathic pain. Diabetes Care 2000;23:365–370.
56 Goroszeniuk T, Hamann W, Kothari S: Percutaneous implantation of the brachial plexus electrode for management of pain syndrome caused by a traction injury. Neuromodulation 2007;10:148–55.
57 Petrovic Z, Goroszeniuk T, Kothari, S: Percutaneous lumbar plexus stimulation in the treatment of intractable pain. Reg Anesth Pain Med 2007;32 (suppl 1):11.
58 Goroszeniuk T: Short-term peripheral neuromodulation trial via stimulating catheter in neuropathic pain treatment. Reg Anesth Pain Med 2003;28 (suppl 1):64.
59 Ather MH, Goroszeniuk T, Sanderson K: The use of paravertebral neurostimulation for thoracic neuropathic pain. Int Monitor 2001;13:68.
60 Kothari S, Goroszeniuk T: Sympathetic plexus stimulation: a novel case study. Reg Anesth Pain Med 2004;29(suppl 2):99.
61 Urmey W, Grossi P: Percutaneous electrode guidance (PEG): a noninvasive technique for prelocation of peripheral nerves to facilitate nerve block. Reg Anesth Pain Med 2002;27:261–267.
62 Goroszeniuk T, Kothari S: Targeted external area stimulation. Reg Anesth Pain Med 2004;29(suppl 2):98.
63 Kothari S, Goroszeniuk T: External neuromodulation as a diagnostic and therapeutic procedure. Eur J Pain 2006;10(suppl 1):S158.
64 Goroszeniuk T: Short neuromodulation trial in neuropathic pain produces varying duration but reproducible pain relief. Proc 4th Congress of EFIC, Prague, 2003, p 326.
65 Khan EI, O'Keeffe JD, Walsh R, Goroszeniuk T: Subcutaneous electrical nerve stimulation (SENS): modality for treatment of neuropathic pain. Anaesthesia 2005;60:305–306.
66 Buchser EE, Martin Y, Koeppel C, Jacob M, Coronado I, Smit A, Chedel D, Durrer A: Subcutaneous peripheral nerve stimulation for refractory low back pain. Proc 11th World Congress on Pain, Sydney, 2005, presentation 1749–P252, p 8.

67 Krutsch JP, McCeney MH, Barolat G, Tamimi MA, Smolenski A: A case report of subcutaneous peripheral nerve stimulation for the treatment of axial back pain associated with postlaminectomy syndrome. Neuromodulation 2008;11:112–115.
68 Wall PD, Gutnik M: Properties of peripheral nerve impulses originating from neuroma. Nature 1974; 248:740–743.
69 Taub A, Campbell JN: Percutaneous local electrical analgesia: peripheral mechanisms; in Bonica JJ (ed): International Symposium on Pain. Adv Neurol. New York, Raven Press, 1974, vol 4, pp 727–732.
70 Chung JM, Fang ZR, Hori Y, Lee KH, Willis WD: Prolonged inhibition of primate spinothalamic tract cells by peripheral nerve stimulation. Pain 1984; 19:259–275.

Kenneth M. Aló, MD
Houston Texas Pain Management
5318 Weslayan #182
Houston, TX 77005 (USA)
E-Mail msmcrae@sbcglobal.net

Slavin KV (ed): Peripheral Nerve Stimulation.
Prog Neurol Surg. Basel, Karger, 2011, vol 24, pp 58–69

Peripheral Nerve Stimulation for the Treatment of Truncal Pain

Kevin D. Cairns[a] · W. Porter McRoberts[b] · Timothy Deer[c]

[a]Florida Spine Specialists, [b]Holy Cross Hospital, Fort Lauderdale, Fla., and [c]Center for Pain Relief, Inc., Charleston, W.Va., USA

Abstract

Neuromodulation practitioners increasingly recognize the potential for peripheral nerve field stimulation (PNfS) to treat pain originating from the trunk. Conditions resulting in truncal pain that may respond to PNfS include cervical and lumbar postlaminectomy syndrome, inguinal neurapraxia, postherpetic neuralgia, and post-thoracotomy pain. The focus of this chapter is to review the mechanism of action in PNfS, patient selection factors, programming strategies, and technical considerations.

Stimulation of the most distal sensory fibers termed peripheral nerve field stimulation (PNfS) is an emerging area of neuromodulation that has been gaining interest in the treatment of truncal pain. Through the pioneering work of Weiner, Slavin, and Kapural, a resurgence in peripheral nerve stimulation for the treatment of headaches and facial pain has renewed interest in stimulating sensory nerves in the periphery [1–3]. Subcutaneous placement of leads in the region of named nerves in the head and neck has been more recently adapted to placement of leads subcutaneously in the trunk. First described by Paucius for treatment of low back pain after surgery, several case studies have discussed the potential for PNfS in the treatment of truncal pain from the lumbar to the cervical region [4, 5]. The difficulty in directly stimulating named peripheral nerves in the trunk limits the application of direct peripheral nerve stimulation (PNS) for truncal pain; however, stimulation of nerve rootlets in the spinal canal using either an anterograde or retrograde technique has been reported for failed back surgery syndrome, post-herpetic neuralgia (PHN), and ilioinguinal neurapraxia [6]. PNfS is different from the conventional direct PNS first reported in 1976 in that PNfS does not require surgical dissection of an identifiable nerve and thus is not limited by location of named nerves when considering treatment [7]. This chapter will focus primarily on PNfS for truncal pain including mechanism of action,

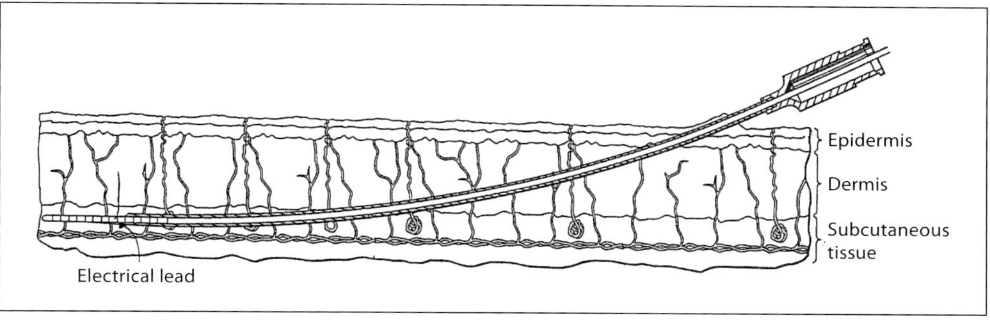

Fig. 1. Lead placement in subcutaneous layer.

technical considerations when implanting leads, patient selection, and programming strategies.

Mechanism of Action

Similar to spinal cord stimulation (SCS), the exact mechanism of action of PNfS is unknown but most likely occurs through the gate control theory of Melzack and Wall [8]. Stimulation of large sensory nerves in the periphery was later demonstrated by Wall and Sweet to alleviate pain based on the clinical application of the gate control theory [9]. Most likely, PNfS alleviates pain by stimulation of A-beta fibers in the subcutaneous layer with subsequent inhibition of A-delta and C fibers (fig. 1). The subcutaneous layer is rich in terminal A-beta sensory terminals and extracellular fluid either in the subcutaneous or subdermal region likely functions as an electrical conduit that facilitates depolarization of these sensory fibers as current follows the path of least resistance. One significant difference between PNfS and spinal cord stimulation is the potential for greater distance between polarities (cathode and anode) in PNfS. Typical SCS contact distances between cathode and anode are less than 10 mm as compared to PNfS distances between cathode and anode being significantly greater. The authors have implanted PNfS leads subcutaneously in the cervical and lumbar region with polarity distances of over 30 inches with dense paresthesia between contacts. Evoked paresthesia across long distances equates to flow of current across longer distances than traditional SCS with likely depolarization of terminal sensory fibers [10]. The neurophysiologic characteristics of terminal sensory A-beta fibers and the impedance characteristics of the extracellular fluid in the subcutaneous and subdermal layers require different programming strategies than SCS. Electrical stimulation in the subcutaneous region may increase the concentration of local endorphins, affect blood flow, altar neurotransmitters, inhibit cell membrane depolarization and thus inhibit nociceptors similar to transcutaneous electrical nerve stimulation (TENS) and temporary percutaneous electrical nerve stimulation (PENS) [7]. Animal studies have suggested that peripheral nerve stimulation may alter the excitation of the central pain processing system thereby alleviating pain [11]. Further work examining the mechanism of action is needed to better understand the neurophysiology and localized changes that occur when current is delivered to the subcutaneous layer (fig. 1).

One potential advantage of PNfS over SCS when treating truncal pain is its ability to target nociceptive pain. Ellrich and Lamp [12] demonstrated that depolarization of the superficial radial nerve significantly decreased laser evoked potentials selectively recording nociceptor stimulation in a group of 15 healthy volunteers. Whether terminal sensory fibers in the subcutaneous region have similar neurophysiologic properties to larger named nerves in the periphery remains to be seen. Given that many pain syndromes targeted in neuromodulation such as FBSS are often mixed pain syndromes, a treatment modality able to potentially target nociceptive pain is advantageous. Treatment of cervical discogenic pain with PNfS as well as disorders not associated with neuropathic pain including abdominal pain further suggest that PNfS may be beneficial as a treatment option for pain of different etiologies [5, 13]. The difficulties of SCS in the long-term treatment of axial back pain are well described and may be related to SCS having a limited ability to treat nociceptive pain as well as the inability of conventional arrays to consistently obtain evoked paresthesia in the trunk [14, 15].

Patient Selection

Patients with different pain generators resulting in truncal pain can benefit from PNfS. Patients considered for PNfS trials have failed traditional interventional spinal procedures such as epidural steroid injections, medial branch blocks, facet joint nerve ablations, SI injections, and in many cases surgery. Conditions resulting in truncal pain that have been reported to respond to PNfS are lumbar postlaminectomy syndrome, axial cervical pain, PHN, inguinal pain, ilioinguinal neurapraxia, and post-thoracotomy pain [4, 5, 16, 17]. Direct nerve stimulation in the lateral recess as well as along the nerve roots has also been described for PHN, post-thoracotomy pain, and ilioinguinal neurapraxia. One of the most common diagnoses treated with PNfS is lumbar post-laminectomy syndrome.

Failed Back Surgery Syndrome

Among the pain generators implicated after spinal surgery are epidural fibrosis, arachnoiditis, spondylolithesis, junctional stenosis, recurrent disc herniation, central pain, and pseudoarthrosis. Patients with truncal pain after surgery often have few interventional options and PNfS offers a nonpharmacologic option to alleviate pain.

Several case series have suggested that PNfS may be effective for truncal pain after surgery. Paicius et al. [4] first reported a series of 6 patients, 5 of whom had prior lumbar surgery with all patients noting greater than 50% pain relief. Verrills et al. [18] reported that among 13 consecutively implanted patients 85% noted greater than 50% pain relief with a mean follow-up period of 7 months. Although long-term data are not available, Krutsch et al. [19] reported a single patient with lumbar FBSS who had 90% improvement at 12 months postimplant. Report of improvement of discogenic pain after cervical surgery has also been reported with 100% relief of a single patient at 9 months follow-up [5]. Retrograde placement of leads near the lumbar and sacral nerve roots has also been reported as a treatment for patients with FBSS although technical challenges and inability to obtain paresthesia in the low back have limited its widespread use. Lead placement for nerve root stimulation can occur by means of anterograde placement leads in the lateral recess stimulating dorsal roots in the vicinity of the dorsal root entry zone as well as retrograde placement of leads targeting a specific nerve root [6].

General considerations when identifying patients for PNfS after lumbar surgery include integrity of large-fiber sensation in the region of pain, anesthesia dolorosa, presence of hardware, and age of the patient. Identifying anesthesia dolorosa is important as placement of leads lateral to the region of anesthesia dolorosa is imperative. Stimulation directly in the region of anesthesia dolorosa often elicits dysesthesia or an absence of evoked paresthesia both resulting in a poor outcome. Similarly, identification of sensory deficit is important as leads should be placed lateral to the area of hypesthesia rather than directly in the area of hypesthesia. In addition, in patients who have had spinal surgery, the authors have noted that it may be important to take into consideration the presence of hardware as placing leads lateral to the hardware or using additional leads may be of benefit. Younger patients may respond better to PNfS than older patients. In a cohort of 23 patients, those over the age of 60 noted an average pain reduction of 2.83 points on the visual analog scale compared to 4.79 in those younger than 60 [20].

Hybrid systems consisting of placement of PNfS leads in the low back in combination with spinal cord stimulator leads may be beneficial when treating patients who have had lumbar surgery with both back and leg pain. One advantage of hybrid stimulation is the ability to target additional areas of pain as well as potentially being able to address the nociceptive and neuropathic components of pain with PNfS and SCS, respectively. Two case series have described overall improvement of pain with concurrent use of a PNfS and SCS hybrid system [21, 22]. Bernstein et al. [22] reported a series of 20 patients with combination SCS/PNfS systems with the majority of patients preferring the hybrid stimulation (stimulation of both SCS and PNfS leads) to either modality in isolation. Four of the 20 patients in this series initially had implanted SCS systems with significant low back pain following SCS implant and subsequently underwent PNfS implant with significant improvement of low back pain. The authors have performed paresthesia mapping on patients with hybrid systems and have noted a significant increase in area of evoked paresthesia above the posterior superior iliac spine (PSIS) with PNfS/SCS hybrid stimulation compared to SCS stimulation alone [unpubl. data]. Further studies looking at outcomes of PNfS in combination with SCS based on location of pain, type of lumbar surgery patient underwent, presence of hardware, MRI findings, and type of pain would be beneficial.

Postherpetic Neuralgia

Case reports suggest stimulating different parts of the peripheral nervous system including dorsal rootlets, direct named nerves, and distal sensory fibers in the subcutaneous region may be beneficial for PHN. Upadhyay et al. [23] reported a patient with percutaneous lead placement over the supraorbital nerve with 100% pain relief in a 55-year-old male with PHN following a vesicular eruption involving distribution of the supraorbital nerve. Dunteman [24] reported less robust results while treating PHN with direct nerve stimulation with mild improvement in less than half of the patients when placing percutaneous leads near the named nerves. Yakovlev and Peterson [25] reported a case of leads placed subcutaneously in an individual with truncal pain involving the right posterior chest wall due to intractable PHN with 100% relief 6 months postimplantation with significant improvement in function. Lead placement along the lateral recess of the spinal canal stimulating dorsal roots has also been reported. The authors originally used this technique for truncal PHN with mixed results and have evolved their approach for PHN to consist of a hybrid system with a single 8-contact lead placed at the lateral recess of the spinal canal corresponding to dermatome of involvement and two 4-contact subcutaneous leads bordering the area of pain in the posterior trunk to maximize chances of a successful trial. PHN may occur from one of three mechanisms: damage to A-delta and C fibers with collateral sprouting occurring from A-beta sensory fibers to nociceptors causing hyperalgesia and allodynia, loss of both large and small neural fibers causing anesthesia dolorosa resulting in hyperpathia and an absence of sensation, and peripheral sensitization with hyperactive primary sensory fibers causing allodynia with primarily intact sensation. Whether choosing a neuromodulation therapy to target different parts of the peripheral nervous system based on the underlying pathophysiologic mechanism in a particular disease syndrome results in different outcomes remains to be seen.

Inguinal Neuropraxia

Approximately 1–2% of patients that undergo hernia surgery have complications of neuralgia that account for the majority of patients with chronic inguinal pain. Stinson et al. [17] reported a case series of 3 patients who noted 75–100% reduction in pain with subcutaneous placement of two 8-contact leads bordering the hernia incision. Interestingly, 1 of the 3 patients had previously failed retrograde placement along the course of the T12 and L1 nerve roots despite 100% evoked paresthesia in the region of pain suggesting the importance of considering different neural targets in neuromodulation. Aló et al. [6] reported successful treatment of ilioinguinal neuropraxia after multiple surgeries with retrograde placement of two 4-contact leads implanted along the T12 and L1 nerve roots. The patient noted painful stimulation initially with a guarded cathode stimulation which improved with a triple cathode and one anode program suggesting the importance of different programming strategies in PNS.

Post-Thoracotomy Pain

PNfS has also been reported for the treatment of post-thoracotomy pain in 2 patients with greater than 50% pain relief and reduced need for pain medications [26]. The authors have combined placement of leads in the lateral recess and subcutaneous region in patients with post-thoracotomy pain with mixed results.

PNfS Technical Considerations

Proper placement of PNfS leads for truncal pain relief requires attention to two fundamental details: lead depth and lead positioning in relation to region of maximal pain. Lead placement in the subcutaneous layer is imperative for proper stimulation of the terminal sensory fibers. Superficial placement of PNfS leads often results in painful dysesthesia noted by patients as a burning and stinging sensation at low sensory thresholds. Placement too deep may result in the lead being inserted into muscle tissue or too far away from terminal sensory afferents to recruit at low energies with patients noting an absence of evoked paresthesia. The subcutaneous layer has the highest density of terminal sensory A-beta afferents and more recently Falco et al. [10] have shown that the subcutaneous layer is amenable as an electrical conduit to create electrical circuits of long distances thereby potentially allowing depolarization of terminal sensory afferents over larger areas.

Most practitioners implant percutaneous 4-contact or 8-contact leads by palpating the distal aspect of the Tuohy needle with advancement to ensure the needle being at the correct depth and also to maintain uniformity in depth. One case has been reported whereby a paddle lead was implanted in the lumbar subcutaneous region following unsuccessful permanent implantation of percutaneous leads with a reported improvement in pain reduction [27]. The advantages of percutaneous lead over paddle during PNfS trial for truncal pain include ease of placement whereby intraoperative stimulation may be performed, circumferential stimulation allowing potential recruitment of additional terminal sensory fibers, ability to minimize local

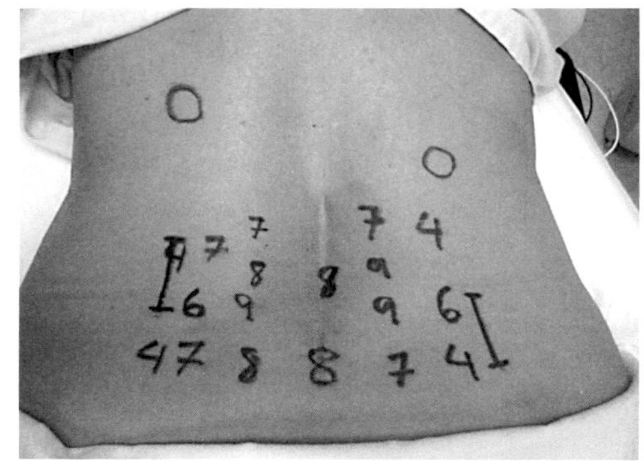

Fig. 2. Marking lumbosacral spine for trial lead implant.

anesthetic minimizing inhibition of sensory fibers during intraoperative stimulation, and wider spacing of contacts within a lead. One potential advantage of paddle lead is the ability to direct stimulation away from the skin minimizing stimulation of A-delta fibers that may cause dysesthesia and ability to potentially target current towards deeper pain generators. The authors prefer percutaneous leads and a 'tenting technique' whereby posterior pressure is applied allowing better separation of the dermal layers from the underlying fascia. Our technique for trial implantation of PNfS leads in the lumbar spine is accomplished in the following manner. The day before both trial and permanent implantation, patients are instructed to mark the area of maximal pain either by marking the region of worst pain or by rating different areas on a scale from zero to ten. On the day of the procedure, this area again is confirmed by palpating the area of pain and having the patient rate the pain from zero to ten. The authors have found this is best accomplished by palpating from outside the region of pain moving centrally and marking the numeric rating scale (NRS) scores directly on the patient (fig. 2). If a patient has pain with certain activities such as walking, standing, etc., they are asked to perform that task to ensure the area of pain is clearly identified. In addition, pinprick sensory testing is performed and attention is paid to whether the patient has signs of allodynia. If allodynia or hypesthesia is noted, the leads are placed just outside of this region. It is the authors' experience that anesthesia dolorosa does not respond to lead placement directly in the area of anesthesia dolorosa but bordering it. The authors have also noted that placing leads at further distances apart is preferable to shorter distances as well. Care must be taken to avoid placing leads over bony protuberances such as the PSIS region which may later cause lead erosion through the skin or placement of leads over the ischium for the same reason.

After prepping and draping the patient in usual sterile fashion a skin wheal is raised 3.5 inches away from the region of maximal pain (noted as a circle in fig. 2). Careful attention is made to minimize the amount of local anesthetic (typically 1–1.5 ml of 1% lidocaine mixed with epinephrine) to avoid spread of anesthetic to the leads that

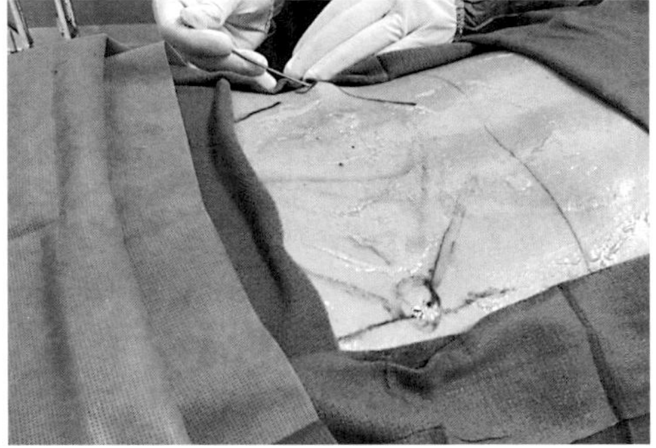

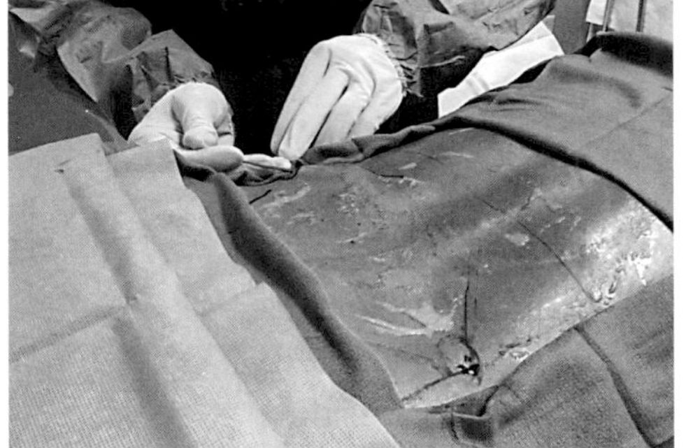

Fig. 3, 4. Tenting techniques for lumbar trial implantation.

may inhibit the patient's perception of paresthesia upon intraoperative trial stimulation. Leads may be staggered to maximize total area of coverage.

Using an 11-blade scalpel, a puncture incision (approximately 5 mm) is made to minimize tissue disruption and the curved Tuohy needle is advanced through the incision. A loss of resistance signifies entrance into the subcutaneous space. The operator then grips the needle hub between the thumb and the index and middle fingers and applies slight posterior pressure. This creates a 'tenting' of the tissue as the distal portion of the needle is raised below the skin surface (fig. 3, 4).

The operator's free hand is used to palpate the skin surface and assess advancement of the needle as denoted by the tenting of the skin. When properly performed, minimal resistance is noted as the tip of the needle is advanced subcutaneously. If there is substantial resistance to advancement of the needle and if skin dimpling is produced, than the lead is in the skin and therefore too superficial and the needle is redirected into a deeper plane. If the needle cannot be palpated, it is too deep in the subcutaneous tissues, and would then be redirected superficially. The stylet is then removed from the introducer needle and the lead is advanced through the needle and the needle is withdrawn over the lead prior to performing intraoperative stimulation.

After performing intraoperative stimulation, the leads are secured to the skin either with an anchoring device or by suturing directly to the lead.

Carayannopoulos et al. [28] describe an ultrasound guided technique for placement of PNS leads for ilioinguinal neuralgia. By visualizing the targeted nerve, a percutaneous approach for placement of trial leads was possible limiting the tissue trauma associated with direct nerve stimulation and allowing parallel placement of electrodes to the targeted nerve. The authors have examined PNfS leads postimplantation with ultrasonography but have not used it as a tool to aid in lead placement. One challenge the authors have identified in placement of leads at a specific depth is that the subcutaneous layer thickness varies as a function of the patient's body mass index. Therefore, ultrasound-guided techniques may best be utilized by identifying different layers rather than placement of the leads at a specific depth given these differences.

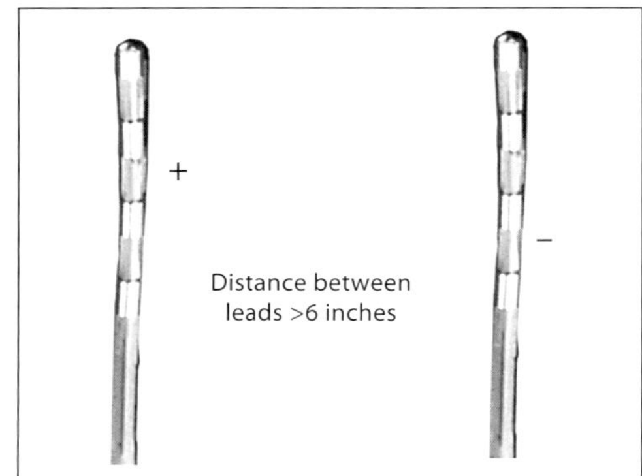

Fig. 5. Wide-spaced bipole array.

PNfS Programming

Programming for PNfS systems is dramatically different from SCS given the differences in the target neural element and different impedance characteristics of the subcutaneous layer compared to the epidural space. Earlier programming techniques used by the authors coupled the two related polarities on the same lead and also using multiple cathodes and anodes on the same lead. Both conventional PNfS programming techniques demanded higher energy requirements for paresthesia and pain relief. In addition, like other implanters, the authors found that by limiting polarities on the same lead the maximum area that could be treated was approximately the size of two business cards. As a result, the authors developed more sophisticated programming techniques which they have found to reduce energy requirements and larger area of paresthesia resulting in better pain relief. Two common programming strategies used by the authors include triple anode single cathode (3A1C) and wide-spaced cross-talk stimulation.

Wide-spaced cross-talk programming refers to an electrode array construct with significantly greater distances between polarities (cathode and anode) on different leads. In a group of 18 patients with chronic pain that were implanted with PNfS systems using a wide-spaced cross-talk programming, patients noted significant pain relief and reduction in pain medications [10] (fig. 5).

Compared to conventional programming involving a cathode/anode array on the same lead where patients note more specific pinpoint stimulation, patients with wide-spaced arrays report a more diffuse 'flow sensation' from one polarity to the other. In general, patients note less painful dysesthesia with wide-spaced arrays with less biting and burning sensation and a larger area of paresthesia compared to conventional programming (polarities on the same lead) and improved pain relief [authors' unpubl. data]. In addition, with lower energy requirements patients better tolerate the stimulation as the incidence of dysesthesia that may occur from activation of painful a delta and c fibers may be minimized. Greater area of paresthesia appears

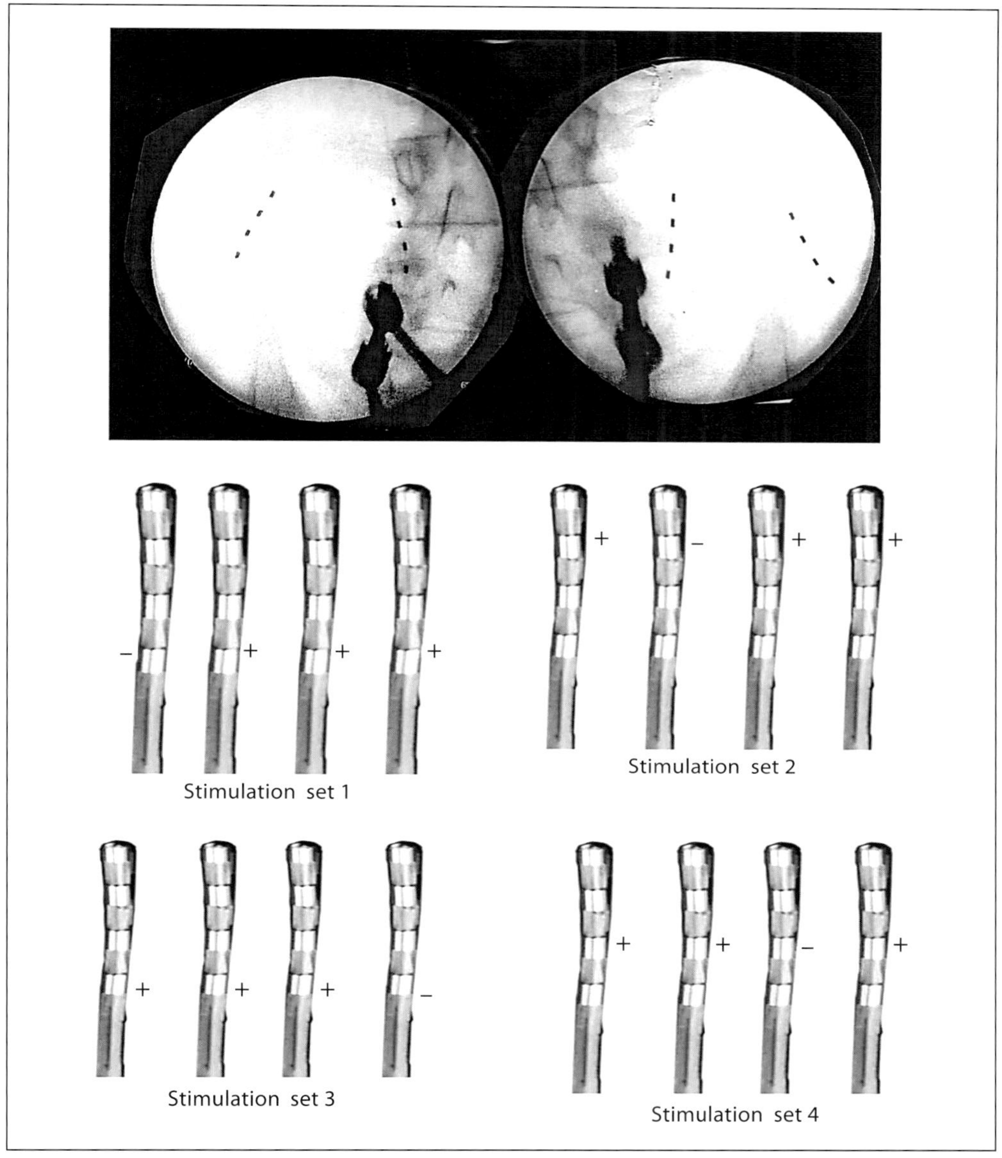

Fig. 6. Four-quattrode lead 3A1C programming array.

to be generated with lower energy requirements using the wider spacing of related polarities.

Triple-anode single-cathode (3A1C) is a novel programming strategy used to create a large area of paresthesia with four-lead PNfS systems. Patients are programmed with four, interleavened stimulation sets each comprising of a single cathode with three anodes: all active electrodes on separate leads. This generates a large area of paresthesia. Programming parameters consist of frequencies of 30 Hz and a pulse width of 200. Patients with 3A1C programming typically report significant pain relief with the use of anodes and cathodes on leads separate from each other resulting in a larger area of paresthesia and improved pain relief than with conventional (cathode and anode on the same lead) programming with an implanted PNfS system (fig. 6).

Patients often report the area between electrodes as one solid area of paresthesia as opposed to four distinctly different and thus smaller areas of paresthesia. Paresthesia does not appear to be diluted as area increases, however increased power is required. The use of an interleavened three anodes and a single cathode array may be a beneficial programming option for patients implanted with four-lead PNfS systems. We hope to encourage clinicians to explore these novel programming technique in hope of achieving a comfortable paresthesia overlap and pain relief for their patients. The need for four peripheral nerve leads appears to be substantiated. Future research is needed regarding the limits of interelectrode distance, the areas of paresthesia generated, the density of paresthesia generated, the pain relief within the paresthesia, the type of pain which is controlled: neuropathic, nociceptive or both, the relation of the paresthesia to the programmed array, e.g. area vs. linear arrays.

References

1 Weiner RL: Occipital neurostimulation for treatment of intractable headache syndromes. Acta Neurochir Suppl 2007;97:129–133.

2 Slavin KV, Colpan ME, Munawar N, Wess C, Nersesyan H: Trigeminal and occipital peripheral nerve stimulation for craniofacial pain: a single-institution experience and review of the literature. Neurosurg Focus 2006;21:E6, 1–5.

3 Kapural L, Mekhail N, Hayek SM, Stanton-Hicks M, Malak O: Occipital nerve electrical stimulation via the midline approach and subcutaneous surgical leads for treatment of severe occipital neuralgia: a pilot study. Anesth Analg 2005;101:171–174.

4 Paicius RM, Bernstein CA, Lempert-Cohen C: Peripheral nerve field stimulation for the treatment of chronic low back pain: preliminary results of long-term follow-up – a case series. Neuromodulation 2007;10:279–290.

5 Lipov EF, Joshi JR, Sanders S, Slavin KV: Use of peripheral subcutaneous field stimulation for the treatment of axial neck pain: a case report. Neuromodulation 2009;12:292–295.

6 Aló K, Yland M, Redko V, Feler C, Naumann C: Lumbar and sacral nerve root stimulation (NRS) in the treatment of chronic pain: a novel anatomic approach and neurostimulation technique. Neuromodulation 1999;2:23–31.

7 Campbell JN, Long DM: Peripheral nerve stimulation in the treatment of intractable pain. J Neurosurg 1976;45:692–699.

8 Melzack R, Wall PD: Pain Mechanisms: a new theory. Science 1965;150:971–979.

9 Wall PD, Sweet WH: Temporary abolition of pain in man. Science 1967;155:108–109.

10 Falco F, Berger J, Vrable A, Onyweu O, Zhu J: Cross talk: a new method for peripheral nerve stimulation: an observational report with cadaveric verification. Pain Physician 2009;12:965–983.

11 Bartsch T, Goadsby PJ: Stimulation of the greater occipital nerve induces increased central excitability of dural afferent input. Brain 2002;125:1496–1509.

12 Ellrich J, Lamp S: Peripheral nerve stimulation inhibits nociceptive processing: an electrophysiological study in healthy volunteers. Neuromodulation 2005;8:225–232.

13 Paicius RM, Bernstein CA, Lempert-Cohen C: Peripheral nerve field stimulation in chronic abdominal pain. Pain Physician 2006;9:261–266.

14 North RB: Spinal cord and peripheral nerve stimulation: technical aspects; in Simpson BA (ed): Pain Research and Clinical Management. Electrical Stimulation and the Relief of Pain. Philadelphia, Elsevier, 2003, vol 15, pp 183–196.

15 Sharan A, Cameron T, Barolat G: Evolving patterns of spinal cord stimulation in patients implanted for intractable low back and leg pain. Neuromodulation 2005;8:40–48.
16 Yakovlev A, Peterson A: Peripheral nerve stimulation in treatment of intractable postherpetic neuralgia. Neuromodulation 2007;10:373–375.
17 Stinson LE, Roderer GT, Cross NE, Davis BE: Peripheral subcutaneous electrostimulation for control of intractable postoperative inguinal pain: a case report series. Neuromodulation 2001;4: 99–104.
18 Verrills P, Mitchell B, Vivian D, Sinclair C: Peripheral nerve stimulation: a treatment for chronic low back pain and failed back surgery syndrome? Neuromodulation 2009;12:68–75.
19 Krutsch JP, McCeney MH, Barolat G, Al Tamimi M, Smolenski A: A case report of subcutaneous peripheral nerve stimulation for the treatment of axial back pain associated with postlaminectomy syndrome. Neuromodulation 2008;11:112–115.
20 Verrills P, Mitchell B, Sinclair C: Peripheral nerve field stimulation: Is age an indicator of outcome? Neuromodulation 2009;12:60–67.
21 Lipov EG, Joshi JR, Slavin KV: Hybrid neuromodulation technique: use of combined spinal cord stimulation and peripheral nerve stimulation in treatment of chronic pain in back and legs. Acta Neurochir (Wien) 2008;150:971.
22 Bernstein CA, Paicius RM, Barkow SH, Lempert-Cohen C: Spinal cord stimulation in conjunction with peripheral nerve field stimulation for the treatment of low back and leg pain: a case series. Neuromodulation 2008;11:116–123.
23 Upadhyay SP, Rana SP, Mishra S, Bhatnagar S: Successful treatment of intractable postherpetic neuralgia (PHN) using peripheral nerve field stimulation. Am J Hosp Palliat Care 2010;27:59–62.
24 Dunteman E: Peripheral nerve stimulation for unremitting ophthalmic postherpetic neuralgia. Neuromodulation 2002;5:32–37.
25 Yakovlev AE, Peterson AT: Peripheral nerve stimulation in treatment of intractable postherpetic neuralgia. Neuromodulation 2007;10:373–375.
26 Al Tamimi M, Davids HR, Langston MM, Krutsch J, Yakovlev A, Barolat G: Successful treatment of chronic neuropathic pain with subcutaneous peripheral nerve stimulation: four case reports. Neuromodulation 2009;12:210–214.
27 Ordia J, Vaisman J: Subcutaneous peripheral nerve stimulation with paddle lead for treatment of low back pain: case report. Neuromodulation 2009;12: 205–209.
28 Carayannopoulos A, Beasley R, Sites B: Facilitation of percutaneous trial lead placement with ultrasound guidance for peripheral nerve stimulation trial of ilioinguinal neuralgia: a technical note. Neuromodulation 2009;12:296–299.

Timothy Deer, MD
The Center for Pain Relief, Inc.
400 Court Street, Suite 100
Charleston, WV 25301 (USA)
Tel. +1 304 347 6141, Fax +1 304 347 6855, E-Mail DocTDeer@aol.com

Slavin KV (ed): Peripheral Nerve Stimulation.
Prog Neurol Surg. Basel, Karger, 2011, vol 24, pp 70–76

Peripheral Subcutaneous Stimulation for Intractable Abdominal Pain

Giancarlo Barolat

Barolat Neuroscience, Denver, Colo., USA

Abstract

Peripheral subcutaneous stimulation has been utilized for a variety of painful conditions affecting the abdominal wall, including sequelae of hernia repair, painful surgical scars, ilio-inguinal neuritis. It has also occasionally been shown to be effective in patients with intractable abdominal visceral pain. Since this is a very recent modality, no large series or prospective studies exist. The results, however, are promising and certainly warrant further investigation.

Chronic abdominal pain can be a result of many conditions affecting both the viscera and the abdominal wall itself. As opposed to the pain due to abdominal-wall-related conditions, abdominal pain caused by visceral pathology is often associated with nausea, feeling of sickness and generalized malaise.

Intraspinal neurostimulation has been found to have a role in the management of some chronic, incurable pain conditions affecting the abdominal region. Spinal cord stimulation has been found to be effective in reducing pain from chronic pancreatitis, irritable bowel syndrome, and intractable pain following multiple hernia operations, to mention a few [1].

Peripheral subcutaneous stimulation is an extension of intraspinal neurostimulation, and has a role in the management of some conditions affecting the abdominal region. Its use in chronic abdominal pain has been limited, particularly as compared to other indications [2–12].

Peripheral subcutaneous stimulation is particularly useful for chronic pain conditions resulting from surgical interventions resulting in pain at the surgical incisions. These conditions are often referred as painful neuromas. Often the patients have undergone many local anesthetic injections as well as surgical revisions of the surgical scar(s). The strategy for peripheral subcutaneous stimulation is no different from similar conditions in other parts of the body. If there are painful surgical scars, the leads can be placed either directly in the painful area(s) of the incisions or, preferably,

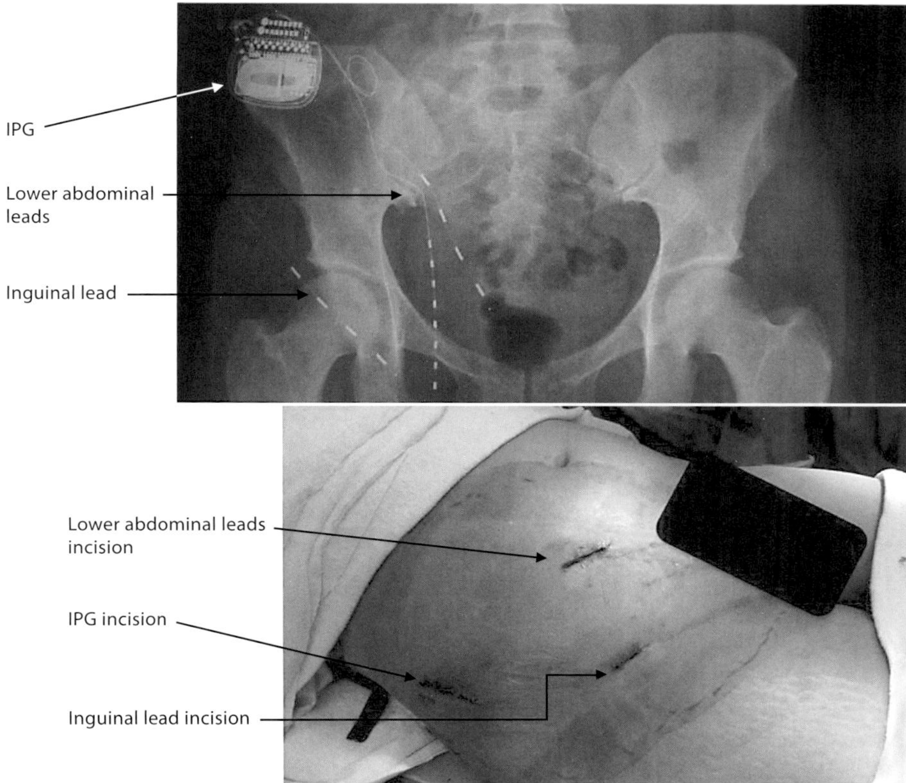

Fig. 1. Chronic severe left inguinal and scrotal pain. Leads staggered with one lead placed just proximal to the scrotal region.

just adjacent to it. In my experience, it is best to have each lead at about 1 cm from the incision and parallel to it. Depending on length of the painful scar, one or two leads might be required on each side. If allodynia is present, the strategy must be modified. The allodynic area must be mapped very carefully, and the leads must be placed in the transition zone between the hypersensitive and the allodynic area. Attention must be paid not to place the leads in the allodynic area, since this could result in both mechanical and electrical aggravation of the allodynia. In rare occasions direct stimulation of the allodynic areas can result in decrease of pain.

Inguinal neuralgia is a well-known complication of hernia repair surgery. The pain can be permanent, constant and excruciating. Most of these patients have undergone innumerable surgical revisions of both the incisional scar and the hernia defect. Rarely, these procedures result in a substantial reduction of the pain or a cure. More often they have only a negligible positive effect on the pain, or even worsen it. Peripheral subcutaneous abdominal stimulation can be very effective in the management of such conditions (fig. 1–3). Unlike a previous belief, the electrode(s) does not need to be placed

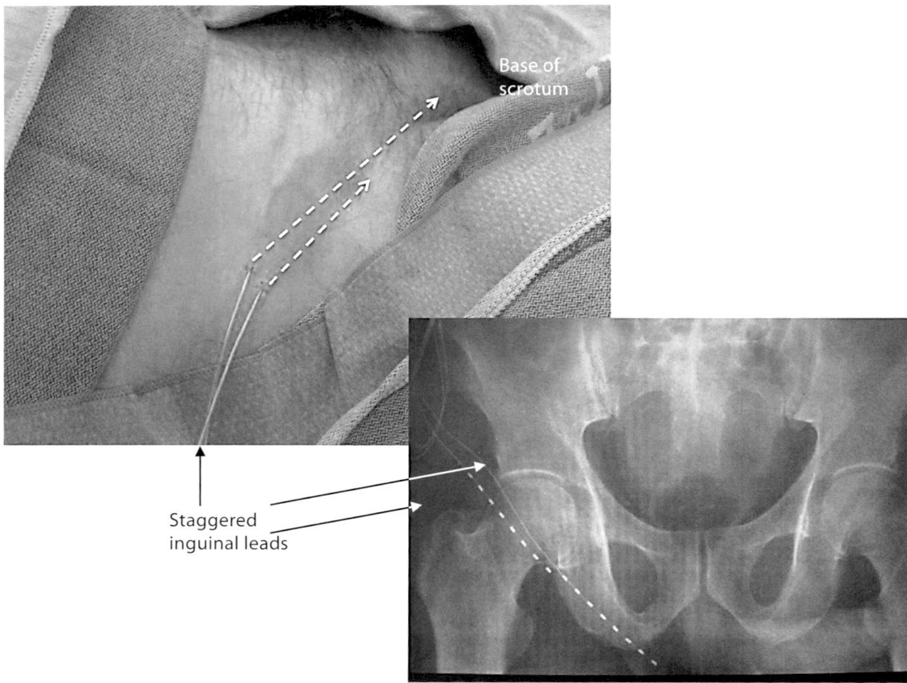

Fig. 2. Chronic left inguinal pain as well as chronic severe lumbar pain. Two leads placed in the left inguinal area and two leads placed in the lumbar area.

exactly on the ilio-inguinal nerve (which in most instances has already been cut or cannot otherwise be found because of being encased in scar tissue). The electrode(s) must be placed exactly in the area of pain. Depending on the size of the painful area, several leads must be necessary. The leads can be placed either sequentially in a longitudinal pattern, if the pain area is narrow and long, or parallel to each other, if the pain area is wider than an inch. In many instances, the pain extends into the scrotal area. This is always a challenge. Placement of leads in the scrotum, in the presence of an intact testicle, can cause mechanical irritation. The author has encountered instances where the scrotal lead had to be removed because of aggravation of testicular irritation. This has not been the author's experience in patients in whom the testicle had been previously removed. In those instances a lead can be advanced, trough the inguinal canal, into the scrotal sac. The use of thinner leads such as the St. Jude Axxess lead might obviate the mechanical irritation caused by the electrode.

Another challenge is when the pain spreads to the peri-vaginal area. Lead advancement to this area may result in painful protrusion (because of the body curvature) and eventually lead to its removal.

I do not recommend inserting leads in the subcutaneous perineal area. If one is trying to address pain in that area, the leads should be placed on the sacral nerve roots.

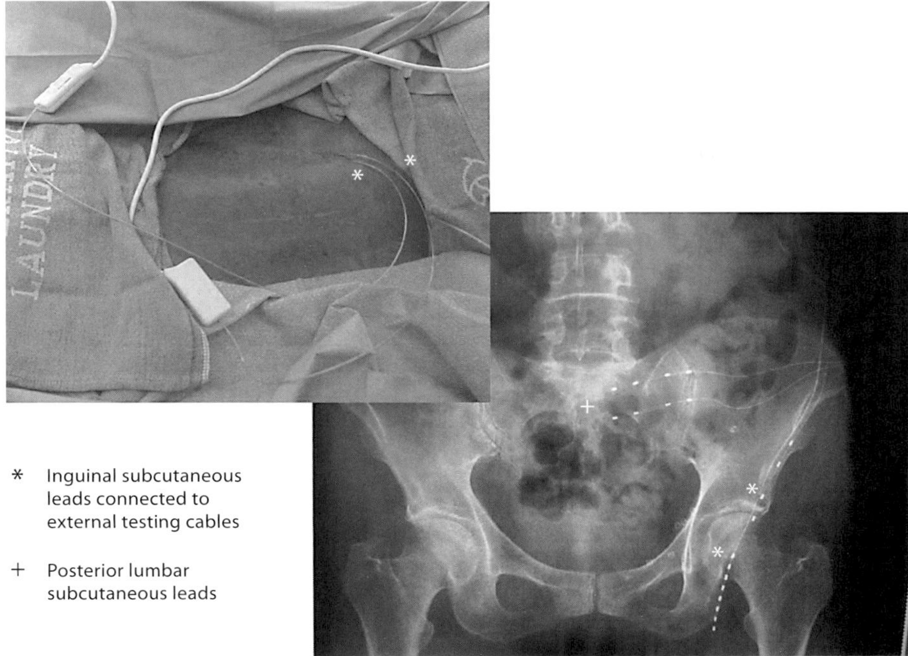

Fig. 3. Severe left inguinal and suprapubic pain. Test trial showed good pain relief. Pulse generator implanted in the right flank. One lead placed in the inguinal region. Two additional leads placed in the suprapubic and upper inguinal region.

Neurostimulation has been found to be effective in abdominal visceral pain, such as the one found in chronic pancreatitis, chronic postcholecystectomy syndrome, etc. [1].

Subcutaneous leads can occasionally be effective in these visceral pain syndromes, although intra-spinal stimulation can usually result in a 'deeper' reach of the stimulation.

Paicius et al. [9] published their experience with three patients who had intractable abdominal pain and had failed nerve blocks, neurolysis, lysis of adhesions and medications.

The first case was a 19-year-old female with a history of right lower quadrant and inguinal pain following right inguinal hernia repair 4 years previously. The patient had no relief following two surgical procedures to release the entrapped right ilioinguinal nerve and removal of scar tissue. Following a trial period, the patient underwent implantation of an octopolar lead in the inguinal region and a pulse generator placed in an abdominal pocket. A 1-year follow-up showed that she had discontinued all her medications and had an average visual analog scale (VAS) score of 0–1.

The second case was a 54-year-old male with a history of liver transplant 4 years prior to presenting for management of severe abdominal and incisional pain with neuroma. He reported right upper and lower abdominal pain beginning just after the transplant, followed by significantly worse pain from the time of an incisional hernia repair six months post transplant. The patient underwent a trial stimulation with two quadripolar cylindrical leads placed subcutaneously over the right costal margin over the site of greatest pain. A third octopolar lead was placed over the liver transplant surgical scar. The patient reported a 90% reduction in overall pain during the trial and underwent subsequent implantation of the system with excellent long-term results.

The third patient was a 39-year-old male with a 3-year history of chronic pancreatitis, who had undergone cholecystectomy, sphincterotomy, and a modified Whipple procedure and placement of multiple stents. He had a history of hospitalizations once or twice a month for management of pancreatitis symptoms. During the subcutaneous trial, the patient had two cylindrical leads placed horizontally in the right upper quadrant of his abdomen. The patient experienced substantial pain relief and subsequently underwent implantation of a system where the leads were placed vertically in the right upper abdominal quadrant. The patient, however, did not experience any substantial pain relief. The leads were repositioned horizontally with good recapture of the pain relief. Based on these observations, the authors believe that, in cases of visceral pain, for optimal coverage, leads should be placed in parallel to the dermatomal distribution of the affected nerves to take advantage of presumed viscerotomal/dermatomal convergence.

Occasionally, peripheral subcutaneous stimulation can be a very viable alternative to intra-spinal stimulation. Figure 4 shows the case of a 35-year-old female with intractable inguinal pain secondary to a chronic pelvic pain syndrome treated by the author. The patient had a nerve root stimulation system implanted, with two percutaneous leads inserted over the S2-S3-S4 nerve roots (fig. 4). The patient had excellent relief from the pain. However, the presence of the leads over the sacral nerve roots caused severe intractable headaches. The patient was torn between the idea of keeping the device and suffer from incapacitating headaches, or have the device removed and suffer from the inguinal pain. The author performed a trial of peripheral subcutaneous stimulation with an octopolar cylindrical lead inserted in the pain area (fig. 4). The patient experienced excellent pain relief. Subsequently, the author performed a surgical procedure where the sacral root leads were removed and the subcutaneous octopolar lead was implanted and connected to the implanted pulse generator. The patient enjoyed the pain relief without the intractable headaches.

The exact role of peripheral subcutaneous stimulation in the management of chronic painful conditions of the abdomen has to be defined. There is a definitive benefit in the management of postherniorraphy pain [13]. There are some encouraging results even in cases of visceral pain.

Peripheral subcutaneous stimulation has potential advantages as a treatment for chronic pain. Advantages include: reversibility, low morbidity with fewer side effects, minimally invasive implantation, percutaneous lead placement, lead insertion with

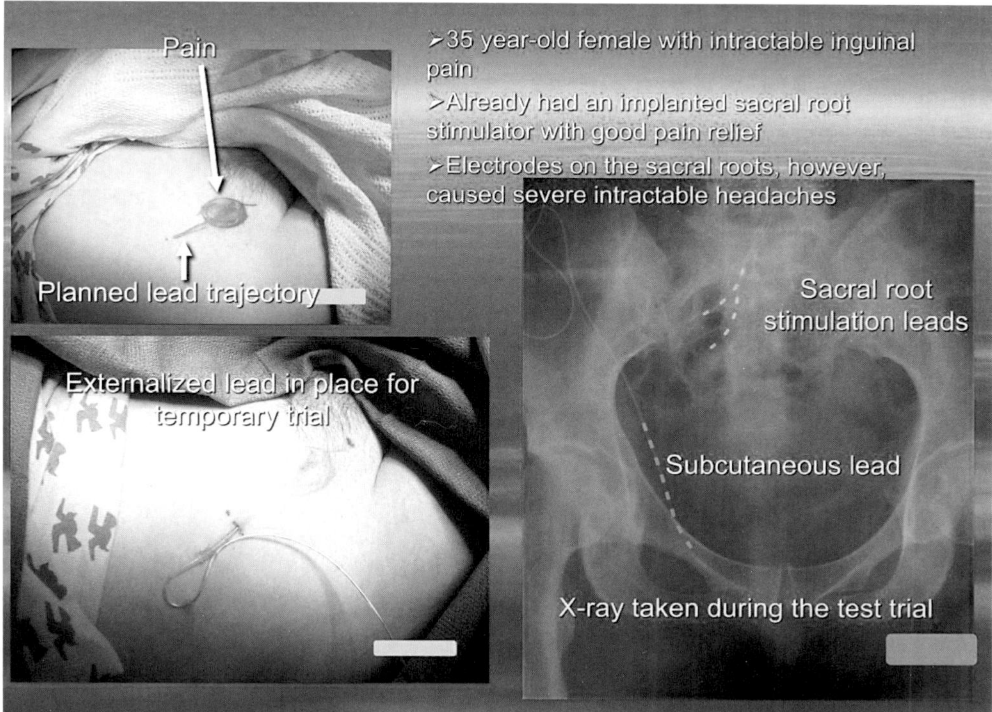

Fig. 4. Severe inguinal pain. Percutaneous leads already in place on the sacral nerve roots. Trial with peripheral subcutaneous stimulation.

the patient awake to confirm proper lead placement, and programmable stimulator systems to improve coverage and effectiveness of stimulation.

This modality is in its infancy, and large well-documented clinical series are necessary to determine which conditions benefit from this modality.

References

1 Kapural L, Nagem H, Tlucek H, Sessler D: Spinal cord stimulation for visceral pain. Pain Medicine 2010;11:347–355.

2 Al Tamimi M, Davids D, Langston M, Krutsch J, Yakovlev A, Barolat G: Successful treatment of chronic neuropathic pain with subcutaneous peripheral nerve stimulation: four case reports. Neuromodulation 2009;3:210–214.

3 Aló K, Holscheimer J: New trends in neuromodulation for the management of neuropathic pain. Neurosurgery 2002;60:690–704.

4 Barolat G: Techniques for subcutaneous peripheral nerve field stimulation for intractable pain; in Krames E, Peckham H, Rezai A (eds): Neuromodulation. Philadelphia, Elsevier, 2009, pp 1017–1020.

5 Bernstein CA, Paicius RM, Barkow SH, Lempert-Cohen C: Spinal cord stimulation in conjunction with peripheral nerve field stimulation for the treatment of low back and leg pain: a case series. Neuromodulation 2008;11:116–123.

6 Krutsch JP, McCeney MH, Barolat G, Al Tamimi M, Smolenski A: A case report of subcutaneous peripheral nerve stimulation for the treatment of axial back pain associated with postlaminectomy syndrome. Neuromodulation 2008;11:112–115.

7 Mobbs RJ, Nair S, Blum P: Peripheral nerve stimulation for the treatment of chronic pain. J Clin Neurosci 2007;14:216–221.

8 Paicius RM, Bernstein CA, Lempert-Cohen C: Peripheral nerve field stimulation for the treatment of chronic low back pain: preliminary results of long-term follow-up: a case series. Neuromodulation 2007;10:279–290.

9 Paicius RM, Bernstein CA, Lempert-Cohen C: Peripheral nerve field stimulation in chronic abdominal pain. Pain Physician 2006;9:261–266.

10 Slavin KV, Nersesyan H, Wess C: Peripheral neurostimulation for treatment of intractable occipital neuralgia. Neurosurgery 2006;58:112–119.

11 Weiner RL, Reed KL: Peripheral neurostimulation for control of intractable occipital neuralgia. Neuromodulation 1999;2:217–221.

12 Yakovlev AE, Peterson AT: Peripheral nerve stimulation in treatment of intractable postherpetic neuralgia. Neuromodulation 2007;10:373–375.

13 Stinson LW, Roderer GT, Cross NE, Davis BE: Peripheral subcutaneous electrostimulation for control of intractable postoperative inguinal pain: a case report series. Neuromodulation 2001;4:99–104.

Giancarlo Barolat, MD
Barolat Neuroscience
Presbyterian/St. Lukes Medical Center
1721 East 19th Street, Suite 434, Denver, CO 80128 (USA)
Tel. +1 303 865 7800, Fax +1 303 9865 7804, E-Mail gbarolat@verizon.net

Slavin KV (ed): Peripheral Nerve Stimulation.
Prog Neurol Surg. Basel, Karger, 2011, vol 24, pp 77–85

Subcutaneous Occipital Region Stimulation for Intractable Headache Syndromes

Richard L. Weiner

Department of Neurosurgery, THR Presbyterian Hospital, Dallas, Tex., USA

Abstract

Subcutaneous occipital nerve region stimulation is becoming an important part of the overall treatment regimen for a number of chronic headache syndromes refractory to nonsurgical, medical management. A combination of improved device technology and methodology, further understanding about appropriate indications and achievement of on-label FDA status should support continued use and success of this neuromodulation modality.

History

Traditional neuromodulation modalities have centered on the indications and methodology of spinal cord (dorsal column) stimulation for a variety of axial and limb chronic pain syndromes refractory to non surgical medical treatments or involved in treating post surgical residual pain. This, despite the fact that the original observations by Sweet and Wepsic [1] for electrical stimulation of nervous system tissue while trying to show clinical correlation with Melzack and Wall's gate control theory of pain [2] were based on stimulation of a peripherally placed cranial nerve branch (trigeminal V2). The subsequent development of peripheral nerve stimulation was, until relatively recently, an acquired taste and infrequently performed because of the need to utilize surgical techniques to perform rather extensive dissections and paddle electrode placement [3] which usually required the collaboration with either a neurosurgeon, plastic surgeon or orthopedic surgeon.

Intraoperative observations made by the author circa 1992 led to the development and increasing popularity of percutaneously placed wire (and paddle) electrodes into the region of peripheral nerves and their tributaries usually within subcutaneous tissues without having to perform extensive surgical dissections. The original observation made in 1992 was that neurostimulation of the subcutaneous tissues within the dermatomal distribution of peripheral nerves and their tributaries produced, in many cases, an agreeable paresthesis of that nerve distribution with pain modulation capabilities. This led to the development and subsequent refinement of implantation methods for percutaneously placed implant devices while also gaining an understanding of intractable pain indications amenable to this treatment modality.

Occipital/suboccipital nerve (ONS) stimulation was the first attempt at proving the validity of the original observation set from 1992. The original group of patients and method published in *Neuromodulation* [4] has fueled a rebirth in peripheral nerve stimulation (PNS) indications and applications throughout the body as well as new terminology including ONS, peripheral nerve field stimulation (PNfS), and subcutaneous stimulation.

Initial Observations

From a historical perspective, the following description summarizes my initial observations ultimately leading to the development of ONS and percutaneous PNS indications and methodology: An obese female patient with a much localized posterior tibial nerve distribution pain syndrome was felt to be a candidate for a surgically placed paddle electrode system available at that time ('Resume' lead, Medtronic, Minneapolis, Minn., USA). Dissection was attempted through a great deal of subcutaneous fatty tissue just above the bifurcation of the nerve at the level of the inferior upper leg posteriorly with the patient in a three-quarter prone position. Needless to say, appropriate surgical landmarks were difficult to confirm, the direction of dissection was difficult to maintain and the nerve was not initially found. An idea was formulated intraoperatively to place a Tuohy needle into the depths of the subcutaneous tissues threading and stimulating a percutaneous wire electrode where the nerve was thought be, thereby, guiding dissection to the nerve. With each stimulation attempt, the patient who was under light sedation, reported paresthesias, some of which appeared to be in the distribution of the posterior tibial nerve. Subsequent dissection along the electrode, however, did not lead to the nerve initially. Though the implant procedure was eventually successful by repositioning and identifying intraoperative landmarks, the intraoperative empirical observation that electrical stimulation of subcutaneous tissues not immediately adjacent to a large, identifiable peripheral nerve, but producing agreeable paresthesias, might be reproducible elsewhere in the body was the impetus for ONS and percutaneous PNS development.

Early ONS Experience

The first ONS patient implants where in late 1993/1994 with relatively rapid improvements in technique design. These cases were initially approached with

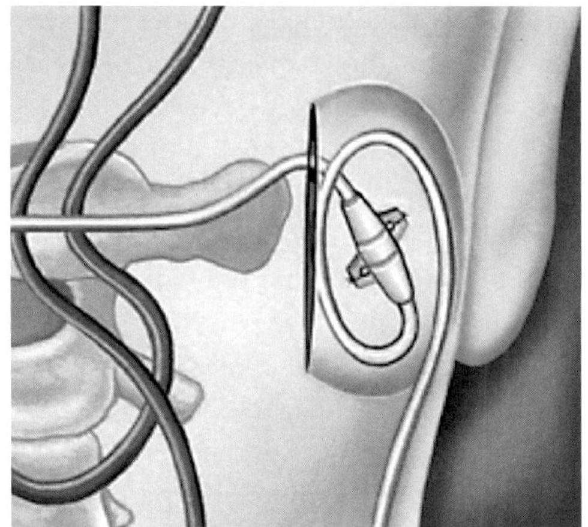

Fig. 1. Lateral incision aiming the electrode to midline.

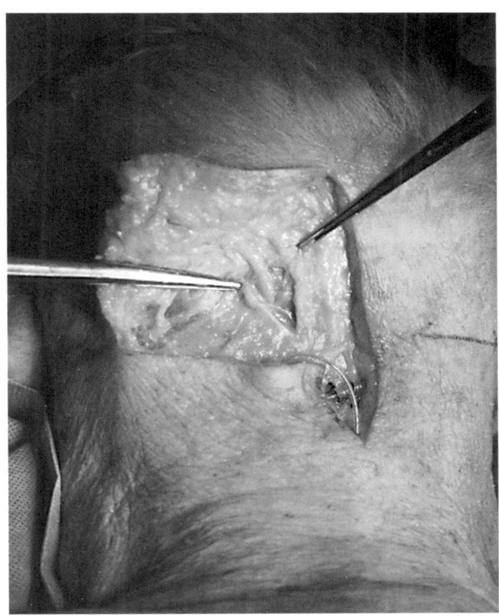

Fig. 2. Occipital nerve and artery becoming superficial into the scalp above the level of a transversely place electrode at C1 posteriorly.

uni- or bilateral laterally placed incisions in the lower suboccipital region, aiming the electrodes towards the midline in a horizontal fashion to capture branches off the greater, lesser and third occipital nerves originating as tributaries from the C2-C3 spinal nerves (fig. 1). The anatomy of this region suggested that these nerves where situated intramuscularly deep to the subcutaneous electrode placements typically at the level of C1 and emerged to innervate the scalp regions somewhat above that level (fig. 2). Therefore, the nerves were not directly being stimulated but there was involvement and transmission of electrical impulses within the subcutaneous tissues adjacent to these nerves. The supine or lateral position with C-arm fluoroscopic guidance developed into an easier use of the prone position with horseshoe frame or lateral position with three-quarters head turn towards prone. Issues with airway control and sedation have led some operators to abandon the prone position but with proper anesthetic control, it remains the most effective position for electrode and implantable pulse generator (IPG) placement. Additionally, a midline posterior vertical incision at the base of the cervicomedullary junction has become standard for initiation of electrode placement.

The initial ONS experience matured very slowly in the mid 1990s as the technique was refined and a number of patients followed long term. An initial series of patients were eventually reported in *Neuromodulation* in April, 1999 [4] with a description of the surgical technique and follow-up data. Numerous presentations, initially in the neurosurgical arena, and subsequently geared towards the pain management field, have led to significant validation and improvements in the techniques and indications for ONS [5–10] (fig. 1, 2).

Indications

The neurosurgical literature in the early days of ONS methodology development tended to diagnose chronic occipital pain as occipital neuralgia and, indeed, many neurosurgeons would see referrals for excision or neurolysis of one or more occipital nerves to treat these pain conditions. The headache neurology community, however, felt that occipital neuralgia was actually a relatively rare diagnosis and that most of these occipital pain syndromes were actually migraine headache variants. In fact, the new International Headache Society international headache classification schemes tries to address these variants including chronic daily headaches, transformed migraine, cervicogenic headaches, C2-mediated occipital headaches, post-traumatic headaches and others [11].

Evolving indications for ONS can be grouped into chronic occipital region pain presentations that appear to involve one or more occipital nerves (greater, lesser, third, etc.) that have failed more conservative medical treatment approaches. Temporary nerve blocks of either the occipital nerves within the posterior scalp or the C2-C3 nerve roots at the foramen can be helpful but not absolute in identifying appropriate ONS candidates.

Frontal headaches in the supraorbital regions can be related to the occipital nerves via referred signals within the trigeminal-cervical vascular nerve complex via the descending tract of V and may respond well to ONS alone or combined ONS and supraorbital subcutaneous neurostimulation.

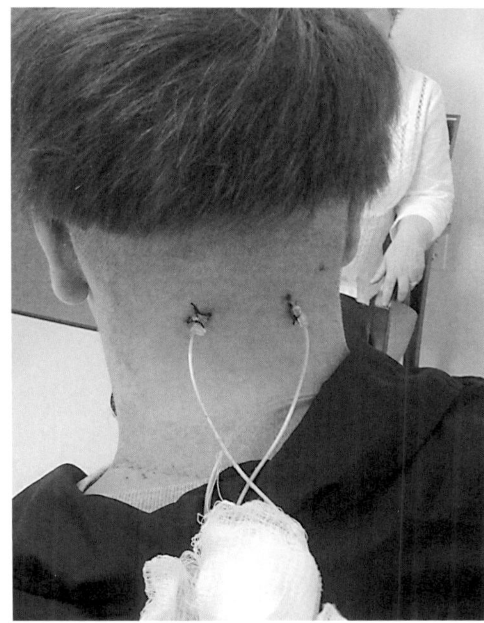

Fig. 3. Temporary electrode placement.

ONS Trial

Experience with neurostimulation of the spinal cord has shown that a trial period of temporary stimulation (varying from 1 to 4 weeks) can enhance the overall success of a permanent implant. Over time, though we have tended to trial our ONS patients, there are occasions when an 'on the table' trial has led to an immediate permanent device placement.

ONS trialing is an extremely simple technique of percutaneous placement of bilateral occipital electrodes under minimal sedation from the neck base, aimed towards the points of maximal occipital tenderness or pain on the side opposite the insertion point (fig. 3).

Techniques

Subcutaneous electrode placement has evolved in terms of electrode choices (percutaneous or wire-type, paddle, Bion; Boston Scientific, Valencia, Calif., USA), anchoring techniques (anchors, glue, suture loop), and location (transverse, angled, vertical) usually from midline incisions at the skull base (fig. 4). As previously mentioned, a prone position with the head flexed in a horseshoe frame offers the best overall way of visualizing the entire occipital/sub occipital region for electrode placement

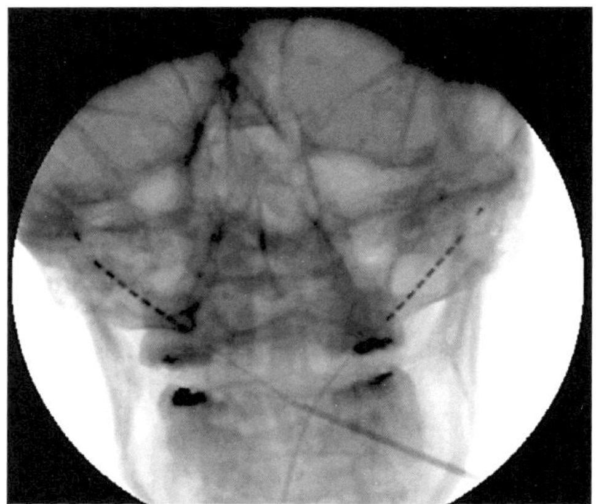

Fig. 4. Angled electrodes.

(fig. 5, 6). Careful sedation techniques are required by a skilled anesthesiologist to ensure success without either airway risk to the patient or inadequate sedation resulting in potential contamination of the operative site.

Generator placement is easiest with electrodes with or without lead extensions into the lower lumbar region just above the buttocks. However, it has been shown that the greatest degree of tension on the system occurs with this placement when the patient bends forward significantly. Placing the IPG either into the upper chest, lateral flank, or abdomen appears to offer less strain on the electrodes and anchors.

Halo PNS

A growing number of patients present with bifrontal and bioccipital pain and have been successfully implanted with dual frontal and dual occipital electrodes at the same sitting utilizing a midline frontal incision just behind the hairline aiming the leads out inferolaterally above the supraorbital nerves, then tunneled posteriorly to the midline sub occipital incision at or just above C1 to join up with bioccipital electrodes placed laterally at that site (fig. 7, 8). All four electrodes are then connected to bifurcated extension cables that are tunneled toward dual channel rechargeable IPGs.

Outcomes

The literature seems to support our early observations that between 60 and 70% of successfully trialed patients achieve long term control of their chronic occipital

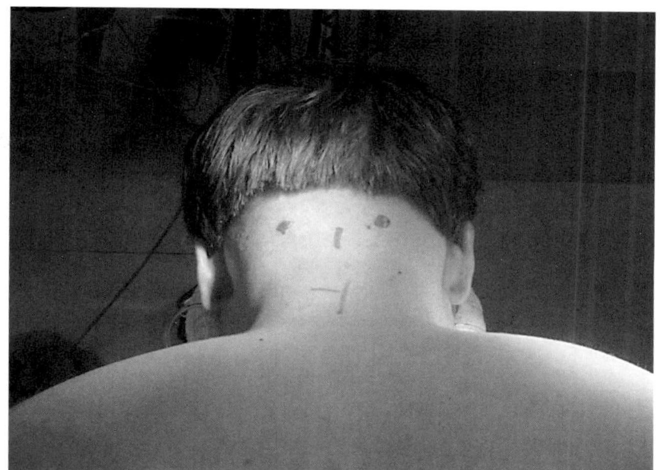

Fig. 5. Prone position with midline incision marked and maximal points of tenderness circled.

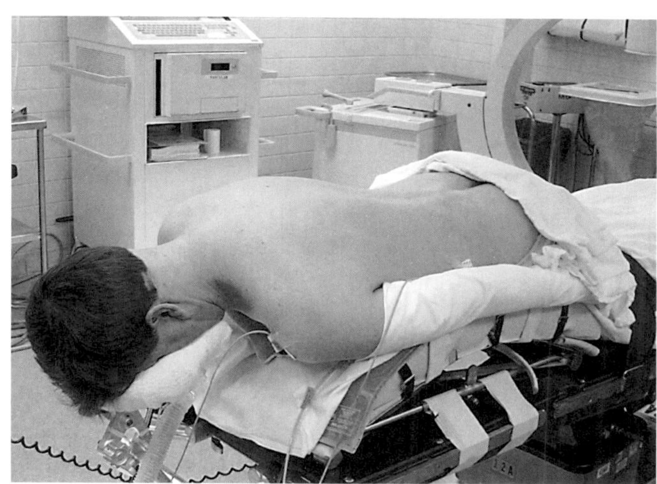

Fig. 6. Prone position in horseshoe frame.

and/or frontal headaches which are usually transformed migraines or chronic daily headaches. Control or success certainly depends on how it is defined and we look for greater than 50% pain reduction (based on visual or verbal scales) and reduction in medication use. Patients, who present with a long history of opioid use, as a rule, do not do nearly as well in the long term.

The main challenges for successful outcomes remain a combination of proper patient selection and education. These devices may not completely ameliorate all pain but can be quite useful as an adjunct to continued medication treatment.

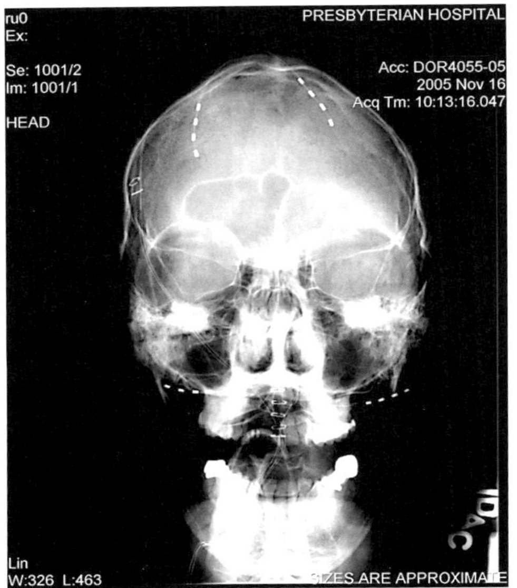

7

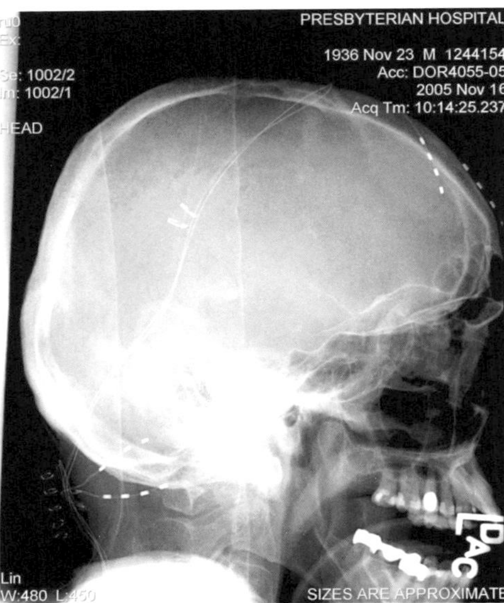

8

Fig. 7. Halo quad lead placement, AP view.
Fig. 8. Halo quad lead placement, lateral view.

Complications

Infection and electrode migration remain high. Migration difficulties are related to anchoring techniques and the fact that these devices were not designed as subcutaneous implant systems. Migration rates as high as 30% have been reported [12, 13]. Infection is also technique-dependent and it is important to remember that contaminated skin flora can be implicated in infections that may sometimes present in a delayed fashion. Wire breakage and IPG malfunction occur much less frequently but it is important not to overstress electrode wiring with tight loops in attempt to prevent migration.

The Future

Interestingly, ONS at this writing has become almost a standard of care for treating intractable occipital headache syndromes in many parts of the world but remains an off-label indication by the FDA. The appropriate clinical studies beyond safety and efficacy data have been difficult to design and implement in the current FDA environment but slow progress is being achieved.

Device design beyond what is currently available will be essential for continued success of the treatment modality. More compact lead and power sources should greatly reduce migration issues and allow placement in multiple areas as needed. Wireless neurostimulator devices with miniaturized components and novel power sources seem immediately on the horizon.

Finally, reimbursement issues will play a role in the survival of neurostimulation as a whole, let alone ONS.

References

1 Sweet WH, Wepsic JG: Treatment of chronic pain by stimulation of fibers of primary afferent neuron. Trans Am Neurol Assoc 1968;93:103–107.
2 Melzack RA, Wall PD: Pain mechanisms: a new theory. Science 1965;150:971–979.
3 Racz GB, Browne T, Lewis R Jr: Peripheral stimulator implant for treatment of causalgia caused by electrical burns. Tex Med 1988;84:45–50.
4 Weiner RL, Reed KL: Peripheral neurostimulation for control of intractable occipital neuralgia. Neuromodulation 1999;2:217–221.
5 Weiner RL: Peripheral nerve neurostimulation. Neurosurg Clin N Am 2003;14:401–408.
6 Popeney CA, Aló KM: Peripheral neurostimulation for the treatment of chronic, disabling transformed migraine. Headache 2003;43:369–375.
7 Johnson MD, Burchiel KJ: Peripheral stimulation for treatment of trigeminal postherpetic neuralgia and trigeminal posttraumatic neuropathic pain: a pilot study. Neurosurgery 2004;55:135–142.
8 Oh MY, Ortega J, Bellotte JB, Whiting DM, Aló K: Peripheral nerve stimulation for the treatment of occipital neuralgia and transformed migraine using a C1–2–3 subcutaneous paddle style electrode: a technical report. Neuromodulation 2004;7:103–112.
9 Kapural L, Mekhail N, Hayek SM, Stanton-Hicks M, Malak O: Occipital nerve electrical stimulation via the midline approach and subcutaneous surgical leads for treatment of severe occipital neuralgia: a pilot study. Anesth Analg 2005;101: 171–174.
10 Slavin KV, Nersesyan H, Wess C: Peripheral neurostimulation for treatment of intractable occipital neuralgia. Neurosurgery 2006;58: 128–132.
11 Headache Classification Subcommittee of the International Headache Society: The International Classification of Headache Disorders, ed 2. Cephalalgia 2004;24(suppl 1):9–160.
12 Jasper JF, Hayek SM: Implanted occipital nerve stimulators. Pain Physician 2008;11:187–200.
13 Falowski S, Wang D, Sabesan A, Sharan A: Occipital nerve stimulator systems: review of complications and surgical techniques. Neuromodulation 2010;13: 121–125.

Richard L. Weiner, MD, FACS
Vice-Chair, Department of Neurosurgery, THR Presbyterian Hospital
Clinical Associate Professor of Neurosurgery, University of Texas Southwestern Medical School
Suite 220, 8230 Walnut Hill Lane, Dallas, TX 75231 (USA)
E-Mail n339rw@gmail.com

Slavin KV (ed): Peripheral Nerve Stimulation.
Prog Neurol Surg. Basel, Karger, 2011, vol 24, pp 86–95

Peripheral Nerve Stimulation for Occipital Neuralgia: Surgical Leads

Leonardo Kapural · James Sable

Pain Management Department, Cleveland Clinic, Cleveland, Ohio, USA

Abstract

Peripheral nerve stimulation (PNS) has been used for the treatment of various neuropathic pain disorders, including occipital neuralgia, for the patients who failed less-invasive therapeutic approaches. Several different mechanisms of pain relief were proposed when PNS is used to treat occipital neuralgia and clinical studies using various types of electrical leads suggested largely positive clinical responses in patients with mostly refractory, severe neuropathic pain. With advancements in cylindrical lead design for PNS and placement/implantation techniques, there are very few clear indications where 'paddle' (surgical) leads could be advantageous. Those include patients who experienced repeated migration of cylindrical lead as paddle lead may provide greater stability, who are experiencing unpleasant recruitment of surrounding muscle and/or motor nerve stimulation and for cases where skin erosions were caused by a cylindrical lead. However, disregarding the type of lead used, multiple clinical advantages of this minimally invasive, easily reversible approach include relatively low morbidity and a high treatment efficacy.

Peripheral nerve stimulation (PNS) is a term generally used to describe techniques for the treatment of neuropathic pain utilizing various types of leads containing electrodes that are positioned around the affected peripheral nerves. Such approaches can be used in the treatment of neuropathic pain of different origins, located in areas that are difficult to reach using spinal cord stimulation (SCS), including the skull, face and occiput. As a rule, the painful area should be limited, pain severe, and the patient should fail other less-invasive therapies and interventions. As new approaches have been developed to more selectively target areas of pain and provide more efficient paresthesia coverage, the list of indications and new modalities of neurostimulation emerged [1].

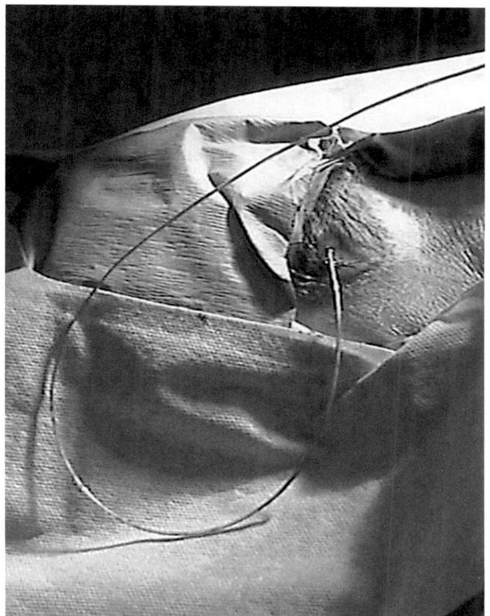

Fig. 1. Currently, most common approach when PNfS trialed for occipital neuralgia is a submastoid approach. Lead (usually cylindrical octopolar lead) is positioned across the occiput via 14 G epidural Tuohy needle. Needle containing flexible, plastic stylette is preferable, as it allows free modeling of its shape, approximating better horizontal curve of the occiput of the individual's head at the C1-C2 level.

Classification and Terminology

Classically, 'PNS is a procedure that targets a single nerve and attempts to produce a paresthesia that spreads along the territory innervated by the stimulated nerve' [2]. Recently, another clinical application of minimally invasive PNS was described [3] where significant open dissection near the peripheral nerve is avoided and near nerve electrode placement achieved. Subsequently in use now are two types of PNS: one minimally invasive approach using cylindrical leads and imaging guidance (ultrasound or CT), and classical nerve dissection where the nerve is exposed and lead placed directly to the nerve stimulated.

Peripheral nerve field stimulation (PNfS) is a somewhat different technique where the goal is to 'produce a field of paresthesia within the peripheral distribution of pain by creating an electrical field around the activated bipoles' [2]. In PNfS, the leads are placed subcutaneously in the area of pain to stimulate the region of the affected nerves or the dermatomal distribution of these nerves (fig. 1, 2). Recently, initial successes of PNfS using cylindrical and paddle leads have been reported in a growing list of clinical settings, primarily in the head and cervical regions [4–8].

Mechanism of Action and History of PNS

Like in SCS, the mechanism of pain suppression provided by PNS is thought to be based on the gate control theory of pain [1]. Chronic and spontaneous afferent

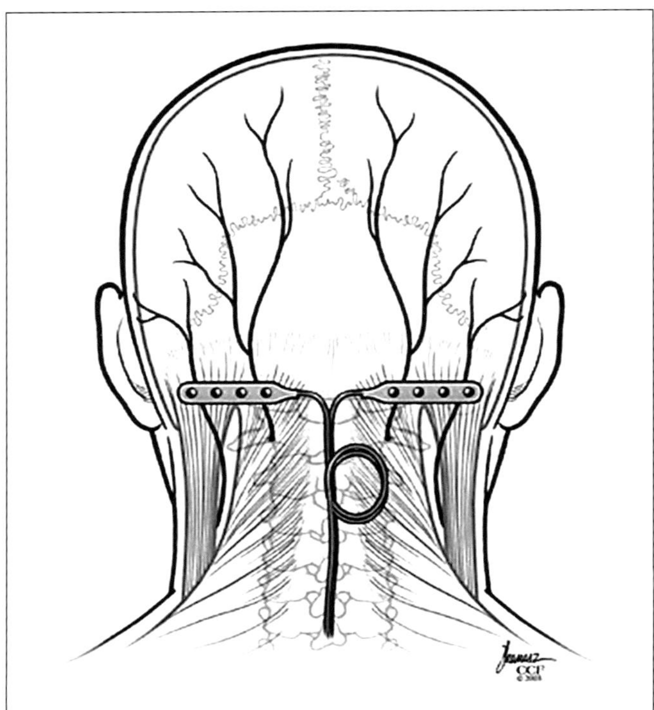

Fig. 2. Schematic of the paddle leads final position when used for the bilateral occipital neuralgia. (Used with permission from [24]).

activity can be inhibited by electrical stimulation of the proximal portion of the affected nerve, suggesting another mechanism through which peripheral nerve stimulation may decrease at least neuropathic pain [9]. Other proposed mechanisms of pain relief include subcutaneous electrical conduction, dermatomal and myotomal electrical stimulation, partial sympathetic blockade and local blood flow alteration [9–11]. Occipital nerve stimulation (ONS) is directed to distal branches of the C2 and C3, which form greater and lesser occipital nerves. As the occipital nerve is a functional part of trigeminocervical complex (TCC), its stimulation may inhibit central nociceptive transmission and provide pain relief from various types of headaches [10, 11].

Over the years, PNS has had lesser therapeutic importance than SCS, for several reasons: lack of scientific investigation, lack of complex trialing, and implantation via surgical exploration of the peripheral nerve with placement of a flat plate multicontact electrode (a paddle electrode) immediately next to it. Such traditional methods of surgically placing the lead continued to be time consuming and reports of nerve injury from electrode insertion or stimulation-related fibrosis made PNS less attractive as a pain-relieving modality [1]. The current FDA-approved electrode for PNS is a homologue of the electrode used for SCS to which a Gortex mesh has been added to allow its fixation to adjacent tissues. Unfortunately, such design does not allow multiple contacts to provide uniform stimulation to a nerve trunk, the diameter of which may vary in size [1]. The PNfS technique of lead insertion in the vicinity of the occipital nerves to treat occipital neuralgia renewed interest in the effectiveness of PNS in general [4–8].

Occipital Neuralgia

Occipital neuralgia is described as 'pain, usually deep and aching, in the distribution of the second cervical dorsal root' according to the International Association for the Study of Pain (IASP) [12]. Symptomatology commonly manifests itself as pain that is lancinating in character, with paroxysmal exacerbations, and is distributed from the inter-nuchal line (between occipital protuberance and mastoid process) with radiations around the hemicranium up to the supraorbital ridge.

The anterior rami of the upper four cervical nerves unite to form the cervical plexus, which supplies the skin and muscles of the neck. The posterior primary ramus of C1 is a motor nerve and supplies multiple muscles. The posterior primary ramus of C2 emerges between the posterior arch of the atlas and the lamina of the axis, curves around the inferior border of the inferior oblique muscle, to which it sends a branch and then divides into a large medial and a small lateral branch. The medial branch is the greater occipital nerve. This pierces semispinalis capitis and then trapezius. This may have profound implications for ONS as closeness of the muscles at the height (and depth) where the leads are positioned may produce unwanted muscle stimulation. The lesser occipital nerve (C2) hooks around the spinal accessory nerve (XI) then ascends along the posterior border of the sternocleidomastoid. It pierces the deep fascia in the upper part of the medial aspect of the posterior triangle. It then splits up into the auricular, mastoid, and occipital branches. The occipital branch is sensory to the skin in the occipital area immediately above and behind the mastoid [13, 14].

The possible sources of cervical spinal pain that might be referred to the head are dictated by the distribution of the upper three cervical spinal nerves. Through their various branches these nerves innervate the joints and ligaments of the median atlanto-axial joint, the atlanto-occipital joint, and lateral atlanto-axial joints, the C2-C3 zygapophyseal joint, the suboccipital and upper posterior neck muscles, the upper prevertebral muscles, the spinal dura mater of the posterior cranial fossa, the vertebral artery, the C2-C3 intervertebral disc, and the trapezius and sternocleidomastoid muscles. All of these structures can be sources of pain and should be considered in the differential diagnosis of cervicogenic headache. In most cases, the cause of the neuralgia is not found. However, there are examples of occipital neuralgia caused by lesions to the nerves [13–15].

Patients with occipital neuralgia usually present with an associated cervicogenic headache. The IASP [12] defines this as 'attacks of moderate or moderately severe unilateral head pain without change of side, ordinarily involving the whole hemicranium, usually starting in the neck or occipital area, and eventually involving the forehead and temporal areas, where the maximal pain is frequently located'. 'The headache usually appears in episodes of varying duration in the early phase, but with time the headache frequently becomes more continuous with exacerbations and remissions. Symptoms and signs such as mechanical precipitation of attacks imply involvement of the neck'.

The reason for globalized pain in occipital neuralgia is explained by convergence between cervical and trigeminal afferents in the spinal cord [16]. Afferents of the trigeminal nerve descend through the spinal tract of the trigeminal nerve. Their collaterals terminate in the pars caudalis of the spinal nucleus of the trigeminal nerve and in the dorsal horns of their respective segment, and send ascending and descending collaterals to adjacent segments. Therefore, at any given cervical segment, second-order neurons that project to higher centers can receive a convergent input from afferents of the trigeminal nerve and the C1, C2, and C3 spinal nerves [13–16].

Indications and Technique for the Implantation of Paddle Leads

The usual indications for PNS using paddle leads are similar to those for SCS procedures. The pain has to be chronic, severe, negatively affecting patient's functionality, and refractory to usual medical treatments. With advancements in cylindrical lead design and placement/implantation techniques, there are very few clear indications where 'paddle' leads could be advantageous when compared to cylindrical. The argument could be made that the placement of paddle leads is associated with less scar tissue formation around the electrode, better field of stimulation, and less of lead migration. Therefore, patients considered for ONS using paddle leads are frequently those who have already had implanted cylindrical leads that migrated and required revisions, sometimes several (fig. 3). The main advantage of plate electrodes is their greater inherent stability, as they are believed to have less propensity to migrate [5, 9, 14]. The lead migration rate for cylindrical leads implanted for ONS can vary between 9 and 33% [17, 18]. Such migration rates are believed to persist over long-term use, and may happen later during its therapeutic use [18]. Although prospective comparison studies related to lead migration are lacking, a large overview of paddle lead use for various indications in the epidural space in the hands of experienced neurosurgeon suggested a significantly lower rate of migration, only 1.1% [19].

Plate electrodes are also more energy efficient. Multiple arrays or different electrode configurations can be constructed with plate electrodes. The insulating side of the plate electrode isolates the contacts from dorsal structures and, using much larger cross-sectional area then a cylindrical electrode, brings the entire contact surface ventrally, closer to the stimulated nerve [20]. Therefore, another indication for the implantation of paddle leads may include patients who are experiencing unpleasant recruitment of surrounding muscle and/or motor nerve stimulation when cylindrical lead is used [21].

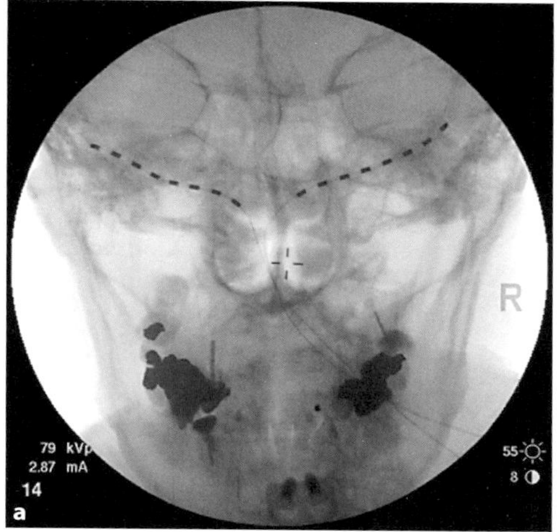

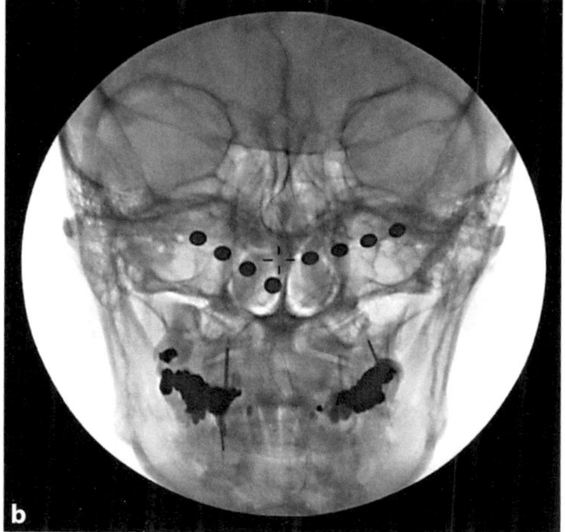

Fig. 3. a, b Same female patient after percutaneous (**a**) and surgical (**b**) permanent lead implantation. Here illustrated indication is currently one of the most common for the implantation of surgical paddle leads. Patient lost adequate stimulation after the cylindrical leads migrated and, in addition, produced localized discomfort in the left occipital area when stimulation turned on. Replacement with surgical paddle leads resulted in restored occipital coverage with more even, stable stimulation.

Finally, another likely indication for the implantation of paddle leads is the presence of repeated skin erosions caused by a cylindrical lead within the delicate area of the posterior neck, which contains minimal subcutaneous fat. During cylindrical lead implantation a Tuohy needle is used to position the lead in the occipital region. As the curve of the occipital region does not perfectly match the curve of a bent Tuohy needle, the needle itself and eventually the lead can terminate at a point much more superficial to the skin at its distal aspect, increasing the risk for skin erosion [22]. Although deeper needle placement may decrease the risk of erosion, it can in turn increase the risk of direct muscle stimulation [21].

Lateral and medial approach to both 'paddle' and cylindrical leads placement have been described (table 1). The technique originally described by Weiner et al. [8], later continued by Slavin et al. [6] and recently detailed by Trentman et al. [23] involved lateral incision close to the mastoid process. Later, midline placement was described and it has been the approach that we use in our institution. Arguments can be made that the midline incision is better due to presence of more subcutaneous fat in the midline of the neck, leaving enough space for anchoring and loop placement (fig. 2) without adding more discomfort to the patient. In addition, if bilateral leads are required, only one small midline incision over the upper neck is used to achieve stimulation of both greater and other occipital nerves. Still, it seems that the frequency of lead migration was higher when midline approach was used with cylindrical leads [18]. It is not clear if the same applies when paddle leads are used via the midline approach [24].

Table 1. Outcomes of the studies where ONS was used for the treatment of various headaches, mainly occipital neuralgia

Study	Technique	Number of patients	Type of lead	Outcome
Oh et al., 2004 [5]	below mastoid	20	paddle	14 patients >90% pain reduction at 6 months' follow-up, 95% improved QoL
Kapural et al., 2005 [25]	midline	6	paddle	VAS decreased at 6 months from 8.66 to 2.5, PDI improvement 49.8 to 14
Johnstone and Sundaraj, 2006 [26]	midline	8	paddle	5/7 with improvement in VAS, 7/8 reduction in opioid use
Magis et al., 2007 [27]	below mastoid	8	paddle	5/8 >90% reduction in pain, 2/8 with 40% improvement in pain
Jones, 2003 [28]	midline	3	paddle	all 3 'excellent' outcome
Weiner, 2006 [29]	various	150	paddle and cylindrical	70–75% >50% improvement (VAS and medication usage)
Weiner et al., 1999 [4]	below mastoid	13	cylindrical	2/3 of patients with >75% pain relief and 1/3 with >50% relief
Hammer and Doleys, 2001 [30]	midline	1	cylindrical	90% improvement in pain 9 months' follow-up
Nörenberg and Winkelmüller, 2001 [31]	below mastoid	3	cylindrical	all three >50% improvement in pain
Popeney and Aló, 2003 [32]	below mastoid	25	cylindrical	100% satisfied at 18 months, 88.7% improvement in MIDAS scores
Rodrigo-Royo et al., 2005 [33]	below mastoid	4	cylindrical	VAS scores to 0 in all patients, global symptom improvement >50% ×4
Slavin et al., 2006 [7]	below mastoid	14	cylindrical	70% adequate pain control, continued employing, decrease in opioid (22 months)
Slavin et al., 2006 [6]	below mastoid	30	cylindrical	22/30 >50% pain reduction trial, 16/22 implants >50% pain reduction
Schwedt et al., 2007 [18]	midline	15	cylindrical	improvement in HIT-6 by 11 and BDI by 20
Burns et al., 2007 [34]	midline	8	cylindrical	20 months' follow-up, 5/8 with >40% improvement in pain
Melvin et al., 2007 [17]	midline	11	cylindrical	VAS, PPI, medication use and number of attacks reduced in >64%
Trentman et al., 2008 [35]	below mastoid	10	cylindrical	all improved, 20 months' follow-up

Described are outcomes of the patients who had paddle lead implants (first 5 rows) and cylindrical lead implants. Please note that descriptive outcomes did not allow comparison between the groups. QoL = Quality of life; PDI = Pain Disability Index.

Similar to the placement of cylindrical lead, patients are positioned prone with support under the chest and forehead, and prepared and draped over the occipital area, neck, and parts of the upper and lower back and left or right upper buttock. Initial incision is made in the nuchal region about 3 cm in length, positioned cranio-caudal for either bilateral or unilateral lead implants. Subcutaneous blunt dissection is then completed from the midline bilaterally at the level of C1-C2 and a pocket created using a 'hockey stick-like' plastic introducer in the shape of the surgical lead. Leads are then positioned and the patient awakened for the intraoperative trial of stimulation. After complete coverage in the painful occipital area has been confirmed by the patient, leads are anchored in position subcutaneously. We usually place a 'strain relief' loop at the implant site (fig. 2). This is loosely sutured at three points to the subcutaneous tissue, the intention being to reduce tension on the lead during flexion. Later, the pulse generator is connected to the two leads by extension cables that were drawn through a subcutaneous tunnel and placed in a pocket in the buttock. We speculated earlier that such a midline approach using 'paddle' leads and extensive anchoring may provide less strain on the lead extension as it occurs only with flexion and is minimal with lateral flexion and rotation of the neck [25].

Clinical Outcomes and Peer-Reviewed Evidence

It needs to be emphasized that the patient group treated using this invasive approach are those patients who were unresponsive to all prior conservative and interventional procedures and uniformly had had uncontrolled occipital headaches despite increasing dosages of membrane stabilizers, antidepressants, and opioids. Clinical outcomes of patient groups receiving paddle leads were illustrated in table 1 and descriptively compared to those patient groups receiving cylindrical leads. Either group of the patients achieved very good outcomes and it is impossible to speculate if the use of either type of electrodes provides better long-term improvements in pain, function or frequency of various headaches, including occipital neuralgia. As the implantation of surgical (paddle) leads causes more tissue injury, it should be reserved for patients with the indications listed above.

Complications

The complication rate for PNS when paddle (surgical) leads are used is generally low, but both minor and major complications have been reported, including local infections, hardware erosions, component disconnections, electrode fractures and displacements, and even sepsis. Perineural fibrosis, described in the past with the use of plate or wraparound electrodes with so-called 'On-Point' PNS electrodes (Medtronic, Minneapolis, Minn., USA) is much less likely with the current ONS application of the paddle leads which essentially serve as PNfS. Still, the most frequent complication of any subcutaneous techniques for ONS is lead migration necessitating electrodes revision [17–19]. Paddle lead implantation may improve lead stability [19], as suggested in multiple reviews and study discussion, although there is no clear evidence in the form of a prospective study to confirm such a claim (please see section on indications for paddle lead implantation).

When clinically compared to spinal cord stimulation, wound dehiscence and infection are associated with lower overall morbidity; however, these complications usually require total system explantation. Another complication that can lead to failure of the system is unpleasant muscle recruitment causing spasm in the neck or occipital region. Recently, a report of a case series suggested that such problem may be less frequent when paddle leads are used [21].

Conclusions

PNS and especially ONS as a treatment modality is seeing a resurgence, with new evidence and widespread use demonstrating effectiveness in attenuating pain and improving function in patients not only with neuralgia that is not controlled with medications, but also in the treatment of migraine and cluster headaches. More research is needed to clearly assess the long-term effectiveness of this treatment. Such use of PNfS does provide multiple clinical advantages, namely, it is easily reversible, minimally invasive, and has relatively low morbidity.

References

1 Stanton-Hicks M: Peripheral nerve stimulation for pain: peripheral neuralgia and complex regional pain syndrome; in Krames ES, Peckham H, Rezai AR (eds): Neuromodulation. Philadelphia, Elsevier, 2009, pp 397–407.

2 Abejon D, Krames ES: Peripheral nerve stimulation or is it peripheral subcutaneous field stimulation; what is in a moniker? Neuromodulation 2009;12:1–4.

3 Huntoon MA, Burgher AH: Ultrasound guided permanent implantation of peripheral nerve stimulation (PNS) system for neuropathic pain of the extremities: original cases and outcomes. Pain Med 2009;10:1369–1377.

4 Weiner RL, Reed KL: Peripheral neurostimulation for control of intractable occipital neuralgia. Neuromodulation 1999;2:217–221.

5 Oh MY, Ortega J, Bellotte JB, Whiting DM, Aló K: Peripheral nerve stimulation for the treatment of occipital neuralgia and transformed migraine using a C1–2–3 subcutaneous paddle style electrode: a technical report. Neuromodulation 2004;7:103–112.

6 Slavin KV, Colpan ME, Munawar N, Wess C, Nersesyan H: Trigeminal and occipital peripheral nerve stimulation for craniofacial pain: a single-institution experience and review of the literature. Neurosurg Focus 2006;21:E5.

7 Slavin KV, Nersesyan H, Wess C: Peripheral neurostimulation for treatment of intractable occipital neuralgia. Neurosurgery 2006;58:112–119.

8 Weiner RL, Aló KM: Occipital neurostimulation (ONS) for treatment of intractable headache syndromes; in Krames ES, Peckham H, Rezai AR (eds): Neuromodulation. Philadelphia, Elsevier, 2009, pp 409–416.

9 Burchiel KJ: Effects of electrical and mechanical stimulation on two foci of spontaneous activity which develop in primary afferent neurons after peripheral axotomy. Pain 1984;18:249–265.

10 Goadsby PJ, Knight YE, Hoskin KL: Stimulation of the greater occipital nerve increases metabolic activity in the trigeminal nucleus caudalis and cervical dorsal horn of the cat. Pain 1997;73:23–28.

11 Bartsch T, Goadsby PJ: Stimulation of the greater occipital nerve induces increased central excitability of dural afferent input. Brain 2002;125:1496–1509.
12 International Association for the Study of Pain: In Merskey H, Bogduk N (eds): Classification of Chronic Pain, ed 2. Seattle, IASP Press, 1994, pp 1–224.
13 Loeser JD: Cranial neuralgias; in Loeser JD (ed): Bonica's Management of Pain, ed 3. Philadelphia, Lippincott, Williams & Wilkins, 2001, pp 855–866.
14 Jasper J, Hayek SM: Implanted occipital nerve stimulators. Pain Physician 2008;11:187–200.
15 Bogduk N: Cervicogenic headache: anatomic basis and pathophysiologic mechanisms. Curr Pain Headache Rep 2001;5:382–386.
16 Piovesan EJ, Kowacs PA, Tatsui CE, Lange MC, Ribas LC, Werneck LC: Referred pain after painful stimulation of the greater occipital nerve in humans: evidence of convergence of cervical afferents on trigeminal nuclei. Cephalalgia 2001;21:107–109.
17 Melvin EA Jr, Jordan FR, Weiner RL, Primm D: Using peripheral stimulation to reduce the pain of C2-mediated occipital headaches: a preliminary report. Pain Physician 2007;10:453–460.
18 Schwedt TJ, Dodick DW, Hentz J, Trentman TL, Zimmerman RS: Occipital nerve stimulation for chronic headache: long-term safety and efficacy. Cephalalgia 2007;27:153–157.
19 Barolat G: Experience with 509 plate electrodes implanted epidurally from C1 to L1. Stereotact Funct Neurosurg 1993;61:60–79.
20 North RB, Lanning A, Hessels R, Cutchis PN: Spinal cord stimulation with percutaneous and plate electrodes: side effects and quantitative comparisons. Neurosurg Focus 1997;15:e3.
21 Hayek SM, Jasper JF, Deer T, Narouze SN: Occipital neurostimulation-induced muscle spasms: implications for lead placement. Pain Physician 2009;12: 867–876.
22 Trentman TL, Dodick DW, Zimmerman RS, Birch BD: Percutaneous occipital stimulator lead tip erosion: report of 2 cases. Pain Physician 2008;11: 253–256.
23 Trentman TL, Slavin KV, Freeman JA, Zimmerman RS: Occipital nerve stimulator placement via a retromastoid to infraclavicular approach: a technical report. Stereotact Funct Neurosurg 2010;88:121–125.
24 Trentman TL, Zimmerman RS: Occipital nerve stimulation: technical and surgical aspects of implantation. Headache 2008;48:319–327.
25 Kapural L, Mekhail N, Hayek S, et al: Occipital nerve electrical stimulation via the midline approach and subcutaneous surgical leads for treatment of severe occipital neuralgia: a pilot study. Anesth Analg 2005;101:171–174.
26 Johnstone CSH, Sundaraj R: Occipital nerve stimulation for the treatment of occipital neuralgia – eight case studies. Neuromodulation 2006;9:41–47.
27 Magis D, Allena M, Bolla M, et al: Occipital nerve stimulation for drug-resistant chronic cluster headache: a prospective pilot study. Lancet 2007;6: 314–321.
28 Jones RL: Occipital nerve stimulation using a Medtronic Resume II electrode array. Pain Physician 2003;6:507–508.
29 Weiner RL: Occipital neurostimulation (ONS) for treatment of intractable headache disorders. Pain Med 2006;7:S137–S139.
30 Hammer M, Doleys DM: Perineuromal stimulation in the treatment of occipital neuralgia: a case study. Neuromodulation 2001;4:47–51.
31 Nörenberg E, Winkelmüller W: The epifascial electric stimulation of the occipital nerve in cases of therapy-resistant neuralgia of the occipital nerve. Schmerz 2001;15:197–199.
32 Popeney CA, Aló KM: Peripheral neurostimulation for the treatment of chronic, disabling transformed migraine. Headache 2003;43:369–375.
33 Rodrigo-Royo MD, Azcona JM, Quero J, Lorente MC, Acín P, Azcona J: Peripheral neurostimulation in the management of cervicogenic headaches: four case reports. Neuromodulation 2005;4:241–248.
34 Burns B, Watkins L, Goadsby PJ: Treatment of medically intractable cluster headache by occipital nerve stimulation: long-term follow-up of eight patients. Lancet 2007;369:1099–1106.
35 Trentman TL, Zimmerman RS, Seth N, Hentz JG, Dodick DW: Stimulation ranges, usage ranges, and paresthesia mapping during occipital nerve stimulation. Neuromodulation 2008;11:56–61.

Leonardo Kapural, MD, PhD
Carolinas Pain Institute
Center for Clinical Research
Winston-Salem, NC 27103 (USA)
Fax +1 216 444 9890, E-Mail lkapural@ccrpain.com

Slavin KV (ed): Peripheral Nerve Stimulation.
Prog Neurol Surg. Basel, Karger, 2011, vol 24, pp 96–108

Occipital Nerve Stimulation: Technical and Surgical Aspects of Implantation

Terrence L. Trentman[a] · Richard S. Zimmerman[b] · David W. Dodick[c]

Departments of [a]Anesthesiology, [b]Neurosurgery, and [c]Neurology, Mayo Clinic, Phoenix, Ariz., USA

Abstract

Occipital nerve stimulation may provide pain relief for patients with otherwise refractory primary headache disorders. While this treatment modality remains an off-label use of spinal cord stimulator technology, a growing body of literature documents surgical techniques, stimulation parameters, complications, and outcome of this novel form of neuromodulation. This chapter will review occipital nerve stimulation, including surgical techniques and complications noted in the literature. A discussion of stimulation parameters used for occipital stimulation will be included. Prospective, blinded studies of occipital nerve stimulation may clarify the role of occipital stimulation in chronic headache management.

Since 1999 there has been a growing interest in neuromodulation of the distal branches of C2-C3 in an effort to treat refractory headache disorders. This is accomplished via implantation of subcutaneous electrodes (wires, or leads) to stimulate peripheral nerves in the occipital region. 'Occipital nerve stimulation' (ONS) is a term generically used to describe the technique.

Subcutaneously implanted occipital nerve stimulators have been used to treat refractory headache disorders including migraine, hemicrania continua, post-traumatic, and cluster headache [1–3]. Other possible indications for ONS are occipital neuralgia [4, 5], transformed migraine [4], C2-mediated headaches [6], and occipital region pain after surgery [7].

In some cases such as intractable chronic cluster headache, ONS may represent a safer pain management technique than other more invasive procedures [8]. It should be noted that, currently, the use of spinal cord stimulation equipment to stimulate the occipital nerves to treat headaches represents off-label (not Food and Drug Administration approved) use of the technology.

For headache management, distal branches of C2-C3 (greater and lesser occipital nerves) are most commonly stimulated. Subcutaneous stimulation of distal branches of the trigeminal nerve has also been described such as supraorbital, supratrochlear, and infraorbital nerve stimulation [9, 10].

The history, mechanisms and outcome of this modality are beyond the scope of this chapter, which will focus on the technical aspects of the procedure with its associated complications such as electrode migration, localized pain, and infection. The surgical technique for both trial and permanent implantation of occipital nerve stimulators will be described, in addition to patient selection considerations and stimulation parameters. Occipital nerve stimulation for occipital neuralgia, in addition to the more common indications of migraine and cluster headache, will be reviewed. The available literature will be summarized and a discussion of future directions will be provided.

Surgical Technique

The anatomy of the nerves of the occipital region has been well described [11–15]. Becser et al. [12] noted great variability in nerve topography between 10 cadavers, both inter- and intraindividually. The greater occipital nerve (GON) was seen to ascend between 5 and 28 mm from the midline at the level of the intermastoid line, while the lesser occipital nerve (LON) was observed between 32 and 90 mm from midline.

Before implantation of spinal cord or occipital nerve stimulators, patients typically undergo a psychological assessment. This is done to evaluate the presence of active drug abuse and/or under or untreated mental health disorders such as anxiety and depression. Also, the patient's ability to make informed consent and use an implanted electronic device is assessed. A pre-operative discussion of the risks of the procedure is of course necessary. Specific risks that should be mentioned include no guarantee of effectiveness, infection, nerve damage, painful direct muscle stimulation, electrode migration with loss of stimulation, electrode fracture, battery failure, eventual need for battery replacement, and hematoma and seroma formation. The complications of occipital stimulators will be discussed more fully below.

Stimulation Trial

There is no available literature to demonstrate the utility of a trial of occipital nerve stimulation before permanent implant, i.e. if a patient experiences at least 50% pain relief during an ONS trial, does this predict long term benefit? Studies are needed to answer this question, as the time and cost associated with the trial is considerable. The appropriate length of an ONS trial and ideal minimal reported pain relief (e.g. 50%) are also unknown. Nonetheless, in our practice candidates for permanent occipital nerve stimulators first undergo a 5- to 7-day trial.

Briefly, the trial is carried out after hair removal with 'clippers' in the occipital region. Sterile preparation of the surgical field is used and antibiotic prophylaxis is given before skin puncture. The patient is placed in the prone or lateral decubitus position and given local anesthesia plus minimal sedation. A Tuohy needle, bent to conform to the curvature of the patient's occiput, is inserted subcutaneously and transversely at the C1 level. An electrode is then inserted through the needle, which is withdrawn leaving the wire in place. Bilateral headaches are treated with bilateral electrodes. Flouroscopy is routinely used to identify anatomic landmarks (C1 arch, mastoid process) and document electrode location. The electrodes are secured with an anchor attached to the skin, and powered with an external power source. Further details of the permanent surgical procedure will be discussed below.

Occipital stimulation techniques that use percutaneous or paddle electrodes do not seek to specifically stimulate the GON or LON. Rather, the electrodes are placed subcutaneously in the occipital region and the fibers of C2-C3 are stimulated. However, it is possible that a contact could be placed immediately adjacent to one of the named nerves. In that scenario, the patient might experience more diffuse paresthesia than would be expected from subcutaneous stimulation. If the patient found the stimulation uncomfortable, the contact array could be changed in an effort to 'program away' from the (presumed) nerve.

In addition to assessing efficacy of the modality in terms of pain control, the trial allows the patient to experience the 'paresthesias' associated with ONS, which are usually described as 'tingling' or 'buzzing' in the occipital region. Rarely, a patient finds the sensation unpleasant and they choose not to pursue a permanent ONS, even if the trial device provided headache relief. Magis et al. [2] noted a patient who found the paresthesias unbearable (postimplant) and eventually had the device removed. Finally, the trial allows the clinician further observation of the patient's behavior and expectations. Some patients expectations of the device are unrealistic, while others may have well entrenched, dysfunctional pain behaviors. As such, they are not good candidates for permanent implantation as long-term outcome will likely be poor [16, 17].

At the end of a successful trial, the implanter has the option of removing the trial electrodes and starting with new components some time later (for the permanent implant). Alternatively, the permanent system can be implanted at the end of the trial using the existing trial electrodes. Although there may be an increased risk of infection when using the trail electrodes for a permanent implant, there is a clear advantage in terms of expense and electrode positioning. If the trial electrodes are removed and the permanent procedure is carried out some time later, there is a chance the patient will not experience the same stimulation they did during the trial, as the permanent electrodes may be in a slightly different location.

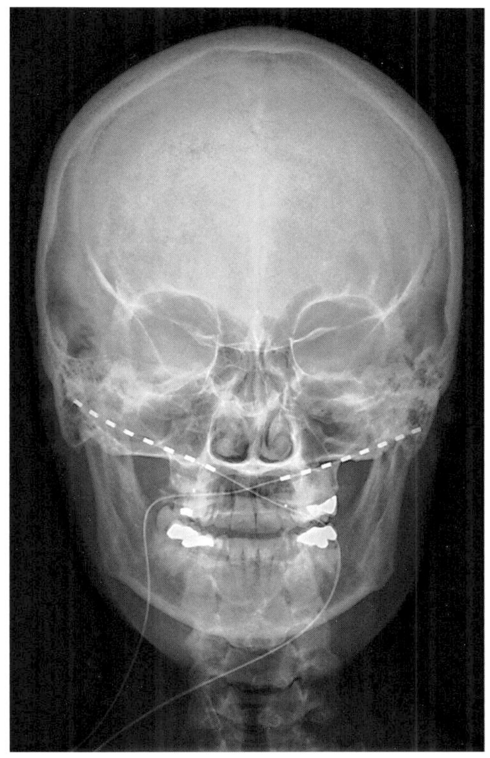

Fig. 1. Intraoperative AP radiograph of bilateral occipital stimulator trial electrodes inserted from a midline approach.

Permanent Implant

In general, 2 surgical approaches have been described for permanent ONS implantation. The first is via a 2-cm midline incision at the C1 level, with the electrode(s) inserted with a lateral trajectory from that point [1, 3, 11, 18–21] (fig. 1). The second is via a lateral (or retromastoid) approach, where the incision is made posterior and inferior to the mastoid process, again at the C1 level [2, 4, 5, 7, 9, 22] (fig. 2). Either percutaneous or paddle electrodes can be used via the midline or lateral approach. In the lateral approach, a single electrode can be inserted across the midline in an effort to provide bilateral stimulation coverage (i.e. contacts of a single electrode are positioned on both sides of the midline), or two electrodes can be used, one with all contacts across the midline and the other completely on the side of the incision (fig. 3). Oh described using either a midline or lateral approach depending on the location of the patient's pain (midline approach for bilateral transformed migraine and lateral approach for unilateral occipital neuralgia) [4]. Kapural et al. [19] noted that the midline approach may be associated with a lower rate of electrode displacement due to electrode strain only with neck flexion, and minimal strain with lateral rotation of the head. However, electrode migration has been associated with the midline approach [1].

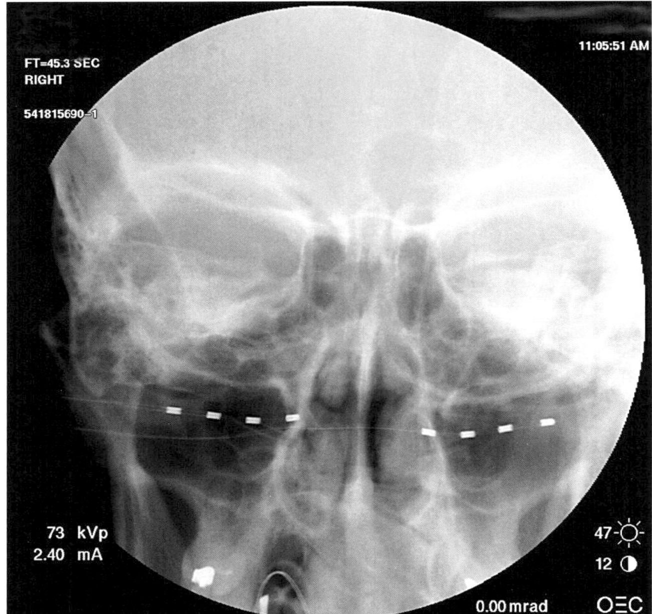

Fig. 2. Intraoperative AP radiograph of symmetrical, bilateral occipital stimulator electrodes inserted from a retromastoid approach. From Trentman et al. [31], with permission.

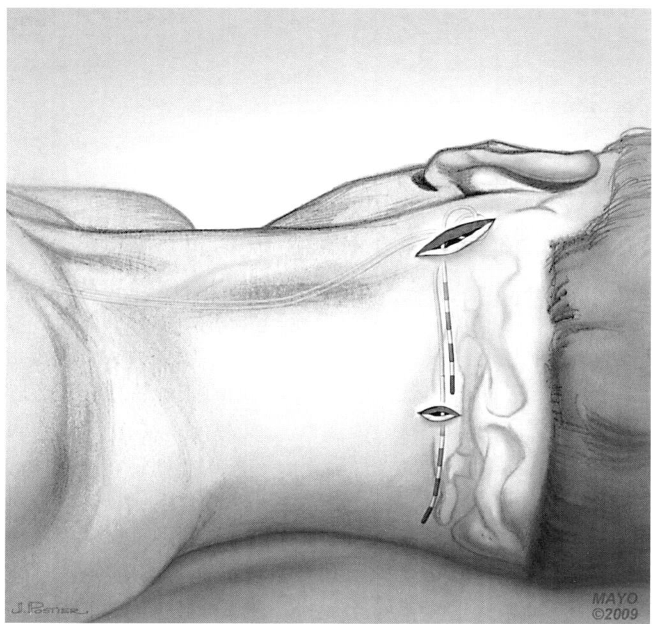

Fig. 3. Illustration of retromastoid approach to ONS permanent implant. From Trentman et al. [31], with permission.

For both midline and lateral incisions, a small pocket is created in the subcutaneous tissues around the incision where the electrode(s) will be looped and anchored. The electrodes are inserted with the goal of placing them in the subcutaneous fat, superficial to the fascia. If the electrodes are too close (or through) the fascia, the patient may experience painful direct muscle stimulation. If they are too superficial, the risk of electrode erosion is increased. The electrodes are tested with the patient awake enough to respond to questioning. If the patient experiences painful stimulation, the wire can be repositioned. We have also had early success with electrode placement under general anesthesia when sedation alone was relatively contraindicated because of co-morbid medical conditions. Our preliminary experience suggests that this may be an acceptable alternative [23].

The paddle electrode requires further dissection of the subcutaneous tissues adjacent to the incision, as it can not be inserted via a needle. The shielded side of the paddle electrode is positioned most superficial (toward the skin) in an effort to direct the current toward the nerves, which emerge from the deep nuchal structures at variable points below the intermastoid line [12]. The paddle style electrode can be sutured to the dense cervical fascia, perhaps decreasing the risk of electrode migration [11]. A technique to distally suture (secure) a percutaneous electrode has also been described [24, 25].

Once the electrode position is satisfactory, a silicone anchor is used with non-absorbable suture to attach the electrode to the fascia. Medical grade silicone glue can be placed between the electrode and the anchor to strengthen the bond. The electrode is looped in the pocket and then tunneled toward an IPG pocket. Depending on the length of electrode selected, the location of the IPG, and the manufacturer, an extension may be needed. A silicone sheath is used to surround and protect the connection between the electrode and the extension when connections are present. As mentioned above, both general [2–4, 11, 22] and local anesthesia (with sedation) [6, 19, 21] have been used successfully during the tunneling and IPG placement for the permanent implant. An anesthetic technique has been described for this procedure [26].

Internal pulse generators have been placed in the buttock, the low abdomen, the midaxillary line, the infrascapular, and the infraclavicular regions [2–4, 6, 7, 11, 18, 19, 21, 22, 24]. One goal is to minimize the mechanical stress on the electrode that may predispose it to migration. The anchor, glue, and loop at the incision site may be protective, but some IPG locations may be associated with less traction on the electrode than others [27]. Pre-operative counseling regarding IPG location should include consideration of the patient's body habitus as well as taking into account any patient preference based on cosmetic concerns.

After completion of the surgical procedure, skull X-rays can be obtained to document final electrode position. These are useful should a future electrode migration or fracture be suspected. The patient controls the ONS with a handheld remote control. It is placed over or near the IPG to turn the device on/off, while reprogramming of the polarity of contacts and other parameters is done by the physician. In our practice, patients are encouraged to minimize head and neck movement and deep bending for at least 6 weeks after surgery. This will hopefully allow a measure of scarring to occur to help hold the device in place. Patients are also advised not to drive a car with the device turned on in the unlikely event they would receive a shock at an inopportune moment potentially causing an accident.

Occipital Nerve Stimulation Programming: Patterns and Parameters

In addition to the contact array, frequency (rate or pulses per second), pulse width, and amplitude are programmable. These parameters are adjusted to patient comfort, as no literature exists to associate specific parameters with outcome. Reported frequencies range from 3 to 130 Hz, pulse width from 90 to 450 ms, and amplitude from 0.1 to 10.0 V [1–3, 5, 6, 18–20, 22]. Hammer and Doleys [7] reported a patient requiring amplitude of 12 V. The stimulator was powered by a radiofrequency system as an implanted battery would be rapidly depleted by this high energy requirement.

We have reported on paresthesia patterns in 10 patients previously implanted with ONS systems [28]. At the beginning of the study, the patient's stimulators were interrogated and found to have a mean pulse width of approximately 400 μs and amplitude of 2.8 ± 2.0 V. The mean rate was 38 ±13 pulses per second. Upon further testing, the subjects were found to have a mean perception threshold of 1.07 V and a mean discomfort threshold of 3.63 V. Therefore, the stimulation range was 1.07–3.63 V.

In our study, paresthesia maps were created based upon patient reported paresthesia distributions during programming of all possible contact combinations. At discomfort threshold, 10% of the patients felt frontal paresthesias whereas essentially 100% of the patients experienced occipital stimulation at perception threshold. In other words, this study suggested that at higher amplitudes, some patients would feel frontal paresthesias with ONS.

The utility of covering all areas of headache pain with paresthesias is unknown, as compared to spinal cord stimulation where the goal is to cover all painful areas with paresthesias. Further study is needed to determine if certain stimulation patterns are associated with better outcome. For instance, are frontal headaches best treated with frontal (e.g. supraorbital) stimulation? Should headache diagnosis (e.g. cluster vs. migraine headache) influence location of stimulation, or is occipital stimulation adequate for all?

Complication Avoidance

A number of complications have been reported after ONS. These can be summarized in categories including electrode migration, infection, lack or loss of effect, localized pain (neck, around system components), and muscle spasm (table 1). Slavin et al. [9]

Table 1. Complications of permanently implanted occipital stimulators

Author	Approach/ components	Location of IPG	Number of patients and laterality of leads	Duration of follow-up	Complications	Disposition/treatment if any
Weiner and Reed, 1999 [5]	L, P	various	13 patients, 17 implants	1.5–6 years	1 migration 1 electrode infection	revised revised
Hammer and Doleys, 2001 [7]	L, P	flank	1 patient, U	9 months	none	
Jones, 2003 [21]	M, S	buttock	3 patients, 1 B	not reported	none	
Popney and Aló, 2003 [20]	M, P	not reported	25 patients, all B	mean 18.3 months	9 migrations 1 infection	revised explant/re-implanted
Gofeld, 2004 [24]	L, P	buttock	1 patient, U	1 week	migration	revised with distal tip fixation
Oh et al., 2004 [4] (see below)	L, S	infra-clavicular	10 patients, occipital neuralgia, all U	see below	cervical pain pain over IPG	explanted explanted
Oh et al., 2004 [4]	M, P in 7/10; M, S in 3/10	buttock	10 patients, transformation migraine, all B	18 patients to 6 months; 1 patient to 4 years	1 infection 1 infection 7 migrations (all P)	antibiotics explant/ reimplantation revised with S
Kapural et al., 2005 [19]	M, S	buttock	6 patients, B	3 months	none	
Rodrigo-Royo et al., 2005 [18]	M, P	buttock	4 patients, 3 U and 1 B	4–16 months	none	
Johnstone and Sudaraj, 2006 [11]	M, S	infraclavicular or low abdomen	7 patients; 5 U and 2 B	6–47 months, mean 25 months	1 infection (IPG) 1 infection (lead)	explant/reimplant for both
Slavin et al., 2006 [9]	L, P	infraclavicular	10 patients, 8 B	5–32 months, mean 22 months	1 infection 1 loss of stimulation 1 pain relief without stimulation	explant explant explant

Table 1. Continued

Author	Approach/ components	Location of IPG	Number of patients and laterality of leads	Duration of follow-up	Complications	Disposition/treatment if any
Magis et al., 2007 [2]	L, S	pectoral	8 patients, U	3–22 months, mean 15.1 months	1 lack of benefit 1 migration 1 migration post fall 1 ONS turned off by magnetic interference 1 chest discomfort with safety belt	explant reprogrammed revision pending
Burns et al., 2007 [3]	M, P	infraclavicular or abdomen	8 patients, B	8–27 months, median 20 months	1 transient excess pain at surgical site 1 patient with migration × 3, muscle stimulation 1 contact failure 1 shock due to wire kink	oral meds and injection revised × 3 revised reprogrammed
Schwedt et al., 2007 [1]	M, P	various	15 patients, 8 B and 7 U	5–42 months, mean 19 months	8 migration 2 neck stiff 1 each IPG site, electrode site, and myofascial pain	revised
Melvin et al., 2007 [6]	M and L; P	abdomen or infrascapular	11 patients; 7 with single octopolar lead; 4 with dual quadripolar electrode	12 weeks	1 lost stimulation/ loose connection 1 migration with neck spasm	revised extension revised
Trentman et al., 2008 [28]	M	Infraclavicular and buttock	1 patient – U 1 patient – B	45 months and 22 months	electrode tip erosion	1 – revised 2 – electrode tip buried

Note that Slavin et al: Neurosurg Focus 2006;21:E6, is omitted as this study describes occipital, supraorbital, and infraorbital stimulators in 22 patients but does not distinguish complications by location of device. S = Surgical or paddle electrode; P = percutaneous or cylindrical electrode; B = bilateral; U = unilateral; M = midline approach; L = lateral or retromastoid approach; revised = new electrode placed.

reported a case of electrode tip erosion, although he did not identify the specific electrode location (occipital vs. supraorbital or infraorbital), while Trentman et al. [29] reported on 2 cases of occipital electrode tip erosion. The electrode was removed and reimplanted 1 month later with return of pain control.

Electrode (lead) migration is arguably the most bothersome and serious complication of ONS. Cervical X-rays typically show electrode migration towards the midline, with the electrode either coiled in the occipital pocket or pulled down toward the IPG. The mechanism of ONS electrode migration is not completely understood. Clearly, the highly mobile neck region places stress on system components that is not encountered in spinal cord stimulation. The remote battery, if placed in a buttock or low abdominal site, will be close to a meter distant from the electrode(s) in a tall patient. Neck movement, flexion and lateral rotation at the waist, and even arm movement can impact the electrodes and extensions.

To avoid complications, there are no outcome studies to guide surgeons as to the best techniques to minimize electrode migration. The use of silicone glue may reduce failure of the anchor/electrode interface. We have prescribed soft collars for patients to wear for 10 days postimplant, in hopes that the collar would remind them to minimize neck movement. Furthermore, we routinely advise patients to minimize head movement, deep bending, and twisting for 6 weeks post implant. Some authors use the retromastoid approach, while others have advocated for the midline approach. Kapural used paddle electrodes via a midline approach, and stated that this approach has several advantages including improved current distribution versus percutaneous electrodes, fewer surges of current, and less frequent electrode dislodgement [19].

Although there is no prospective, in vivo data to guide decision making regarding location of the IPG, we have recently examined this question in an in-vitro model [27]. Pathway length changes for simulated retromastoid or midline electrode placements were measured in volunteers during various movements like flexion and extension of the neck and low back. We concluded that the retromastoid to infraclavicular pathway was associated with the least electrode pathway length change, and that this may result in fewer electrode migrations. The low abdominal IPG site was also an acceptable alternative, while the buttock site was associated with the greatest electrode pathway length change (fig. 4).

Use of Occipital Stimulation for Occipital Neuralgia

Occipital neuralgia has multiple potential etiologies including trauma, osteoarthritis, C2 nerve root compression, and Chiari malformation [30]. When conservative therapies, including anti-inflammatory drugs, injections, and physical therapy modalities are ineffective, ONS has been described.

Currently, limited data are available regarding ONS for occipital neuralgia. Most of the literature focuses on primary headache disorders such as migraine, chronic

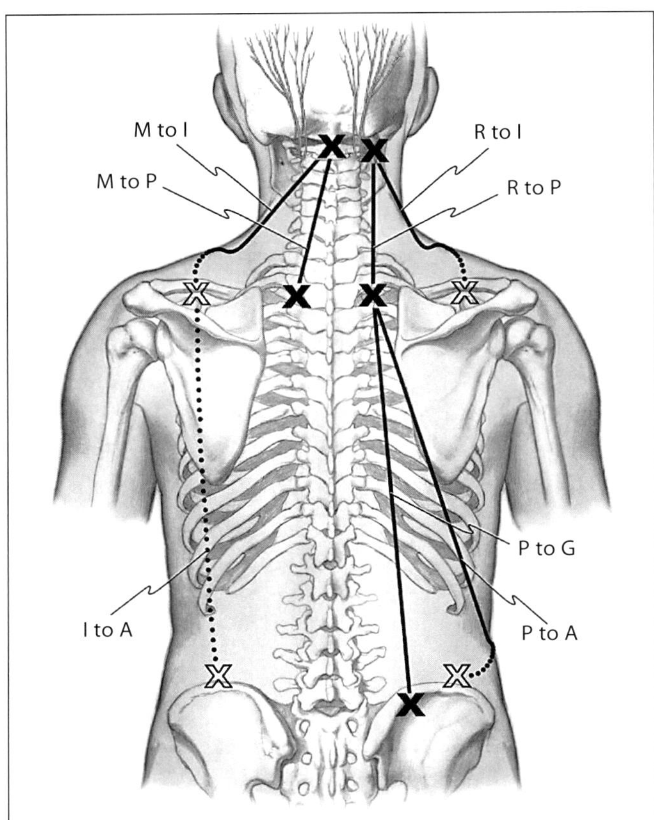

Fig. 4. Pathways measured during volunteer movement. M to P = Midline occipital to periscapular pathway; R to P = retromastoid to periscapular pathway; M to I = midline occipital to infraclavicular pathway; P to G = periscapular to gluteal pathway; P to A = periscapular to low abdomen pathway; I to A = infraclavicular to low abdomen pathway. Dotted lines and open X's represent anterior pathways and attachment sites. Solid lines and X's are posterior. From Trentman et al. [27], courtesy of Wiley-Blackwell publishing.

cluster headache, and hemicrania continua. Weiner and Reed's [5] landmark paper described treatment of medically intractable occipital neuralgia with ONS. In 12 of 13 patients, they demonstrated a good-to-excellent response (>50% pain relief) over an 18-month to 6-year time frame. The 13th patient underwent ONS explant due to symptom resolution.

As noted above, Oh et al. [4] reported on 10 patients with occipital neuralgia who underwent ONS with paddle style electrodes. Eight of the patients obtained excellent (>90%) relief at 1 month and 7 had excellent relief at 6-month follow-up. One patient requested ONS explant because of cervical pain with stimulation, while another patient developed pain at the pulse generator site and had the system explanted.

In a case report, Hammer and Doleys [7] described a patient with occipital neuralgia refractory to surgical interventions and injections. Pain relief was obtained when they threaded an electrode under a neuroma apparently created by a C2 nerve transection.

Future Directions

Occipital nerve stimulation is emerging as a treatment modality for refractory headache disorders. However, many questions remain unanswered. There is a clear need for prospective, placebo-controlled, blinded studies to evaluate the efficacy of neuromodulation of the occipital nerves. In terms of surgical considerations, the case series and small studies currently available do not definitively answer questions such as the ideal approach to the occipital nerves, the best electrode, and the best location for the IPG. Correlating stimulation trial results and long term outcome has been studied in SCS but not yet in ONS.

Electrode (lead) migration will likely continue to be a major complication of ONS as long as electrodes are tethered to connective tissue and powered by remote batteries. Future developments may provide miniaturized, local power sources that will ideally eliminate mechanical stress on the stimulator system. Improved anchoring systems and surgical techniques may also minimize device fracture, movement, and localized pain.

References

1 Schwedt TJ, Dodick DW, Hentz J, Trentman TL, Zimmerman RS: Occipital nerve stimulation for chronic headache: long-term safety and efficacy. Cephalalgia 2007;27:153–157.

2 Magis D, Allena M, Bolla M, De Pasqua V, Remacle JM, Schoenen J: Occipital nerve stimulation for drug-resistant chronic cluster headache: a prospective pilot study. Lancet Neurol 2007;6:314–321.

3 Burns B, Watkins L, Goadsby PJ: Treatment of medically intractable cluster headache by occipital nerve stimulation: long-term follow-up of eight patients. Lancet 2007;369:1099–1106.

4 Oh MY, Ortega J, Bellotte JB, Whiting DM, Alo KM: Peripheral nerve stimulation for the treatment of occipital neuralgia and transformed migraine using a C1–2–3 subcutaneous paddle style electrode: a technical report. Neuromodulation 2004;7:103–112.

5 Weiner RL, Reed KL: Peripheral neurostimulation for the control of intractable occipital neuralgia. Neuromodulation 1999;2:217–221.

6 Melvin EA Jr, Jordan FR, Weiner RL, Primm D: Using peripheral stimulation to reduce the pain of C2-mediated occipital headaches: a preliminary report. Pain Physician 2007;10:453–460.

7 Hammer M, Doleys DM: Perineuromal stimulation in the treatment of occipital neuralgia: a case study. Neuromodulation 2001;4:47–51.

8 Leone M, Franzini A, Broggi G, Bussone G: Hypothalamic stimulation for intractable cluster headache: long-term experience. Neurology 2006;67:150–152.

9 Slavin KV, Colpan ME, Munawar N, Wess C, Nersesyan H: Trigeminal and occipital peripheral nerve stimulation for craniofacial pain: a single-institution experience and review of the literature. Neurosurg Focus 2006;21:E6.

10 Johnson MD, Burchiel KJ: Peripheral stimulation for treatment of trigeminal postherpetic neuralgia and trigeminal posttraumatic neuropathic pain: a pilot study. Neurosurgery 2004;55:135–141; discussion 141–132.

11 Johnstone CS, Sundaraj R: Occipital nerve stimulation for the treatment of occipital neuralgia – eight case studies. Neuromodulation 2006;9:41–47.

12 Becser N, Bovim G, Sjaastad O: Extracranial nerves in the posterior part of the head. Anatomic variations and their possible clinical significance. Spine 1998;23:1435–1441.

13 Bogduk N: The clinical anatomy of the cervical dorsal rami. Spine 1982;7:319–330.

14 Bogduk N: The anatomy of occipital neuralgia. Clin Exp Neurol 1981;17:167–184.

15 Natsis K, Baraliakos X, Appell HJ, Tsikaras P, Gigis I, Koebke J: The course of the greater occipital nerve in the suboccipital region: a proposal for setting landmarks for local anesthesia in patients with occipital neuralgia. Clin Anat 2006;19:332–336.

16 Doleys DM: Psychological factors in spinal cord stimulation therapy: brief review and discussion. Neurosurg Focus 2006;21:E1.
17 Doleys DM: Psychological assessment for implantable therapies. Pain Digest 2000;10:16–23.
18 Rodrigo-Royo MD, Azcona JM, Quero J, Lorente MC, Acin P, Azcona J: Peripheral neurostimulation in the management of cervicogenic headache: four case reports. Neuromodulation 2005;8:241–248.
19 Kapural L, Mekhail N, Hayek SM, Stanton-Hicks M, Malak O: Occipital nerve electrical stimulation via the midline approach and subcutaneous surgical leads for treatment of severe occipital neuralgia: a pilot study. Anesth Analg 2005;101:171–174.
20 Popeney CA, Alo KM: Peripheral neurostimulation for the treatment of chronic, disabling transformed migraine. Headache 2003;43:369–375.
21 Jones RL: Occipital nerve stimulation using a Medtronic resume II electrode array. Pain Physician 2003;6:507–508.
22 Slavin KV, Nersesyan H, Wess C: Peripheral neurostimulation for treatment of intractable occipital neuralgia. Neurosurgery 2006;58:112–119; discussion 112–119.
23 Trentman TL, Zimmerman RS, Dodick DW, Dormer CL, Vargas BB: Occipital nerve stimulator placement under general anesthesia: initial experience with 5 cases and review of the literature. J Neurosurg Anesthesiol 2010;22:158–62
24 Gofeld M: Anchoring of suboccipital lead: case report and technical note. Pain Pract 2004;4: 307–309.
25 Lou L: Uncommon areas of electrical stimulation for pain relief. Curr Rev Pain 2000;4:407–412.
26 Lim HB, Hunt K: Anesthetic management for surgical placement of greater occipital nerve stimulators in the treatment of primary headache disorders. J Neurosurg Anesthesiol 2007;19:120–124.
27 Trentman TL, Mueller JT, Shah DM, Zimmerman RS, Noble BM: Occipital nerve stimulator lead pathway length changes with volunteer movement: an in vitro study. Pain Pract 2010;10:42–48.
28 Trentman TL, Zimmerman RS, Seth N, Hentz J, Dodick DW: Stimulation ranges, usage ranges, and paresthesia mapping during occipital nerve stimulation. Neuromodulation 2008;11:56–61.
29 Trentman TL, Dodick DW, Zimmerman RS, Birch BD: Percutaneous occipital stimulator lead tip erosion: report of two cases. Pain Physician 2008;11: 253–256.
30 Anthony M: Headache and the greater occipital nerve. Clin Neurol Neurosurg 1992;94:297–301.
31 Trentman TL, Slavin KV, Freeman JA, Zimmerman RS: Occipital nerve stimulator placement via a retromastoid to infraclavicular approach: a technical report. Stereotact Funct Neurosurg. 2010;88: 121–125.

Terrence L. Trentman, MD
Department of Anesthesiology
5777 E Mayo Blvd
Phoenix, AZ 85054 (USA)
Tel. +1 480 342 1800, Fax +1 480 342 2319, E-Mail trentman.terrence@mayo.edu

Slavin KV (ed): Peripheral Nerve Stimulation.
Prog Neurol Surg. Basel, Karger, 2011, vol 24, pp 109–117

Peripheral Neuromodulation for Migraine Headache

Damien J. Ellens[a] · Robert M. Levy[a–c]

Departments of [a]Neurological Surgery, [b]Physiology and [c]Radiation Oncology, Feinberg School of Medicine, Northwestern University, Chicago, Ill., USA

Abstract

Extremely high prevalence among general population along with the high percentage of treatment-refractory cases makes migraine headaches one of the potentially largest indications for neuromodulation. Cranial peripheral nerve stimulation targeting the occipital nerve(s) alone or in combination with others appears to be both safe and efficacious for the treatment of medically intractable migraine headaches. Although initial reports of occipital nerve stimulation for migraine headaches were very encouraging, this clinical benefit was not clearly confirmed in larger-scale prospective randomized trials. Moreover, the exact mechanism of neuromodulation effect in migraine treatment remains unclear. Significant further investigation needs to be performed to optimize our knowledge concerning patient selection, stimulation targets and parameters and device programming, and further improve clinical results. At present, neurostimulation for migraine headache pain is performed in the United States on an 'off-label' basis, but based upon our experience and the increasing evidence in the medical literature, we look forward to its approval by the FDA in the near future so that patients suffering from severe, medically intractable headache pain may gain access to these potentially important therapies.

Almost 40 million Americans suffer from intractable migraine, chronic daily headache, cervicogenic and secondary headache syndromes including occipital neuralgia [1]. About 5% of these patients suffer daily or near daily headaches, including transformed migraine and chronic daily headaches, resulting in significant loss of quality of life related to narcotic dependence, restriction in daily activities, failed personal and career objectives and an overwhelming sense of despair and hopelessness [2].

The term 'chronic daily headache' refers to a group of nonparoxysmal headaches, including those associated with overuse of pain-relieving medications, that present on a daily or near daily basis with a duration of greater than 4 hours a day and lasting longer than 6 months [3]. Roughly 2.2 million Americans, about 0.5–6% of the population, are afflicted by chronic daily headaches [4]. Episodic migraine headaches cost

American employers 13 billion USD a year from absenteeism, with direct treatment costs running over USD 1 billion annually [5].

Pharmacotherapy for migraine headaches includes those medications that offer acute pain relief (abortives) and those used for migraine prevention. Pharmacologic options for acute pain relief include nonsteroidal anti-inflammatory agents, triptans, opioids, ergot compounds and sedatives. Medications effective in headache prevention include anticonvulsants, antidepressants, beta-blockers and serotonin antagonists. Since migraines are often triggered by environmental or emotional factors, recognition and avoidance of precipitating agents like caffeine, stress and a number of foods can provide significant relief and decrease the need for medications. Alternative nonpharmacological migraine treatment options include acupuncture, biofeedback, massage and diet control.

Ablative and decompressive neurosurgical techniques have been tried in patients with migraine headaches. In the past, neurosurgeons performed occipital neurolysis and neurectomy for the treatment of headache pain. Such techniques may result in delayed neuropathic pain in the sensory distribution of the affected occipital nerve(s). Ganglionectomy at the second cervical level was reported to be 80% effective at a 3-year follow-up in posttraumatic second cervical pain syndromes [6]. Nontraumatic pain in this region was not, however, significantly relieved by ganglionectomy, and the procedure is not without risk. Second cervical nerve decompression was also reported to be nearly 80% effective in providing pain relief at 2 years [7]. Posterior rhizotomy at the first, second or third cervical level performed by ventrolateral dorsal root entry zone lesioning is sometimes effective but is highly invasive and has a significant risk [8]. Neurolysis of the greater occipital nerve is often effective initially in controlling pain, but patients commonly report significant recurrence within 2 years [9]. Peripheral nerve stimulation using a cuff electrode was found to be effective in 6 patients with occipital neuralgia [10]. Direct stimulation of the greater occipital nerve has also been shown to be very effective in relieving painful peripheral neuropathy [11].

The use of implanted neurostimulation for the treatment of migraine headache is a relatively recent development. When Weiner and Reed [12] first reported their use of percutaneously implanted occipital nerve stimulation electrodes, the stated indication for this treatment was that of occipital neuralgia. However, subsequent evaluation of 8 of these patients by positron emission tomography demonstrated patterns most consistent with chronic migraine headaches [13]. Subsequently, other reports found occipital nerve stimulation efficacious for the treatment of several headache disorders including migraine headaches [14, 15], cluster headache [16, 17], hemicrania continua [18] and true occipital neuralgia [19].

Surgical Procedure

The standard surgical procedure for occipital nerve stimulation has been significantly refined since its first description [12]. Multiple authors have contributed to the technical development of neurostimulator electrode placement describing the use of both cylindrical and paddle-type leads [14, 15, 20, 21].

For the stimulation trial procedure, percutaneous-type cylindrical leads are used almost exclusively. Trial lead placement is performed with the patient in the supine position with the head turned sharply away from the side of pain. After the injection of local anesthetic at a point 1 cm caudal and 1 cm medial to the tip of the mastoid process, a bent Tuohy needle is advanced under fluoroscopic guidance into the subcutaneous space toward the posterior cervical midline. The needle is advanced until the tip of the needle projects over the odontoid process of C2 on antero-posterior fluoroscopic images. The stylet of the needle is removed and replaced with a multi-contact cylindrical lead; centering the contacts over the expected location of the occipital nerve(s). A purse-string suture is placed around the exit site of the Tuohy needle through the skin and the needle is carefully withdrawn and removed. Physiologic testing is then performed and the lead position is adjusted until the patient reports stimulation-induced paresthesias throughout the distribution of the nerve. The purse-string suture is then secured around the exit of the lead through the skin and the wound is dressed.

If trial stimulation is successful, permanent surgical implantation is usually undertaken. The surgical technique using percutaneous-type cylindrical neurostimulation leads involves making a vertical incision about 2 cm long down to the cervicodorsal fascia, either 1 cm caudal and 1cm medial to the tip of the mastoid process (for the lateral to medial approach) or at the posterior midline at the level of C1 (for the medial to lateral approach). For the former approach, the patient is positioned supine with their head turned sharply away from the side of their pain; for the latter approach, the patient is placed in the prone position. A subcutaneous pocket above the fascia is developed to accommodate the fixation hardware and for placement of a redundant loop of the electrode wire.

A Tuohy needle is gently bent to a curve similar to the curvature of the neck, and is then passed under fluoroscopic guidance transversely into the subcutaneous plane across the course of the occipital nerve(s) to the posterior cervical midline. At this level, the greater and lesser occipital nerves are located within the cervical musculature and overlying fascia. Single (for unilateral) or dual (for bilateral) four or eight electrode leads may be used; these can be placed from midline toward either side, or across the entire cervical curvature from one side to the other, or by using bilateral incisions.

Once the lead is adequately positioned, the lead is fixed to the underlying fascia using two silicone anchors secured with nonabsorbable suture material [22]. A strain relief loop is made in the lead wire to help prevent migration by decreasing electrode traction during normal patient movement. The lead is then tunneled to a pulse generator implanted over the chest wall.

While many authors prefer this transverse lead orientation which provides the possibility of stimulating the greater, lesser and potentially third occipital nerves, some favor a vertical lead trajectory which allows for stimulation along the peripheral branches of the occipital nerve. Another variation in technique employs subcutaneous placement of paddle-type leads, with the electrode contacts oriented down towards the fascia, which provide unidirectional stimulation and greater current densities.

Mechanism of Action

There are two prevailing theories with respect to the potential mechanism of action of peripheral nerve stimulation in the relief of migraine headache pain. The first of these invokes modulation of the same gait-control mechanism implicated in the mechanism of action of spinal cord or peripheral nerve stimulation for somatic neuropathic pain [23]. The second suggests that retrograde activation of the C2 and C3 nerve roots, resulting from occipital nerve stimulation, modulates the brainstem nuclei involved in the trigeminal-vascular system thus inhibiting or aborting migraine headaches. The group of Goadsby and Weiner [13] evaluated 8 patients with chronic migraine treated with bilateral suboccipital stimulation using positron emission tomography (PET). Patients underwent PET imaging during three phases: (1) with their stimulators at optimum pain relief settings with the patients experiencing stimulation-induced paresthesias, (2) with the stimulator off and the patient experiencing pain without stimulation induced paresthesias, and (3) with the stimulator partially active with intermediate levels of pain and paresthesia. Significant blood flow changes were seen in the dorsal rostral pons, anterior cingulate cortex and cuneate nucleus; this pattern suggested stimulation induced modification of the brainstem trigeminal vascular system implicated in migraine headaches. Interestingly, the areas of activity during stimulation were, in fact, similar to the pattern seen in episodic migraine.

Independent Clinical Trials

In a study of 13 occipital neuralgia patients implanted with percutaneous occipital leads followed for 18 months to 6 years, 12 patients continued to report good to excellent response and required minimal oral analgesic medications [12]. Upon independent evaluation of the clinical vignettes of these patients, it was suggested that these patients rather suffered from migraine headaches. In a subsequent report of 25 patients with occipital neuralgia treated with occipital percutaneous neurostimulation leads, with an average follow-up of 18 months, 88% showed a positive response, with an overall 50% reduction in headache days [14]. Slavin et al. [19] reported 10 patients with occipital neuralgia treated with percutaneous occipital stimulation; 70% reported good pain control at 22 months, with between 60 and 90% pain relief; patients also decreased their use of analgesics and continued employment.

Oh et al. [15] reported 20 patients suffering from transformed migraine headaches treated with occipital paddle type neurostimulation leads. All patients had greater than 75% pain relief at 1 month. 80% reported greater than 75% pain relief at 6 months, and 95% reported both improvement in their quality of life and their willingness to undergo the procedure again.

Eight patients with drug-resistant chronic cluster headaches were treated with suboccipital neurostimulation on the side of the headache and reported by Magis et al. [17]. At a mean follow-up of 15 months, 2 patients were pain free, 3 had 90% reduction in headaches, and 2 patients had 40% improvement. In another study, 10 of 14 patients with intractable chronic cluster headache treated with bilateral occipital nerve stimulation reported significant improvement [16].

Industry-Sponsored Clinical Trials

As of 2010, neurostimulation for the treatment of migraine headache is not approved by the Food and Drug Administration. As such, it is used by physicians on an 'off label' basis. While this is both reasonable and appropriate, industry is not allowed to market or promote the use of their products for 'off-label' indications. In light of this limitation, and the significant potential of neuromodulation for the treatment of migraine headache, all three of the major equipment manufacturers in this sector (Medtronic, Minneapolis, Minn., St. Jude Medical, Plano, Tex., and Boston Scientific, Valencia, Calif., USA) have sponsored research trials to investigate the safety and efficacy of their neurostimulation products for the treatment of migraine headaches. Thus far, these corporate sponsored trials have been the largest and best designed studies of neuromodulation for headache.

Medtronic

The Occipital Nerve Stimulation for the Treatment of Intractable Migraine (ONSTIM) trial, sponsored by Medtronic, was a preliminary study to determine whether a well designed placebo controlled trial could provide insights into the potential risks and benefits of occipital nerve stimulation in patients with migraine headache. These insights could then be used for the design of a phase III pivotal trial which, if it met its primary endpoint(s), might lead to FDA approval of this therapy. This trial collected electronic diary data from patients enrolled at 9 centers over 3 months who reported 15 or more headaches per month and were not responsive to conventional medical therapies. Patients were randomized into three groups: in one group, patients received a neurostimulator and had the ability to control the level of stimulation, in the second group, patients received a neurostimulator as part of a device control group, and the third group received standard medical management. A positive response was defined as at least 50% reduction in the number of headache days per month, and/or a 3 or more point reduction in pain intensity on a 0- to 10-point pain scale. The ONSTIM trial further collected three years of safety data on enrolled patients.

The results of this multicenter, randomized, blinded controlled feasibility trial were recently published [24]. Of note is that all subjects eligible for the trial received an occipital nerve block and randomization required a positive response to the nerve block. Seventy-five of 110 enrolled subjects were assigned to a treatment group and complete data were available for 66 of these patients. Three-month responder rates were 39% for the group receiving active occipital nerve stimulation, 6% for the surgical control group, and 0% for the group receiving medical management only. There were no adverse device events reported while lead migration occurred in 12 of 51 (24%) of subjects.

St. Jude Medical

St. Jude Medical Neuromodulation has sponsored an Investigation Device Exemption pivotal trial to evaluate occipital nerve stimulation in chronic migraine patients. 150 patients were randomized from 15 centers, with success defined as a 50% reduction in pain and no increase in headache frequency or duration. Other headache measures included the Migraine Disability Assessment (MIDAS) questionnaire, Headache Index, Pain and Distress Score and patient satisfaction. Patients were randomized in a 2:1 ratio to either a stimulation trial followed by device implantation and active stimulation for 12 weeks or a stimulation trial followed by device implantation but sham stimulation for 12 weeks. After 12 weeks, subjects were unblinded but continued to be followed for 1 year. Data collection from this study has been completed and we await publication of the data.

Boston Scientific

Boston Scientific performed a prospective, randomized, double-blind, placebo-controlled trial of occipital nerve stimulation for drug refractory migraine named the PRISM (Precision Implantable Stimulator for Migraine) trial. The results of the PRISM study were presented at the 14th Congress of the International Headache Society and the 51st Annual Scientific Meeting of the American Headache Society in September, 2009 [25]. 132 patients who met the 2004 International Classification of Headache Disorders (ICHD-2) criteria for migraine were enrolled. All patients had failed therapy with a least two acute and two preventive medications, and all had 6 days or more per month of migraine headaches lasting 4 or more hours with moderate to severe pain. Prior to permanent implant, all subjects underwent percutaneous trial stimulation.

During the 12-week blinded period, patients were randomized in a 1:1 ratio to receive bilateral active stimulation or sham stimulation. At 12 weeks, all patients were converted to active stimulation. The primary endpoint of the study, change from baseline in migraine days per month, was evaluated at 12 weeks 125 subjects; there was no significant difference between groups (–5.5 vs. -3.9 days/month; $p = 0.29$). In patients who responded positively to a percutaneous trial, however, stimulation reduced migraine days per month by 8.8 days, as compared with 0.7 days in those whose trial failed to provide relief ($p < 0.001$). Two-year follow-up data showed that the most frequent adverse events were device infection, non-target area sensory phenomena and pain at the implant site.

The Northwestern Experience

Having a similar experience to that reported in the ONSTIM trial, with only about 40% of migraine headache patients having a significant response to occipital nerve stimulation, we began several years ago to look for possible explanations and alternative solutions. In our experience, patients whose pain was located within the sensory distribution of the occipital nerve(s), or those who identified that their headache pain originated from the occipital nerve(s) tended to respond overwhelmingly to occipital nerve stimulation. Those patients whose migraine pain fell outside these areas, however, tended to respond poorly. We thus began to question the hypothesis that occipital nerve stimulation was helping migraine headache pain by retrograde modulation of the trigeminal vascular system. We proposed that neurostimulation for migraine headache pain acted in a manner similar to that of peripheral nerve stimulation for somatic pain; that is, through a 'pain gate control' mechanism [23] where the degree of pain relief correlates directly with the degree of overlap of the pain with stimulation induced paresthesias [26].

To further investigate this proposal, we began to carefully map out the topography of patient's usual migraine headache pain. We then identified those specific cranial and peripheral nerves whose sensory distribution covered these areas of pain and proposed cranial peripheral nerve stimulation of any and all of those involved nerves. These nerves have included the greater and lesser occipital nerves as well as the supraorbital, auriculotemporal, infraorbital, supratrochlear and infratrochlear nerves. We then embarked on a trial of cranial peripheral nerve stimulation in patients who had failed aggressive medical therapy including comprehensive pharmacologic trials, selective nerve root blocks, and psychological therapies.

In a prospective, nonrandomized group of 50 patients, 45 of whom were diagnosed with chronic daily headache or chronic migraine, data collected by non-interested third parties revealed that 83% of patients reported a good to excellent relief at two year follow-up with an additional 9% reporting satisfactory pain relief of 30% or more. All 92% of these patients indicated their retrospective willingness to have the device implanted based upon their 2-year experience and their unwillingness to have the devices removed [unpubl. data]. This approach is not without its complications. While infection and lead erosion are uncommon problems, lead migration or fracture occurred in up to 66% of patients [unpubl. data]. Fewer lead revisions have been seen in patients after adopting more aggressive fixation techniques and with the use of larger percutaneous leads, but this remains a problem that suggests the need for hardware specifically designed for this application.

Conclusion

Cranial peripheral nerve stimulation, whether of the occipital nerve(s) alone or in combination with others, appears to be both safe and efficacious for the treatment of medically intractable migraine headache. Significant further investigation needs to be performed to optimize our knowledge concerning patient selection, stimulation targets and parameters and device programming and further improve clinical results. At present, neurostimulation for migraine headache pain is performed in the United States on an 'off-label' basis, but based upon our experience and the increasing evidence in the medical literature, we look forward to its approval by the FDA in the near future so that patients suffering from severe, medically intractable headache pain may gain access to these potentially important therapies.

References

1 Silberstein SD, Lipton RB, Goadsby PJ: Headache in Clinical Practice, ed 2. London, Martin Dunitz, 2002.

2 Weiner RL, Aló KM. Occipital neurostimulation for treatment of intractable headache syndromes; in Krames E, Peckham PH, Rezai AR (eds): Neuromodulation. London, Elsevier, 2009, vol 2, pp 409–416.

3 Newman LC, Lipton RB, Solomon S, Stewart WF: Daily headaches in a population sample: results from the American Migraine Study (abstract). Headache 1994;34:295, abstr 6.

4 Spierings EL, Schroevers M, Honkoop PC, Sorbi M: Presentation of chronic daily headache: a clinical study. Headache 1998;38:191–196.

5 Lipton RB, Humelsky S, Stewart W: Epidemiology and impact of headache; in Silberstein SD, Lipton RB, Nalessio D (eds): Wolff's Headache and Other Head Pain, ed 7. Oxford, Oxford University Press, 2001, pp 85–107.

6 Lozano AM, Vanderlinden G, Bachoo R, Rothbart P: Microsurgical C-2 ganglionectomy for chronic intractable occipital pain. J Neurosurg 1998;89: 359–365.

7 Pikus HJ, Phillips JM: Outcome of surgical decompression of the second cervical root for cervicogenic headache. Neurosurgery 1996;39:63–71.

8 Dubuisson D: Treatment of occipital neuralgia by partial posterior rhizotomy at C1–3. J Neurosurg 1995;82:581–586.

9 Bovim G, Fredriksen TA, Stolt-Nielsen A, Sjaastad O: Neurolysis of the greater occipital nerve in cervicogenic headache: a follow-up study. Headache 1992;32:175–179.

10 Picaza JA, Hunter SE, Cannon BW: Pain suppression by peripheral nerve stimulation: chronic effects of implanted devices. Appl Neurophysiol 1977–1978; 40:223–234.

11 Waisbrod H, Panhans C, Hansen D, Gerbeshagen HU: Direct nerve stimulation for painful peripheral neuropathies. J Bone Joint Surg (Br) 1985;67: 470–472.

12 Weiner RL, Reed KL: Peripheral neurostimulation for control of intractable occipital neuralgia. Neuromodulation 1999;2:217–221.

13 Matharu MS, Bartsch, Ward N, Frackowiak RSJ, Weiner R, Goadsby PJ: Central neuromodulation in chronic migraine patients with suboccipital stimulators: a PET study. Brain 2004;127:220–230.

14 Popeney CA, Aló KM: Peripheral neurostimulation for the treatment of chronic, disabling transformed migraine. Headache 2003;43:369–375.

15 Oh MY, Ortega J, Bellotte JB, Whiting DM, Aló K: Peripheral nerve stimulation for the treatment of occipital neuralgia and transformed migraine using a C1–2–3 subcutaneous paddle style electrode: a technical report. Neuromodulation 2004;7:103–112.
16 Burns B, Watkins L, Goadsby PJ: Treatment of medically intractable cluster headache by occipital nerve stimulation: long-term follow-up of eight patients. Lancet 2007;369:1099–1106.
17 Magis D, Allena M, Bolla M, De Pasqua V, Remacle JM, Schoenen J: Occipital nerve stimulation for drug-resistant chronic cluster headache: a prospective pilot study. Lancet Neurol 2007;6:314–321.
18 Burns B, Watkins L, Goadsby PJ: Treatment of hemicrania continua by occipital nerve stimulation with a Bion device: long-term follow-up of a crossover study. Lancet Neurol 2008;7:1001–1012.
19 Slavin KV, Nersesyan H, Wess C: Peripheral neurostimulation for treatment of intractable occipital neuralgia. Neurosurgery 2006;58:112–119.
20 Weiner RL: The future of peripheral nerve stimulation. Neurol Res 2000;22:299–304.
21 Aló KM, Holsheimer J: New trends in neuromodulation for the management of neuropathic pain. Neurosurgery 2002;50:690–704.
22 Franzini A, Messina G, Leone M, Broggi G: Occipital nerve stimulation (ONS). Surgical technique and prevention of late electrode migration. Acta Neurochir (Wien) 2009;151:861–865.
23 Melzack RA, Wall PD: Pain mechanisms: a new theory. Science 1965;150:971–979.
24 Saper JR, Dodick DW, Silberstein SD, McCarville S, Sun M, Goadsby PJ: Occipital nerve stimulation for the treatment of intractable chronic migraine headache: ONSTIM feasibility study. Cephalalgia 2010 [Epub ahead of print].
25 Lipton RB, Goadsby PJ, Cady RK, Aurora SK, Grosberg BM, Freitag FG, Silberstein SD, Whiten DM, Jaax KN: PRISM Study: occipital nerve stimulation for treatment-refractory migraine. Headache 2010;50:515.
26 North RB, Nigrin DJ, Fowler KR, Szymanski RE, Piantadosi S: Automated 'pain drawing' analysis by computer-controlled, patient-interactive neurological stimulation system. Pain 1992;50:51–57.

Robert Levy, MD, PhD
Department of Neurological Surgery
Feinberg School of Medicine, Northwestern University
676 North St. Clair Street Suite 2210, Chicago, IL 60611 (USA)
E-Mail rml199@northwestern.edu

Slavin KV (ed): Peripheral Nerve Stimulation.
Prog Neurol Surg. Basel, Karger, 2011, vol 24, pp 118–125

Occipital Neuromodulation for Refractory Headache in the Chiari Malformation Population

Sudhakar Vadivelu · Paolo Bolognese · Thomas H. Milhorat · Alon Y. Mogilner

Harvey Cushing Institutes of Neuroscience and the Department of Neurosurgery, Hofstra-North Shore LIJ School of Medicine, Manhasset, N.Y., USA

Abstract

Chronic occipital and suboccipital headache is a common symptom in patients with Chiari I malformation (CMI). These headaches may persist despite appropriate surgical treatment of the underlying pathology via suboccipital decompression, duraplasty and related procedures. Occipital stimulation has been shown to be effective in the treatment of a variety of occipital headache/pain syndromes. We present our series of 18 patients with CMI and persistent occipital headaches who underwent occipital neurostimulator trials and, following successful trials, permanent stimulator placement. Seventy-two percent (13/18) of patients had a successful stimulator trial and proceeded to permanent implant. Of those implanted, 11/13 (85%) reported continued pain relief at a mean follow-up of 23 months. Device-related complications requiring additional surgeries occurred in 31% of patients. Occipital neuromodulation may provide significant long-term pain relief in selected CMI patients with persistent occipital pain. Larger and longer-term studies are needed to further define appropriate patient selection criteria as well as to refine the surgical technique to minimize device-related complications.

Chronic headache in the occipital and suboccipital region is one of the most common complaints in patients with Chiari I malformation (CMI). These headaches may persist despite appropriate surgical treatment of the underlying pathology via posterior fossa decompression, duraplasty, cranioplasty, and occipito-cervical fusion. Peripheral stimulation in the occipital region, known as occipital nerve stimulation (ONS), described in detail in other chapters in this publication, has been shown to be effective in the treatment of occipital pain syndromes of various etiologies. This chapter reviews our center's early experience with the use of neurostimulation in the CMI population.

Chiari Malformation: Etiology and Associated Symptomatology

In 1891, an anatomical depiction of cerebellar ectopia was noted by Hans Chiari with presumptive association to hydrocephalus and without elaboration on symptomatology [1]. Other first hypotheses during this time included that of Charles-Prosper Ollivier d'Angers who suggested embryological variations could represent an etiology for spinal cord level – cerebrospinal fluid (CSF) deformities such as syringomyelia and spina bifida [2]. Magnetic resonance imaging a century later led to improved diagnosis of this condition. Milhorat et al. [3] described the clinical findings in a large series of CMI patients, of which suboccipital headache was the most common symptom, as seen in 81% of patients. The patients describe the headache as 'a heavy, crushing, or pressure-like sensation at the back of the head that radiated to the vertex and behind the eyes and inferiorly to the neck and shoulders'. The pathogenesis of these occipital headaches remains unclear – overcrowding of the posterior fossa with [3–5] or without [5] prominent cerebellar ectopia may alter CSF dynamics and lead to accentuated headaches as a manifestation of pathologic increases in intracranial pressure. The commonly seen accentuation of these headaches with cough, Valsalva maneuver and other activities associated with increasing intracranial pressure would support that theory, although it should be noted that not all patients report worsening of their headaches with such maneuvers [5]. McGirt et al. [4] suggested that occipital headaches in the Chiari population are strongly associated with hindbrain CSF flow abnormalities, while frontal and generalized headaches are not.

Within the last decade, several reports have suggested a genetic association to connective tissue disorders supported by evidence of a possible hereditary component [6, 7]. In these cases, the radiographic findings associated with CMI, namely downward herniation of the cerebellar tonsils, may result not from a congenitally small posterior fossa but rather from a functional craniocervical settling secondary to these connective tissue disorders. Although surgical treatment of clinically significant CMI has traditionally involved decompression of the posterior fossa contents, in patients with craniocervical settling secondary to connective tissue disorders, a posterior fossa decompression may not only fail to improve the symptoms and even exacerbate craniocervical instability, and thus a stabilization procedure such as a craniocervical fusion may be indicated [7].

Despite appropriate surgical repair via decompression, duraplasty, cranioplasty, and, in select patients, occipital-cervical fusion, there remains a small subset of patients in whom occipital headaches may persist or even progress despite resolution of other CMI associated symptoms. It is thought that in some patients, post-surgical phenomena such as post-operative dural adhesions, as well as inadvertent damage to the greater or lesser occipital nerves, may also contribute to persistence of chronic headache. In this subset of patients, treatment of these symptoms remains challenging.

Neurostimulation

Slavin et al. [8] were the first to report the use of ONS in 3 patients with persistent chronic occipital headache following Chiari decompression who were from a subset of 14 patients with different pain etiologies undergoing ONS. Current indications for ONS include refractory occipital neuralgia, chronic migraine, as well as trigeminal autonomic cephalalgias such as cluster headache [9]. A single case report noted success of ONS in a case of refractory pain after occipital cervical fusion with dramatic reduction in VAS scores (9/10 to 1/10) at 1 year of follow-up [10].

Many believe that the success of occipital nerve stimulation can be explained via the gate control theory of Melzack and Wall [11], in which stimulation of large A-ß fibers inhibits nociceptive conduction in the smaller A∂ and C fibers at the level of the dorsal horn of the spinal cord. Functional imaging studies in patients successfully treated with ONS for chronic migraine have documented a central neuromodulatory effect in regions of the brainstem, thalamus and cortex [12]. Nonetheless, the mechanism of pain relief via occipital neuromodulation remains unclear.

Since 2006, collaboration between the Chiari Institute and the Center for Functional and Restorative Neurosurgery at our institution has resulted in a case series of CMI patients with persistent occipital headaches referred for ONS treatment.

Methods

Patient Selection

General referral criteria included patients with the clinical and radiographic diagnosis of CMI, persistent and disabling occipital headaches despite appropriate corrective surgery, and comprehensive multidisciplinary pain management. Patients were selected for an ONS trial if their primary pain was in the occipital/suboccipital region – those with the primary complaints of frontal, temporal, or vertex headache were not selected for ONS. It should be noted, however, that 12 of the 18 patients also reported significant secondary frontal headaches. Success of occipital nerve block was not a requirement for patient selection.

Surgical Technique

Percutaneous Trial

All patients underwent a percutaneous trial, lasting from 3 to 7 days, for assessment of successful pain relief. Patients with unilateral pain underwent a single percutaneous lead placement, while dual leads were used for cases of bilateral pain. The trials were performed under local anesthesia with intravenous sedation using a variety of agents including midazolam, diprivan, and dexmedetomidine hydrochloride. Prophylactic antibiotics were given at the start of the case and throughout the duration of the outpatient trial. In all our cases, we used a lateral-to-medial approach to cannulation and electrode placement [13]. Patients were positioned semilaterally or prone, depending on the nature of the pain (unilateral or bilateral) and the presence of an occipital-cervical fusion, in which case the prone position was used for a bilateral placement. Because a portion of our CMI cohort had undergone a posterior fossa decompression, cranioplasty, occipital cervical fusion, and/or ventriculoperitoneal shunt, great care was taken to keep the needles and implants away from the hardware.

The initial needle insertion was done once the local landmarks were identified. After sterile prepping, draping, and infiltration of the needle entry point with local anesthetic, the spinal needle was slightly bent and then used to cannulate the subcutaneous layer of the scalp. Fluoroscopy was used continuously to control advancement of our cannula and lead position in respect to the odontoid process and the arch of C1. Eight contact leads manufactured by Medtronic, Boston Scientific, or St. Jude Neuromodulation were used. The lead was inserted through the needle and then the needle was partially withdrawn for the testing. When lead placement was deemed satisfactory, the needle and guidewire were removed, and 3–0 nylon suture in a purse-string fashion was placed around the externalized electrode to secure it in place. The leads were connected to an external programmer, and the stimulation settings were then optimized in the recovery room once all sedation had worn off.

Permanent Implant

Those patients who reported a minimum of 50% pain improvement using a visual analogue scale (VAS) during the trial period underwent permanent placement. After intubation and receiving general anesthesia, patients were placed either in the supine position with the head rotated away from the side of interest, or in the lateral or prone position, depending on the location of generator placement. Most patients returned for the permanent implant with their trial leads in place. An initial X-ray was taken to identify the placement of the trial implant just prior to removal. Once the trial leads were removed, the operative site was prepped and draped. For bilateral placement, a 5-mm midline incision was made down to the subcutaneous layer, and a lead was placed through the needle from the midline incision towards the contralateral mastoid process. A 4-cm retromastoid incision was then made vertically and dissection performed into a suprafascial plane. The spinal needle was then used to pass the initial lead to the retromastoid incision, and the second lead was then placed from lateral to medial, again under fluoroscopic guidance with the trial image used as comparison. The leads were then anchored to the retromastoid fascia with anchors provided by the equipment manufacturers. For generator placement in the chest region, a standard 4-cm infraclavicular incision was made, followed by a subcutaneous pocket. The leads were tunneled down subcutaneously to this infraclavicular region and plugged directly into the implantable pulse generator. For an abdominal or buttock placement, depending on the size of the patient, extension leads were used when necessary. The generator at this point was checked for impedance and programmed. All incisions were irrigated, closed primarily, and covered with sterile dressings.

Results

The charts of all patients undergoing an occipital nerve stimulator trial with the diagnosis of Chiari malformation were reviewed. Eighteen patients, 16 female, 2 male, average age 34 years (range 16–54 years), underwent percutaneous occipital nerve stimulator trials (table 1). The pain was bilateral in all but 2 patients, and all but 2 patients had undergone prior posterior fossa decompression. During the trial period, a pain reduction greater than 50% by visual analogue scale (VAS) was noted in 13 of 18 patients (72%) who proceeded to permanent implant. Of the 13 patients implanted, 2 patients

Table 1. Demographics, history and outcomes of 18 patients with the diagnosis of CMI who underwent occipital nerve stimulator trials at our institution

Patient no.	Age/gender	Previous medical history	Occipital pain location	Trial result	Last follow-up	Duration of follow-up months
1	30/F	CM, EDS	bilateral	success	continued pain relief	51
2	43/M	CM, EDS, hydrocephalus	bilateral	success	continued pain relief	50
3	42/M	CM, posterior fossa arachnoid cyst	bilateral	success	system explanted due to lack of efficacy	N/A
4	36/F	CM, EDS, FM	right	success	system explanted due to lack of efficacy	N/A
5	54/F	CM, FM, RLS	right	success	expired from unrelated cause	N/A
6	18/F	CM, EDS	bilateral	failure	no implant	N/A
7	40/F	CM	bilateral		single lead migration, not revised	12
8	16/F	CM	bilateral	failure	no implant	N/A
9	39/M	CM, hydrocephalus	bilateral	failure	no implant	N/A
10	42/F	CM, EDS	bilateral	success	continued pain relief	26
11	32/F	CM, syringomyelia	bilateral	success	continued pain relief	26
12	38/F	CM	bilateral	success	continued pain relief	14
13	47/F	CM	bilateral	success	continued pain relief	16
14	39/F	CM	bilateral	success	continued pain relief	12
15	22/F	CM	bilateral	success	continued pain relief	11
16	33/F	CM	bilateral	success	continued pain relief	12
17	24/F	CM	bilateral	failure	no implant	N/A
18	17/F	CM, EDS	bilateral	failure	no implant	N/A

CM = Chiari malformation; EDS = Ehler-Danlos syndrome; FM = fibromyalgia; RLS = restless leg syndrome.

Table 2. Surgical complications

Patient no.	Complication
1, 12	lead migration
1	infection at generator site
5	lead tip erosion
10	discomfort at the generator site requiring revision

reported loss of efficacy of the device, without any evidence of lead migration or device malfunction, at 6 and 7 months following implantation, and the devices were explanted as per patient requests. Of the remaining 11 patients implanted, one expired of an unrelated medical condition 1 year after permanent implant. The remaining 10 continue to report >50% relief at latest follow-up (mean 23 months, range 11–51 months).

Complications

The surgical complications in our case series were similar in nature and in frequency to those reported in the literature for occipital nerve stimulation. There were no complications from the trial procedures. Complications requiring one or more surgical revision occurred in 4 of the 13 patients implanted (31%) (table 2). Lead migration, a frequent event in the ONS literature, occurred in 2 of the 13 patients implanted. At the time of revision in one of those patients, a defect was found in the lead anchor (Titan, Medtronic) involving the inner metal tubing slipping out from the silastic outer covering of the anchor. This was later confirmed by the manufacturer to be a defect in the anchor itself, which was then recalled from clinical use and subsequently re-released in a modified version. Use of the modified anchor has not been associated with any subsequent lead migrations in this case series or in other cases of peripheral stimulation or epidural spinal cord stimulation performed at this center.

Unique to our patient population is the high percentage of patients with prior surgeries in the occipital region, including craniectomies, cranioplasties, and occipital-cervical fusion with hardware. Initial experience with standard horizontal placement of the electrodes (parallel to the arch of C1) resulted in lead tip erosion in one patient, where the tip was superficial to the occipital fusion plate. Given that event, subsequent leads were never placed over the fusion hardware but rather more lateral and, in one patient with laterally placed plates, we placed the lead in a vertical rather than a horizontal fashion (fig. 1).

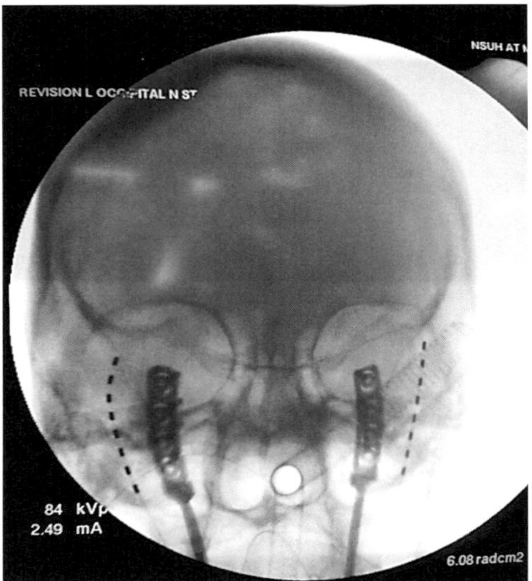

Fig. 1. Vertically placed occipital nerve stimulation leads in a patient with an occipital cervical fusion.

In one patient, an infection occurred at the site of the implantable pulse generator, necessitating removal and re-implantation 3 months later.

Discussion

Given the success of ONS in treating a variety of clinical syndromes that present with occipital and suboccipital headache, it is reasonable to apply this technique to the CMI population in which such headaches are a frequent complaint. This patient population is entirely a postsurgical one, in that all of these patients have had one or more surgeries aimed at treating the underlying malformation but yet remain disabled by severe headache.

The presence of prior surgery in all of these patients posed a number of technical problems not usually present in other ONS populations. Multiple prior incisions and the presence of hardware including fusion constructs and shunt tubing required greater attention to placement of the incisions, lead tips, extension leads, and generators. Nonetheless, given that ONS is a low-risk entirely subcutaneous procedure, there was no permanent morbidity in any patient from these procedures.

Whereas we attempted to select patients in whom occipital headaches were the primary symptom, the frequent co-existence of constant headaches in the frontal region suggests that some of failures in this series may be due to suboptimal pain relief in the regions not covered by ONS. Indeed, 1 patient in this series (patient 17) who failed the occipital stimulator trial ultimately underwent a bilateral supraorbital stimulator trial and subsequent permanent device implantation with good results at 2 years of follow-up.

Conclusion

Occipital nerve stimulation appears to be successful in treating a subset of patients with Chiari I malformation with refractory occipital headaches. The unique characteristics of these patients, many of whom have undergone multiple surgical procedures, have necessitated occasional modifications to the surgical technique to minimize device-related complications, which remain frequent but not serious.

References

1 Chiari H: Über Veränderungen des Kleinhirns infolge Hydrocephalie des Grosshirns. Dtsch Med Wochenschr 1891;17:1172–1175.
2 Koehler PJ: Chiari's description of cerebellar ectopy (1891): with a summary of Cleland's and Arnold's contributions and some early observations on neural-tube defects. J Neurosurg 1991;75:823–826.
3 Milhorat TH, Chou MW, Trinidad EM, Kula RW, Mandell M, Wolpert C, Speer MC: Chiari I malformation redefined: clinical and radiographic findings for 364 symptomatic patients. Neurosurgery 1999;44:1005–1017.
4 McGirt MJ, Nimjee SM, Floyd J, Bulsara KR, George TM: Correlation of cerebrospinal fluid flow dynamics and headache in Chiari I malformation. Neurosurgery 2005;56:716–721.
5 Sansur CA, Heiss JD, DeVroom HL, Eskioglu E, Ennis R, Oldfield EH: Pathophysiology of headache associated with cough in patients with Chiari I malformation. J Neurosurg 2003;98:453–458.
6 Boyles AL, Enterline DS, Hammock PH, et al: Phenotypic definition of Chiari type I malformation coupled with high-density SNP genome screen shows significant evidence for linkage to regions on chromosomes 9 and 15. Am J Med Genet A 2006;140:2776–2785.
7 Milhorat TH, Bolognese PA, Nishikawa M, McDonnell NB, Francomano CA: Syndrome of occipitoatlantoaxial hypermobility, cranial settling, and Chiari malformation type I in patients with hereditary disorders of connective tissue. J Neurosurg Spine 2007;7:601–609.
8 Slavin KV, Nersesyan H, Wess C: Peripheral neurostimulation for treatment of intractable occipital neuralgia. Neurosurgery 2006;58:112–119.
9 Goadsby PJ: Neuromodulatory approaches to the treatment of trigeminal autonomic cephalalgias. Acta Neurochir Suppl 2007;97:99–110.
10 Ghaemi K, Capelle HH, Kinfe TM, Krauss JK: Occipital nerve stimulation for refractory occipital pain after occipitocervical fusion: expanding indications. Stereotact Funct Neurosurg 2008;86:391–393.
11 Melzack R, Wall PD: Pain mechanisms: a new theory. Science 1965;150:971–979.
12 Matharu MS, Bartsch T, Ward N, Frackowiak RS, Weiner R, Goadsby PJ: Central neuromodulation in chronic migraine patients with suboccipital stimulators: a PET study. Brain 2004;127:220–230.
13 Trentman TL, Slavin KV, Freeman JA, Zimmerman RS: Occipital nerve stimulator placement via a retromastoid to infraclavicular approach: a technical report. Stereotact Funct Neurosurg 2010;88:121–125.

Alon Y. Mogilner, MD, PhD
Section of Functional and Restorative Neurosurgery
Department of Neurosurgery
North Shore – LIJ Health System, 865 Northern Boulevard, Great Neck, NY 11021 (USA)
Tel. +1 516 570 4430, Fax +1 516 570 4460, E-Mail Amogilner@nshs.edu

Slavin KV (ed): Peripheral Nerve Stimulation.
Prog Neurol Surg. Basel, Karger, 2011, vol 24, pp 126–132

Peripheral Nerve Stimulation in Chronic Cluster Headache

Delphine Magis · Jean Schoenen

Headache Research Unit, University Department of Neurology, CHR Citadelle, Liège, Belgium

Abstract

Cluster headache is well known as one of the most painful primary neurovascular headache. Since 1% of chronic cluster headache patients become refractory to all existing pharmacological treatments, various invasive and sometimes mutilating procedures have been tempted in the last decades. Recently, neurostimulation methods have raised new hope for drug-resistant chronic cluster headache patients. The main focus of this chapter is on stimulation of the great occipital nerve, which has been the best evaluated peripheral nerve stimulation technique in drug-resistant chronic cluster headache, providing the most convincing results so far. Other peripheral nerve stimulation approaches used for this indication are also reviewed in detail. Although available studies are limited to a relatively small number of patients and placebo-controlled trials are lacking, existent clinical data suggest that occipital nerve stimulation should nonetheless be recommended for intractable chronic cluster headache patients before more invasive deep brain stimulation surgery. More studies are needed to evaluate the usefulness of supraorbital nerve stimulation and of vagus nerve stimulation in management of cluster headaches.

Cluster headache is well known as one of the most painful primary neurovascular headaches. Episodic cluster headache, as defined by the 2nd Edition of the International Classification of Headache Disorders (ICHD-II 3.1.1) [1], is characterized by attacks of unilateral periorbital pain associated with ipsilateral autonomic signs (ptosis, miosis, conjunctival injection, tearing, rhinorrhea, nasal congestion) occurring in bouts (clusters) of weeks or months, separated by headache-free intervals of variable length (months or years). Chronic cluster headache (CCH, ICHD-II 3.1.2) is a disabling condition affecting 10% of cluster headache patients [2]. Patients are considered as 'chronic' when attacks occur during at least 1 year without remissions or with remissions lasting less than 1 month [1]. Beside acute therapies – sumatriptan injection, oxygen inhalation or zolmitriptan nasal spray in decreasing order of efficacy –, CCH sufferers most often require one or more preventive drugs to be relieved, the most effective being steroids (oral or as suboccipital infiltrations), verapamil, lithium carbonate and methysergide.

Unfortunately, about 1% of CCH patients become refractory to all existing pharmacological treatments. Criteria defining drug-resistant chronic cluster headache (drCCH) were proposed recently [3]. Intractable CCH is a dreadful condition which ruins the patients' social, family and professional life, and may push some of them to commit suicide as the ultimate pain-relieving solution. Hence, various invasive and sometimes mutilating procedures have been attempted in the last decades, targeting the trigeminal or cranial parasympathetic pathways, among them radiofrequency lesions, glycerol injections or balloon compressions of the Gasserian ganglion, stereotactic radiosurgery or root section of the trigeminal nerve, trigeminal tractotomy, lesions of the nervus intermedius or greater superficial petrosal nerve, blockade or radiofrequency lesions of the pterygopalatine ganglion, and microvascular decompression of the trigeminal nerve combined with nervus intermedius section [4]. None of these sometimes mutilating procedures gave long-term satisfactory results.

More recently, neurostimulation methods have raised new hope for drCCH patients. The most convincing studies performed up to now concerned hypothalamic deep brain stimulation (DBS). Its effect can be spectacular (62.5% pain-free rate in Leone et al.'s series [5], 50% in Schoenen et al.'s [6]) and rapid in onset. Minor and manageable adverse effects are due to the stimulation of the hypothalamus and neighboring areas (oculomotor disturbances, dizziness, panic attacks) or to the local tissue irritation at the site of stimulator implantation. Unfortunately, as with the implantation of stimulation electrodes in other sites, hemorrhage may occur. DBS-induced hemorrhage may be minor and asymptomatic, but it was massive and fatal in 1 CCH patient [6]: less-risky, efficient procedures were therefore warranted. Hence, peripheral nerve stimulation (PNS) was considered to help these patients.

We will mainly focus our chapter on stimulation of the great occipital nerve, which has been the best evaluated PNS technique in drCCH, providing the most convincing results so far.

Occipital Nerve Stimulation

Rationale

Peripheral neurostimulation is a non-destructive and minimal invasive way to control drug-resistant pain. Experimental studies have demonstrated that trigeminal and cervical afferents converge on second-order nociceptors in the spinal trigeminal nucleus [7]. Suboccipital injections of steroids and/or local anesthetics in the region of the greater occipital nerve have shown efficacy in cluster headache [8]. Finally, there were anecdotal reports of clinical benefit with occipital nerve stimulation (ONS) in various types of intractable headache including some cluster patients [9]. In line with these observations, ONS studies were undertaken in drCCH patients.

Available Efficacy Studies
Two open-label trials [10–12] and 9 case reports [13–15] with encouraging results have been published up to now (February 2010). Burns et al. [11, 12] implanted 14 drCCH patients. Efficacy on attack frequency and intensity was assessed according to an estimate of percentage change and subjective satisfaction made by the patients. The first patient was implanted unilaterally and improved, after which the attacks shifted side; hence, all subsequent patients were implanted bilaterally. After a mean follow-up of 17 months, 3 patients described a marked improvement ≥ 90%, 3 a moderate improvement of 40–60%, and 4 a mild improvement of 20–30%.

We performed the other large study [10] and published on 8 drCCH patients followed prospectively at baseline and after implantation using headache diaries. We found a mean 79.9% reduction of attack frequency and 50% of intensity; 2 patients became pain-free, and 3 had an improvement around 90%. Since publication, we have a useful follow-up for another patient and a maximal follow-up of 32 months. The therapeutic score is slightly lower with a mean attack frequency reduction of 54% and intensity decrease of 47%. Our patients were implanted unilaterally on the cluster side and only a transient side shift of attacks occurred in 2 patients. All of our patients were treated with several preventive medications at high doses before ONS. After ONS, all of them were able to reduce preventive medication, but not to interrupt it completely.

We have presently included 15 drCCH patients with a mean follow-up around 29 months [16]. Unfortunately, 1 patient had an immediate postoperative infection of the material which had to be removed. Nine of the 14 remaining patients are totally pain-free (64%), 2 patients have an improvement in frequency exceeding 90%, and 1 patient a 89% amelioration. Two patients are not responding or describe mild improvement, though the latter is rather satisfied by ONS. Intensity of residual attacks is not improved by ONS. Four patients (29%) were able to reduce their prophylaxis. Subjectively, 9 patients are very satisfied by ONS and 1 patient is moderately satisfied.

Finally, a few ONS-treated drCCH patients were also reported by Schwedt et al. [13]. In 1 patient there was a 70% of attack frequency and intensity, with persisting autonomic attacks, in 3 others a 33% improvement in headache days and 20% had improvement in intensity. Trentman et al. [15] reported 6 cases of cluster headache patients treated with ONS using a completely different device, among them 3 showed an excellent response.

Adverse Events
Only mild and reversible side effects are reported with ONS.

Batteries run flat rather rapidly because of the high stimulation intensities compared to deep brain stimulation (range 2.4–10 V in our study). In our recent follow-up of up to 5 years, battery depletion is found in 8/14 patients, i.e. 57%. However, recurrent battery replacement (up to 2 per year in 1 patient) can now be avoided by the availability of rechargeable systems.

The other major adverse event is local infection of the device. In our group of 15 patients, 1 had an acute postoperative infection whereas 2 other patients developed delayed infectious signs after 21 and 38 months, respectively. The origin of this late appearing infection is unknown; it could be due to cutaneous erosion (mainly in thin subjects) or hematogenous contamination.

Local discomfort, such as neck stiffness, pain at the myofascial incision or the stimulator sites, was a common adverse effect. ONS-induced paresthesias in the territory of the greater occipital nerve (GON) are felt by all patients and may vary in intensity with head and neck position. They are used to assess lead positioning preoperatively if local anesthesia is used [11], and to select or adjust the stimulation parameters. Their disappearance is often the first sign of a flat battery. In our study, 2 patients found the stimulation-induced paresthesias unbearable and decided to switch their stimulators off after 4 months [10]; however, 1 of them was objectively improved by ONS. If general anesthesia is required for technical reasons, or for the patient's comfort, the surgeon has to rely on anatomical landmarks [10]. Hence, close contact of the lead with the GON may be lacking, which probably explains why high stimulation intensities are needed in several patients.

In our experience, ONS is also associated with clinical peculiarities like side shift and isolated autonomic paroxysms in around 50% of responders. However, we confirm our first observation that contralateral attacks in implanted drCCH patients remain infrequent (a few per year on average) and do not appear to bother patients at all. Our interpretation for the occurrence of autonomic paroxysms without pain is that ONS does not act on the pathology's generator but is only a symptomatic treatment (see below).

Similar to hypothalamic DBS, there are no known prognostic factors for ONS efficacy. In particular, the response to GON blocks with steroids and local anesthetics does not seem to be predictive of the therapeutic effect of ONS [10, 13]. There is at present no placebo-controlled trial of ONS because blinding of the patients is difficult to achieve due to the paresthesias. An alternative might be to use low-voltage stimulations barely producing paraesthesias as a control. However, the lowest effective stimulation intensity able to produce an effect of ONS has not been determined yet. It is, nonetheless, unlikely that the clinical improvements of drCCH found with ONS are due to a placebo effect or to the natural evolution of the disease, since in most patients responding to the neurostimulation severe attacks resumed rapidly after cessation of the stimulation due to an empty battery [10].

Mode of Action

The neurobiological mechanisms by which ONS can improve drCCH remain to be elucidated. We found no change in pain thresholds after ONS [10], which argues against a direct nonspecific analgesic effect. As mentioned above, one rationale for ONS in headaches was the experimental evidence of convergence of cervical and trigeminal nociceptive afferents on second-order nociceptors in the trigeminal nucleus caudalis

[7]. The nociception-specific blink reflex, mediated by a polysynaptic network in the medulla, increased with duration of ONS in our study [10] which could be due to sensitization in the trigeminal nucleus caudalis and is probably not related to the clinical effect of ONS. A more likely explanation for the therapeutic effect of ONS in drCCH is the induction of slow neuromodulatory changes in centers belonging to the pain matrix or playing a pathogenic role in the disorder. For instance, in a functional imaging study of ONS in chronic migraine, activity of an area in the dorsal rostral pons, known to be activated during migraine attacks, was modulated proportionally to the pain, whereas activity in the left pulvinar was correlated with ONS-induced paresthesias [9]. Such slow plastic changes might explain why the therapeutic effect after ONS takes some time to appear.

Interestingly, the preliminary results of a study in which we explored cerebral metabolism with 18-fluoro-deoxyglucose PET scanning in 10 drCCH patients before and after implantation [17], show a metabolic normalization in various regions of the so-called pain neuromatrix after several months of ONS, and a lack of short-term changes induced by the stimulation, supporting the hypothesis that ONS acts through slow neuromodulatory processes. Moreover, ONS responders exhibit a selective activation of perigenual cingular cortex, a pivotal structure in the endogenous opioid system, suggesting that ONS may restore balance within dysfunctioning pain-control centers. That ONS is nothing but a symptomatic treatment is illustrated by the persistent hypothalamic hypermetabolism which could explain why autonomic attacks may persist despite pain relief and why cluster attacks recur shortly after stimulator arrest after several months of ONS [17].

Other Neurostimulation Methods

Supraorbital Nerve Stimulation

Narouze and Kapural [18] published the case of a drCCH patient successfully treated with supraorbital nerve stimulation (SNS). After a convincing 7-day trial with a percutaneous quadripolar electrode, the subject received a permanent implant of the lead and attacks fully disappeared after 2 months of continuous stimulation. The patient was still pain free 12 months later and was able to stop all preventive treatment. Switching off the stimulator led to attack recurrence within 24 h. SNS was also useful for aborting attacks. As for ONS, one hypothesis to explain the effect of SNS is the induction of slow neuromodulatory processes at the level of the spinal trigeminal nucleus [18].

Vagus Nerve Stimulation

Lastly, neurostimulation of the vagus nerve (VNS) with a device similar to the one used to treat refractory epileptic patients may be an interesting option in drCCH. A few case reports presented at meetings suggest that in epileptics who are also migraineurs,

VNS may markedly improve both the epilepsy and the migraine. Mauskop [19] reported modest improvement in 2 drCCH patients with VNS. In the first patient who also had major depression, VNS reduced cluster headache attack frequency but he remained depressive and in need of various antidepressant drugs. The second subject had a significant decrease in MIDAS score after VNS, but was dependent on fentanyl patches, with a poor general functional level due to comorbidity with anxiety, fatigue, low back pain and depression. The time to obtain an effect in patient 1 was 2 months and neck pain was the only reported side effect. More recently, Franzini et al. [20] reported the case of a drCCH patient successfully treated with hypothalamic DBS, in whom a head trauma provoked attack worsening. They then performed VNS in this patient, which together with DBS reduced his attack frequency by 50% [20].

Conclusions

Peripheral neurostimulation offers new hope for patients suffering from drug-resistant chronic cluster headache. Available studies are limited to a relatively small number of patients and placebo-controlled trials are lacking.

ONS offers the advantage to be a riskless and efficient procedure. Hence, two recent trials of a total of 29 patients show that ONS is an effective treatment for drCCH: 90% or more improvement in 14 patients, among them 9 are pain-free. These long-term results are similar to those of the more invasive hypothalamic DBS. Only minor local adverse effects are reported. However, preliminary physiopathological studies and clinical observations suggest that ONS does not act on the disease generator but is just a symptomatic treatment. At present, ONS should nonetheless be recommended for intractable CCH patients before hypothalamic DBS.

More studies are needed to evaluate the usefulness of SNS and VNS in the management of cluster headaches.

References

1 The International Classification of Headache Disorders, ed 2. Cephalalgia 2004;24(suppl 1):9–160.

2 Sjaastad O, Bakketeig LS: Cluster headache prevalence: VAGA study of headache epidemiology. Cephalalgia 2003;23:528–533.

3 Goadsby PJ, Schoenen J, Ferrari MD, Silberstein SD, Dodick D: Towards a definition of intractable headache for use in clinical practice and trials. Cephalalgia 2006;26:1168–1170.

4 Matharu MS, Boes CJ, Goadsby PJ: Management of trigeminal autonomic cephalgias and hemicrania continua. Drugs 2003;63:1637–1677.

5 Leone M, Franzini A, Broggi G, Bussone G: Hypothalamic stimulation for intractable cluster headache: long-term experience. Neurology 2006;67: 150–152.

6 Schoenen J, Di Clemente L, et al: Hypothalamic stimulation in chronic cluster headache: a pilot study of efficacy and mode of action. Brain 2005;128: 940–947.

7 Bartsch T, Goadsby PJ: Increased responses in trigeminocervical nociceptive neurons to cervical input after stimulation of the dura mater. Brain 2003;126: 1801–1813.

8 Ambrosini A, Vandenheede M, Rossi P, et al: Suboccipital injection with a mixture of rapid- and long-acting steroids in cluster headache: a double-blind placebo-controlled study. Pain 2005;118: 92–96.
9 Matharu MS, Bartsch T, Ward N, Frackowiak RS, Weiner R, Goadsby PJ: Central neuromodulation in chronic migraine patients with suboccipital stimulators: a PET study. Brain 2004;127:220–230.
10 Magis D, Allena M, Bolla M, De Pasqua V, Remacle JM, Schoenen J: Occipital nerve stimulation for drug-resistant chronic cluster headache: a prospective pilot study. Lancet Neurol 2007;6:314–321.
11 Burns B, Watkins L, Goadsby PJ: Treatment of medically intractable cluster headache by occipital nerve stimulation: long-term follow-up of eight patients. Lancet 2007;369:1099–1106.
12 Burns B, Watkins L, Goadsby PJ: Treatment of intractable chronic cluster headache by occipital nerve stimulation in 14 patients. Neurology 2009;72: 341–345.
13 Schwedt TJ, Dodick DW, Trentman TL, Zimmerman RS: Occipital nerve stimulation for chronic cluster headache and hemicrania continua: pain relief and persistence of autonomic features. Cephalalgia 2006; 26:1025–1027.
14 Schwedt TJ, Dodick DW, Hentz J, Trentman TL, Zimmerman RS: Occipital nerve stimulation for chronic headache–long-term safety and efficacy. Cephalalgia 2007;27:153–157.
15 Trentman TL, Rosenfeld DM, Vargas BB, Schwedt TJ, Zimmerman RS, Dodick DW: Greater occipital nerve stimulation via the Bion microstimulator: implantation technique and stimulation parameters. Clinical trial: NCT00205894. Pain Physician 2009; 12:621–628.
16 Magis D, Gerardy PY, Remacle JM, Schoenen J: Sustained efficacy of occipital nerve stimulation in drug-resistant chronic cluster headache after up to 5 years treatment. J Headache Pain 2010;11(suppl 1): 15(abstr).
17 Magis D, Bruno MA, Gerardy PY, Fumal A, Hustinx R, Laureys S, Schoenen J: Central neuromodulation in cluster headache patients treated with occipital nerve stimulators: a PET study. Acta Neurol Belgica 2010;110(suppl 1):7(abstr).
18 Narouze SN, Kapural L: Supraorbital nerve electric stimulation for the treatment of intractable chronic cluster headache: a case report. Headache 2007;47: 1100–1102.
19 Mauskop A: Vagus nerve stimulation relieves chronic refractory migraine and cluster headaches. Cephalalgia 2005;25:82–86.
20 Franzini A, Messina G, Leone M, Cecchini AP, Broggi G, Bussone G: Feasibility of simultaneous vagal nerve and deep brain stimulation in chronic cluster headache: case report and considerations. Neurol Sci 2009;30(suppl 1):S137–S139.

Prof. Jean Schoenen
Headache Research Unit, Department of Neurology
Liège University, CHR Citadelle
Boulevard du 12eme de Ligne, 1, BE-4000 Liège (Belgium)
Tel. +32 4223 8663, Fax +32 4225 6451, E-Mail jschoenen@ulg.ac.be

Slavin KV (ed): Peripheral Nerve Stimulation.
Prog Neurol Surg. Basel, Karger, 2011, vol 24, pp 133–146

Peripheral Nerve Stimulation for Fibromyalgia

Mark Plazier[a–c] · Sven Vanneste[a,b] · Ingrid Dekelver[d] · Mark Thimineur[e] · Dirk De Ridder[a–c]

[a]Brai[2]n, [b]TRI and Departments of [c]Neurosurgery and [d]Physical Therapy and Revalidation, University Hospital Antwerp, Antwerp, Belgium; [e]Interventional Pain Medicine, Derby, Conn., USA

Abstract

Fibromyalgia is a condition marked by widespread chronic pain, accompanied by a variety of other symptoms, including sleep and fatigue disorders, headaches, disorders of the autonomic nervous system, as well as cognitive and psychiatric symptoms. It occurs predominantly in women and is often associated with other systemic or autoimmune diseases. Despite its serious socioeconomical burden, the treatment options remain poor. In this chapter, the authors discuss the possibilities of using greater occipital nerve stimulation as a treatment for fibromyalgia, based on available clinical studies. Greater occipital nerve stimulation has already been used successfully to treat occipital neuralgia and various primary headache syndromes. Testable hypothetical working mechanisms are proposed to explain the surprising effect of this treatment on widespread bodily pain.

Introduction

Fibromyalgia

Fibromyalgia is a disease characterized by widespread musculoskeletal pain. It is lacking a clear pathophysiology and doesn't influence specific laboratory tests nor causes specific abnormalities on physical examination. Hence, the diagnosis of fibromyalgia remains a pure clinical diagnosis. The American College of Rheumatology (ACR) proposed diagnostic criteria in 1990. These criteria include a history of widespread pain, lasting for more than three months, affecting all quadrants of the body. Furthermore, 18 tender points were defined which elicit a painful sensation by applying a force of 4 kg. These points include myofascial structures at the occipital area, the neck area, chest area, back area, the elbows and knees. Eleven of these 18 trigger points should elicit pain in order to consider the diagnosis of fibromyalgia [1].

Besides pain, fibromyalgia is accompanied by a variety of other symptoms which is why it is called a syndrome. The most common of these associated symptoms are headaches, sleeping disorders, fatigue, irritable bowel syndrome and cognitive dysfunction [2, 3]. Other symptoms include nocturnal jaw tightness, morning stiffness, paresthesias of arms and legs, urinary urgency, esophageal dysmotility, dryness of mouth and eyes, allergic complaints, and cold and swollen hands [4–6]. Psychiatric disorders are frequently encountered in fibromyalgia patients as well, such as depression and anxiety disorders [7].

Fibromyalgia not only frequently mimics other diseases but also is often associated with them. These include lupus erythematosus (20%), Sjögren syndrome (20%), rheumatoid arthritis (30%), inflammatory bowel disease (7–49%), hepatitis C (9%), HIV (12%), Lyme (8%), and diabetes mellitus (11%). This complicates its diagnosis.

The prevalence of fibromyalgia is as high as 2.9–4% in a general population and it mainly affects women in a 9:1 ratio. The mean age of onset is between 20 and 55 years [6, 8].

Because of this high prevalence and the multisymptomatic characteristics health care utilization in fibromyalgia patients is extensive, resulting in a high socioeconomic burden. Fibromyalgia has a large financial impact on both direct medical costs consisting of treatment costs and patient care and indirect costs due to work loss. Several estimations of these costs have been published. Berger et al. [9] estimate the mean total healthcare costs in a study sample of 33,176 patients at USD 9,573 per patient over 12 months in the United States. Boonen et al. [10] report an average annual disease-related cost per patient of EUR 7,813 in a Dutch population.

The pathophysiology of fibromyalgia is poorly understood. Several theories have been proposed in order to explain this condition. Amongst them sleep disturbances, a general hyperactivity of the nociceptive system, sympathetic hyperreacitivity and hormonal disturbances have been proposed [11–14]. More and more evidence points to an abnormal function of the central nervous system. Patients are characterized by a more pronounced sensation of mechanical and heat pain and this form of hyperalgesia is caused by a supraspinal central nervous system etiology [15, 16]. Furthermore, various functional brain-imaging studies have shown cortical and subcortical augmentation of pain processing and an increased sympathetic and decreased parasympathetic tone [13, 16–19].

The treatment of fibromyalgia is mainly symptomatically and comprises combinations of pharmaceutical, psychological and physical approaches [20, 21]. Besides pain medication, antidepressant medication has been proven to be effective in fibromyalgia as well as medication used in the treatment of neuropathic pain such as gabapentin and pregabalin [22–26]. The US Food and Drug Administration has approved the use of pregabalin for the treatment of fibromyalgia.

Combining pharmaceutical treatment with psychological therapy, such as cognitive behavioral therapy, and physical treatment, such as aerobic exercise, seems to be the most effective. The American Pain Society published guidelines for the management of fibromyalgia patients in 2005 [27]. The European League Against Rheumatism (EULAR) formulated recommendations and evidence-based guidelines for its treatment as well [28]. Still, the search for new and more effective treatment possibilities continues. One of these new treatment possibilities consists of peripheral nerve stimulation of the greater occipital nerve by implantation of an occipital nerve stimulator [29; (Plazier, unpubl. data)].

Greater Occipital Nerve Stimulation

The greater occipital nerve is a branch of the dorsal ramus of the 2nd cervical nerve. This particular nerve provides sensory innervation to the occipital scalp, together with the lesser occipital nerve. Anastomoses between the first, second, third and fourth cervical nerves form the upper cervical plexus.

Stimulation of this nerve has been shown to be effective in the treatment of occipital neuralgia and primary headache syndromes. Picaza et al. [30] performed the first surgical stimulation of this nerve for the treatment of occipital neuralgia in 1977. A variety of primary headache syndromes tend to respond to occipital nerve stimulation [31, 32] as well, raising the question how this form of peripheral nerve stimulation exerts its effects.

The greater occipital nerve has connections with the trigeminal nerve at the level of the cervico-trigeminal complex located at the dorsal horn of the cervical spinal cord. Le Doaré et al. [33] revealed this connection in a rat model by measuring the FOS expression at the dorsal horn and the nucleus caudalis after infiltrating the cervical musculature with a nociceptive agent. This connection has been shown in cats and humans as well [34, 35].

Results in headache treatment are promising with success rates between 70 and 100% [36] (table 1).

However, none of these studies have been performed in a placebo-controlled way due to the fact that paresthesias are felt at higher stimulation amplitudes. In a study published by Thimineur and De Ridder [29], in which greater occipital nerve stimulation was applied in fibromyalgia patients suffering from migraine, the results revealed not only an improvement in headache-associated pain, but in widespread bodily pain as well.

Greater Occipital Nerve Stimulation in Fibromyalgia

Thimineur and De Ridder [29] implanted 12 patients with an occipital nerve stimulator for chronic daily headache, all of whom also fulfilled the criteria for fibromyalgia. Two Quatrode® (St. Jude Medical Neuromodulation, Plano, Tex., USA) leads were placed bilaterally, subcutaneously at the occipital scalp, approximately 2 cm above the inion at an imaginary line drawn between the top of the ears. In this group of patients the severity of headache-associated pain, diffuse bodily pain and associated symptoms such as sleep disturbance, fatigue and depression were monitored. The patients were stimulated with a rechargeable internal pulse generator (IPG) at

Table 1. Occipital nerve stimulation for headache syndromes

Study	Indication	Responders	Effect
Melvin et al. (2007)	occipital headache (n = 11)	11/11	67%
Popeney et al. (2003)	migraine (n = 25)	20/25	88.7% improvement MIDAS
Oh et al. (2004)	occipital neuralgia (n = 20)	18/20	90%
Weiner et al. (1999)	occipital neuralgia (n = 13)	13/13	100% good to perfect
Matharu et al. (2004)	migraine (n = 8)	8/8	100% good to perfect
Kapural et al. (2005)	cervicogenic headache (n = 6)	6/6	70%
Rodrigo-Royo et al. (2005)	occipital neuralgia (n = 4)	4/4	100%
Slavin et al. (2006)	occipital neuralgia (n = 10)	10/10	> 50%
Magis et al. (2007)	cluster headache (n = 8)	7/8	50%
Schwedt et al. (2007)	cluster headache (n = 3), hemicrania (n = 6), migraine (n = 8), post-trauma (n = 2)	15/19	52%
Burns et al. (2007)	cluster headache (n = 8)	6/8	64%
Picaza et al. (1977)	occipitale neuralgia (n = 6)	3/6	100% good to perfect
Schwedt et al. (2006)	hemicrania continua (n = 2)	1/2	70%
Ghaemi et al. (2008)	postcervical fusion pain (n = 1)	1/1	90%
Amin et al. (2008)	supraorbital neuralgia (n = 10)	10/10	77%
Burns et al. (2009)	cluster headache (n = 14)	10/14	52%

6, 12, 18, 24 and 30 Hz, with a pulse width of 50 µs and amplitudes between 5 and 25.5 mA.

Apart from a significant improvement in headache-associated pain, the scores for bodily pain (VAS), depression (BDI), fatigue (FIS) and quality-of-life (SF-36) also improved in a significant way. A reduction of fibromyalgia-related widespread bodily pain of approximately 60% was obtained. Although these results are exciting,

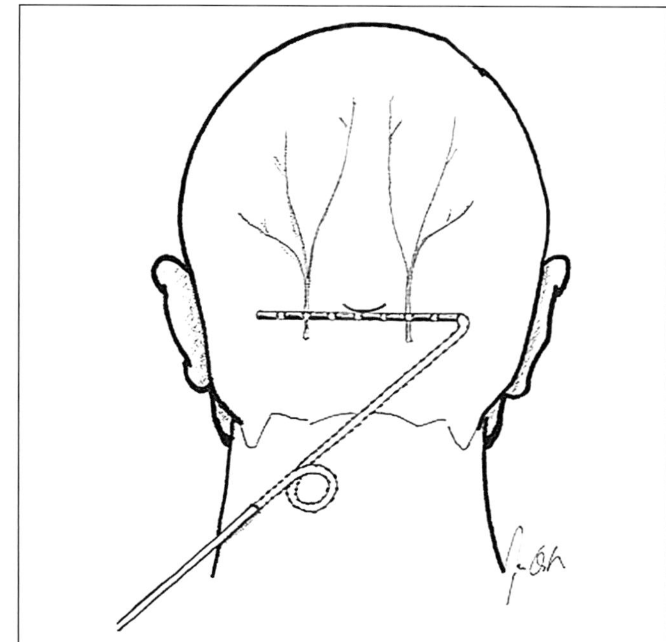

Fig. 1. Schematic drawing of an implanted occipital nerve trial lead. The lead is placed just below the inion at the origins of the branches of the greater occipital nerve. Notice the sharp angle of the lead to prevent migration.

one must keep in mind that this study lacked placebo control. The placebo response encountered in most available pain treatments may get as high as 35% [37]. Except for the lack of placebo control, one might suggest that the improvement in headache-related pain might have influenced the other scores as well.

These results motivated the authors to perform a second study in which the effects of greater occipital nerve stimulation on fibromyalgia related symptoms were evaluated in a placebo controlled way [Plazier et al., unpubl. data].

Eleven patients were included in the study protocol, all suffering from fibromyalgia and diagnosed in accordance with the ACR-90 criteria [1]. The patients were implanted with an Octrode® (St. Jude Medical Neuromodulation) lead, which was inserted transversely crossing the midline of the occipital scalp, just below the inion (fig. 1).

Implantation was followed by a trial period, consisting of 10 weeks, and subsequently by an open-labeled follow-up period of 6 months after permanent implantation.

During the trial and the follow-up period after permanent implantation, various scales for pain (VAS, Pain Catastrophizing Scale, Pain Vigilance and Awareness Questionnaire), mood (Beck Depression Inventory II), fatigue (modified Fatigue Impact Scale) as well as the fibromyalgia impact scale and the amount of positive trigger points were monitored.

The patients were stimulated at individually selected frequencies (6, 10, 12, 18 and 40 Hz), based on optimal pain suppression. Stimulation was performed with a pulse width of 300 μs at alternating positive and negative poles by a rechargeable internal pulse generator.

For 10 weeks, the 11 implanted patients were stimulated in a placebo-controlled cross-over design. This design existed of two arms: (1) sham stimulation (stimulation at the absolute minimal amplitude of the stimulation device, which is considered as noneffective stimulation, and so as sham stimulation), and (2) stimulation at subsensory threshold levels, which prevented the sensation of paresthesias at the occipital scalp area. Both arms of this study were using parameters below the sensory threshold. This resulted in a placebo-controlled study, whereas the effective (2) and noneffective (1) arms were intractable for the patients. Afterwards, all 11 patients got the opportunity to get implanted with a permanent IPG. Two patients were not satisfied with their response to stimulation and so eventually 9 patients were implanted with an IPG.

During the trial period, a significant decrease in fibromyalgia-related pain (approximately 40%) and pain catastrophizing scores were noted. However, mood and fatigue scores were not influenced in a significant way by applying occipital nerve stimulation.

After the trial period the results remained stable for a period of 6 months with a decrease in pain of approximately 45% as well as a significant decrease in the amount of positive trigger points and the overall score on the fibromyalgia Impact Questionnaire.

These results confirm the previously obtained results by Thimineur and De Ridder [29] in a placebo-controlled manner, and suggest that occipital nerve stimulation could become part of the treatment modality for fibromyalgia-related pain. However, how this kind of stimulation works is entirely unknown.

It is proposed that the central nervous system plays a critical role in the pathophysiology of fibromyalgia. Neuroendocrine, autonomic nervous system and neuroimmunological factors might also be involved in the widespread bodily pain [13, 17, 18, 38]. Thus, it is expected that stimulation of the greater occipital nerves modulates these systems in one or another way.

The greater occipital nerve afferents enter the C2 segment of the spinal cord at the level of the nucleus caudalis of the trigeminal nerve forming the trigeminocervical complex. The nucleus caudalis projects to the thalamus, which relays sensory input to the cortex [33, 34, 39, 40]. Furthermore, animal studies have shown connections between neurons of the C2 spinal cord and the hypothalamus [41], the thalamus [42, 43], the periaqueductal grey (PAG) [42], the caudate nuclei [44], the amygdala and orbitofrontal cortex [43] as well as the cerebellum [45]. Thus, the C2 spinal cord is connected to many other brain structures directly.

Greater Occipital Nerve Stimulation and the Brain

A few studies have been performed analyzing the influence of greater occipital nerve stimulation on the brain function. Matharu's group performed PET scans in 8 patients implanted with a greater occipital nerve stimulator for chronic migraine.

These scans were performed in three different states: (1) stimulator at optimal settings (pain-free, experiencing paresthesia), (2) stimulator off (experiencing pain), and (3) stimulator partially activated (intermediate pain and paresthesia). This study revealed significant changes in the regional cerebral blood flow in the dorsal rostral pons, anterior cingulate cortex (ACC) and the cuneus, correlated to pain scores. Changes in the ACC and the left pulvinar correlated to paresthesia scores [46]. As these structures are well known to be involved in the brain pain matrix [47], these data might suggest that stimulation of the greater occipital nerve results in a modulation of brain activity in pain related cortical and subcortical structures. This might be a direct or indirect effect; however, these changes in cerebral blood flow might be solely related to the changes in pain sensation and paresthesias and not the direct product of the stimulation. In order to provide an answer to these questions, the effects of greater occipital nerve stimulation in healthy subjects might be useful.

The authors performed a functional MRI on a healthy subject, one of the co-authors (D.D.R.), implanted with an occipital nerve stimulator. Analysis of the data revealed significant increases in BOLD signal in the thalami, hypothalami, orbitofrontal cortex, premotor cortex, peri-aqueductal gray matter, inferior parietal cortex and cerebellum. During stimulation, deactivation could be found in primary areas like the primary motor (M1), visual (V1) and somatosensory areas (S1) as well as in the secondary somatosensory area (S2) and the amygala [Kovacs et al., in press]. The results of Matharu's study showed a correlation between paresthesias and changes in blood flow in the ACC and left pulvinar. This might suggest that the sensation of paresthesias might be, at least partially, responsible for the changes in brain activity. However, in the fMRI study we performed stimulation at both supra-sensory threshold levels (inducing paresthesias at the occipital scalp) and at the sub-sensory threshold level. Both conditions resulted in altered BOLD signals, which might suggest that occipital nerve stimulation alters brain activity as a direct result of the stimulation. Hence, this study suggests that greater occipital nerve stimulation exerts its effect at the level of the central nervous system (fig. 2).

Results from an EEG source localization study (LORETA) [48] support these findings in fibromyalgia patients implanted with an occipital nerve stimulator [Plazier et al., unpubl. data]. EEG data were acquired in 9 patients in two conditions: (1) during stimulation (pain suppression), and (2) without stimulation (no pain suppression). Making use of the LORETA-Key software package [48], which permits solving the inverse problem and to localizing EEG activity to cortical structures, statistical analysis revealed differences in brain activity in several pain-matrix-related structures, amongst them the cingulate cortex (fig. 3).

Both fMRI and EEG data suggest that one of the mechanisms involved in fibromyalgia-related bodily pain suppression is based on changes of activity in the central nervous system. Four different hypothetical pathophysiological mechanisms can be proposed on how occipital nerve stimulation might exert its effect in fibromyalgia.

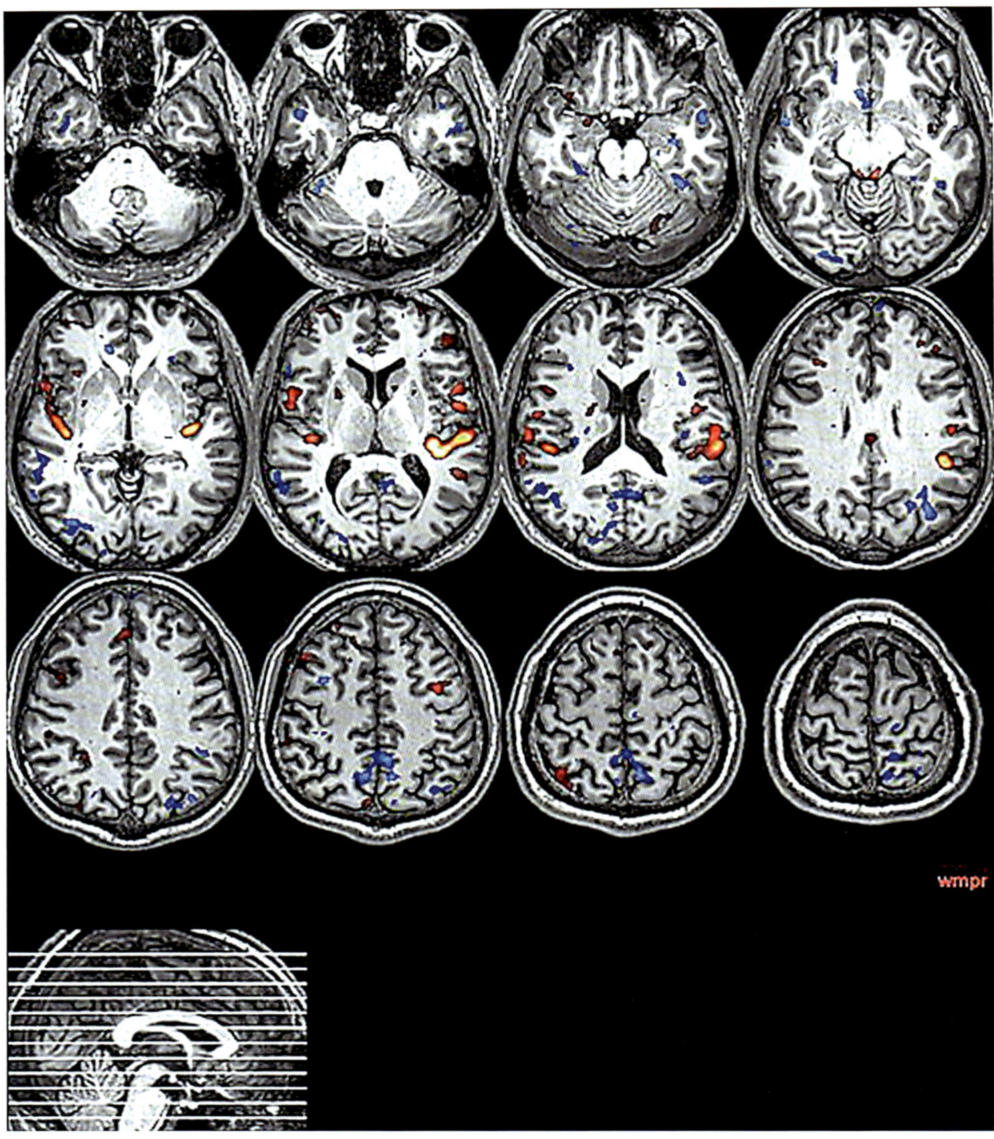

Fig. 2. Global BOLD activation and deactivation for occipital nerve stimulation for all stimulation frequencies combined (image by Silvia Kovacs and Stefan Sunaert, KU Leuven, Belgium).

Hypotheses Concerning the Working Mechanism of Occipital Nerve Stimulation in Fibromyalgia

Just as the general pathophysiology of fibromyalgia remains unknown, the mechanism by which greater occipital nerve stimulation exerts its effect is still unclear, one can only state possible hypotheses about why greater occipital nerve stimulation is

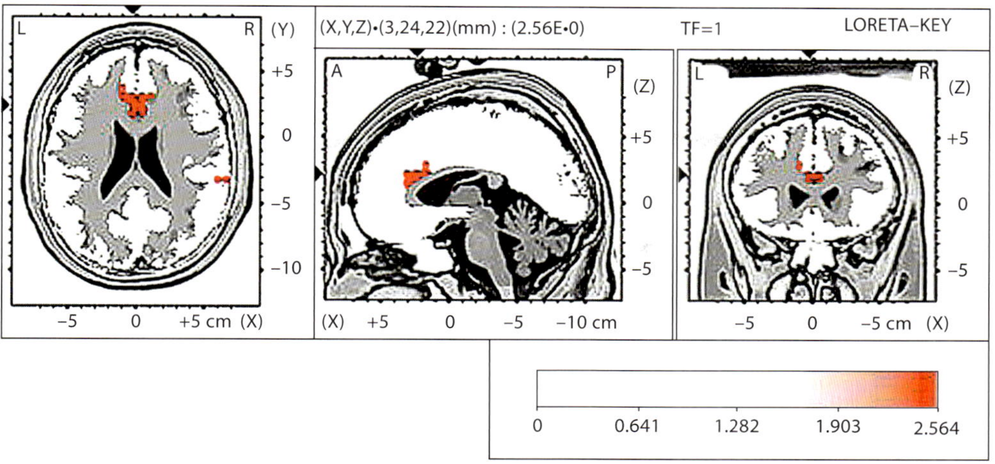

Fig. 3. LORETA source localization of high-frequency EEG activity (24–28 Hz) at the cingulate cortex during occipital nerve stimulation compared to no stimulation. All voxels presented are significant at the $p < 0.05$ interval.

beneficial in the treatment of fibromyalgia. Several possible explanations can be proposed based on the data presented here.

1 Direct modulation of spinothalamic pathways at the level of C2 in the spinal cord can suppress bodily pain.
2 C2 stimulation can modulate autonomic nervous system involvement in fibromyalgia.
3 C2 modulation acts indirectly via the mesolimbic dopaminergic system as suggested by the first fMRI study performed during C2 stimulation.
4 A combination of the three above-mentioned mechanisms.

(1) Direct Modulation of Spinothalamic Pathways at the Level of C2 in the Spinal Cord Can Suppress Bodily Pain [29]

The stimulation may exert influence on the lateral spinothalamic pathways, as the largest population of cells of origin of the spinothalamic pathways (35%) are found at the level of C2-C3 (in the Old World monkey) [49]. Interrupting the C1-C2 anterolateral spinothalamic tract of the spinal cord is a well-known neurosurgical technique, causing contralateral loss of pain sensation below the level of the lesion [50, 51]. Evidence, using spinal cord and thalamic stimulation, has been presented that C1-C2 spinal neurons (in the primate) mediate an inhibitory effect of viscerosomatic input on spinothalamic neurons [52]. This suggests not only lesioning but also electrical stimulation might exert a suppressing effect on the spinothalamic input below the level of electrical input. The generalized pain suppressive effect of the C2 stimulation might mediate its effect via modulation of the lateral spinothalamic cell bodies and nerve fibers of C2.

In Kovacs study [unpubl. data], the primary sensory cortices, inclusive of the somatosensory cortex are deactivated during C2 stimulation, suggesting that pain perception might be decreased, as the primary somatosensory cortex shows a general increase of activity in neural pain syndromes [53, 54].

(2) C2 Stimulation Can Modulate Autonomic Nervous System Involvement in Fibromyalgia
A considerable amount of publications demonstrate involvement of the autonomic nervous system in the pathophysiology of fibromyalgia [5, 18, 55], many based on Heart Rate Variability measurements. A general increase in sympathetic tone [5, 13, 56–58] and potential decrease in parasympathetic tone [57–59] have been proposed. The structures of the brain which regulate the autonomic nervous system consist of structures such as the autonomic centers at the brainstem (sympathetic locus coeruleus, and parasympathetic nucleus tractus solitarius), the subgenual and dorsal part of the anterior cingulate, the insulae, amydala and hypothalamus. Most of these structures are connected monosynaptically to the neurons at the C2 spinal cord [41]. Furthermore, some neurons in the C2 spinal cord respond to sympathetic [60] or parasympathetic [61] stimulation or to both sympathetic and parasympathetic stimulation [60, 62]. And many of these structures are involved in the sensation of pain as well [63, 64]. According to the imaging studies described above, the activity in these structures can be altered by greater occipital nerve stimulation, which provides a theoretical basis to hypothesize that greater occipital nerve stimulation might influence the sympathetic and parasympathetic tone. A simple way to prove or disprove this hypothesis is to perform HRV studies in implanted patients.

(3) C2 Modulation Acts Indirectly Via the Mesolimbic Dopaminergic System
Because dopamine is implicated in both pain modulation and affective processing, it can be hypothesized that fibromyalgia may involve a disturbance of dopaminergic neurotransmission [65]. It has been shown that healthy subjects release dopamine in basal ganglia during painful stimulation, whereas fibromyalgia patients do not. In healthy subjects, the amount of dopamine release correlates with the amount of perceived pain, but in fibromyalgia patients it does not [65]. This has been confirmed by a PET study demonstrating that fibromyalgia might be characterized by a disruption of dopaminergic neurotransmission [66]. Voxel-based morphometry has shown that dopamine metabolism changes might contribute to the associated changes in gray matter density. Fibromyalgia is characterized by gray matter changes bilaterally in the parahippocampal gyri, in the right posterior cingulate cortex, and left anterior cingulate cortex [67]. As our EEG study shows changes in the anterior cingulate, it is possible that occipital nerve stimulation interferes with dopaminergic modulation of this area, which is implicated in the pathophysiology of fibromyalgia. The reward system uses both dopamine and opioid receptors, with dopamine related more to motivational aspects and opioids more to pleasure related aspects [68–70]. In fibromyalgia

both systems seem to dysfunction, as altered endogenous opioid analgesic activity has been demonstrated in the nucleus accumbens, the dorsal ACC and the amygdala [71]. This could explain why opioids often are less beneficial in fibromyalgia patients than in controls. Hypothetically occipital nerve stimulation can interfere with the opioid system via the direct connections between the C2 spinal cord and the amygdala or the indirect modulation of the ACC.

(4) A Combination of the Three Above-Mentioned Mechanisms
Future studies will have to elucidate whether 1, 2 or all 3 of the proposed mechanisms are involved in the improvement of fibromyalgia using occipital nerve stimulation.

Conclusion

Fibromyalgia has a serious impact on society because of its high prevalence and the high direct and indirect medical costs. Since there is no generally accepted pathophysiology of this condition, treatment options remain limited.

Peripheral nerve stimulation, by means of greater occipital nerve stimulation, seems to be a promising addition in the treatment of fibromyalgia and besides the therapeutic value, it is an interesting tool to provide information about the pathophysiology of fibromyalgia.

The mechanism of action of greater occipital nerve stimulation is not completely clear and its effectiveness in syndromes as fibromyalgia might suggest that is has direct and indirect effects on cerebral structures via neurons at the level of the C2 spinal cord. This raises some hypotheses about the possible working mechanism of occipital nerve stimulation in fibromyalgia. It is clear that further research is needed and that it should focus on differences in brain activity, which can be demonstrated by functional imaging studies.

References

1 Wolfe F, Smythe HA, Yunus MB, et al: The American College of Rheumatology 1990 criteria for the classification of fibromyalgia: report of the multicenter criteria committee. Arthritis Rheum 1990;33: 160–172.

2 Theadom A, Cropley M: Dysfunctional beliefs, stress and sleep disturbance in fibromyalgia. Sleep Med 2008;9:376–381.

3 Bennett RM, Jones J, Turk DC, Russell IJ, Matallana L: An internet survey of 2,596 people with fibromyalgia. BMC Musculoskelet Disord 2007;8:27.

4 Clauw DJ: Fibromyalgia: more than just a musculoskeletal disease. Am Fam Physician 1995;52:843–851, 853–854.

5 Vaerøy H, Qiao ZG, Mørkrid L, Førre O: Altered sympathetic nervous system response in patients with fibromyalgia (fibrositis syndrome). J Rheumatol 1989;16:1460–1465.

6 Wolfe F, Ross K, Anderson J, Russell IJ, Hebert L: The prevalence and characteristics of fibromyalgia in the general population. Arthritis Rheum 1995;38: 19–28.

7 Arnold LM, Bradley LA, Clauw DJ, Glass JM, Goldenberg DL: Evaluating and diagnosing fibromyalgia and comorbid psychiatric disorders. J Clin Psychiatry 2008;69:e28.

8 Branco JC, Bannwarth B, Failde I, et al: Prevalence of fibromyalgia: a survey in five European countries. Semin Arthritis Rheum 2010;39:448–453.

9 Berger A, Dukes E, Martin S, Edelsberg J, Oster G: Characteristics and healthcare costs of patients with fibromyalgia syndrome. Int J Clin Pract 2007; 61:1498–1508.

10 Boonen A, van den Heuvel R, van Tubergen A, Goossens M, Severens JL, van der Heijde D, van der Linden S: Large differences in cost of illness and wellbeing between patients with fibromyalgia, chronic low back pain, or ankylosing spondylitis. Ann Rheum Dis 2005;64:396–402.

11 Moldofsky H: The significance of the sleeping-waking brain for the understanding of widespread musculoskeletal pain and fatigue in fibromyalgia syndrome and allied syndromes. Joint Bone Spine 2008;75:397–402.

12 Staud R: Evidence of involvement of central neural mechanisms in generating fibromyalgia pain. Curr Rheumatol Rep 2002;4:299–305.

13 Martinez-Lavin M: Fibromyalgia as a sympathetically maintained pain syndrome. Curr Pain Headache Rep 2004;8:385–389.

14 Neeck G, Riedel W: Hormonal pertubations in fibromyalgia syndrome. Ann NY Acad Sci 1999;876: 325–338; discussion 339.

15 Kosek E, Ekholm J, Hansson P: Sensory dysfunction in fibromyalgia patients with implications for pathogenic mechanisms. Pain 1996;68:375–383.

16 Gracely RH, Petzke F, Wolf JM, Clauw DJ: Functional magnetic resonance imaging evidence of augmented pain processing in fibromyalgia. Arthritis Rheum 2002;46:1333–1343.

17 Petzke F, Clauw DJ, Ambrose K, Khine A, Gracely RH: Increased pain sensitivity in fibromyalgia: effects of stimulus type and mode of presentation. Pain 2003;105:403–413.

18 Cohen H, Neumann L, Kotler M, Buskila D: Autonomic nervous system derangement in fibromyalgia syndrome and related disorders. Isr Med Assoc J 2001;3:755–760.

19 Kooh M, Martínez-Lavín M, Meza S, Martín-del-Campo A, Hermosillo AG, Pineda C, Nava A, Amigo MC, Drucker-Colín R: Simultaneous heart rate variability and polysomnographic analyses in fibromyalgia. Clin Exp Rheumatol 2003;21:529–530.

20 Scascighini L, Toma V, Dober-Spielmann S, Sprott H: Multidisciplinary treatment for chronic pain: a systematic review of interventions and outcomes. Rheumatology (Oxford) 2008;47:670–678.

21 Busch AJ, Schachter CL, Overend TJ, Peloso PM, Barber KA: Exercise for fibromyalgia: a systematic review. J Rheumatol 2008;35:1130–1144.

22 Dadabhoy D, Clauw DJ: Therapy Insight: fibromyalgia – a different type of pain needing a different type of treatment. Nat Clin Pract Rheumatol 2006;2: 364–372.

23 Häuser W, Bernardy K, Uçeyler N, Sommer C: Treatment of fibromyalgia syndrome with antidepressants: a meta-analysis. JAMA 2009;301:198–209.

24 Russell IJ, Mease PJ, Smith TR, Kajdasz DK, Wohlreich MM, Detke MJ, Walker DJ, Chappell AS, Arnold LM: Efficacy and safety of duloxetine for treatment of fibromyalgia in patients with or without major depressive disorder: results from a 6-month, randomized, double-blind, placebo-controlled, fixed-dose trial. Pain 2008;136:432–444.

25 Serra E: Duloxetine and pregabalin: safe and effective for the long-term treatment of fibromyalgia? Nat Clin Pract Neurol 2008;4:594–595.

26 Lyseng-Williamson KA, Siddiqui MA: Pregabalin: a review of its use in fibromyalgia. Drugs 2008;68: 2205–2223.

27 Goldenberg DL, Burckhardt C, Crofford L: Management of fibromyalgia syndrome. JAMA 2004;292:2388–2395.

28 Carville SF, Arendt-Nielsen S, Bliddal H, et al: EULAR evidence-based recommendations for the management of fibromyalgia syndrome. Ann Rheum Dis 2008;67:536–541.

29 Thimineur M, De Ridder D: C2 area neurostimulation: a surgical treatment for fibromyalgia. Pain Med 2007;8:639–646.

30 Picaza JA, Hunter SE, Cannon BW: Pain suppression by peripheral nerve stimulation: chronic effects of implanted devices. Appl Neurophysiol 1977;40: 223–234.

31 Vogel HB: Occipital nerve stimulation for chronic headache. Cephalalgia 2007;27:1288.

32 Weiner RL: Occipital neurostimulation for treatment of intractable headache syndromes. Acta Neurochir Suppl 2007;97:129–133.

33 Le Doaré K, Akerman S, Holland PR, Lasalandra MP, Bergerot A, Classey JD, Knight YE, Goadsby PJ: Occipital afferent activation of second order neurons in the trigeminocervical complex in rat. Neurosci Lett 2006;403:73–77.

34 Bartsch T, Goadsby PJ: Increased responses in trigeminocervical nociceptive neurons to cervical input after stimulation of the dura mater. Brain 2003;126:1801–1813.

35 Piovesan EJ, Di Stani F, Kowacs PA, Mulinari RA, Radunz VH, Utiumi M, Muranka EB, Giublin ML, Werneck LC: Massaging over the greater occipital nerve reduces the intensity of migraine attacks: evidence for inhibitory trigemino-cervical convergence mechanisms. Arq Neuropsiquiatr 2007;65: 599–604.

36 Jasper JF, Hayek SM: Implanted occipital nerve stimulators. Pain Physician 2008;11:187–200.
37 Hrobjartsson A, Gotzsche PC: Is the placebo powerless? An analysis of clinical trials comparing placebo with no treatment. N Engl J Med 2001;344: 1594–1602.
38 McLean SA, Williams DA, Stein PK, Harris RE, Lyden AK, Whalen G, Park KM, Liberzon I, Sen A, Gracely RH, Baraniuk JN, Clauw DJ: Cerebrospinal fluid corticotropin-releasing factor concentration is associated with pain but not fatigue symptoms in patients with fibromyalgia. Neuropsychopharmacology 2006;31:2776–2782.
39 Busch V, Frese A, Bartsch T: The trigemino-cervical complex: integration of peripheral and central pain mechanisms in primary headache syndromes. Schmerz 2004;18:404–410.
40 Bartsch T, Goadsby PJ: Stimulation of the greater occipital nerve induces increased central excitability of dural afferent input. Brain 2002;125:1496–1509.
41 Newman HM, Stevens RT, Apkarian AV: Direct spinal projections to limbic and striatal areas: anterograde transport studies from the upper cervical spinal cord and the cervical enlargement in squirrel monkey and rat. J Comp Neurol 1996;365:640–658.
42 Mouton LJ, Klop EM, Holstege G: C1-C3 spinal cord projections to periaqueductal gray and thalamus: a quantitative retrograde tracing study in cat. Brain Res 2005;1043:87–94.
43 Burstein R, Potrebic S: Retrograde labeling of neurons in the spinal cord that project directly to the amygdala or the orbital cortex in the rat. J Comp Neurol 1993;335:469–485.
44 Pfaller K, Arvidsson J: Central distribution of trigeminal and upper cervical primary afferents in the rat studied by anterograde transport of horseradish peroxidase conjugated to wheat germ agglutinin. J Comp Neurol 1988;268:91–108.
45 Matsushita M, Xiong G: Uncrossed and crossed projections from the upper cervical spinal cord to the cerebellar nuclei in the rat, studied by anterograde axonal tracing. J Comp Neurol 2001;432:101–118.
46 McLean SA, Williams DA, Stein PK, Harris RE, Lyden AK, Whalen G, Park KM, Liberzon I, Sen A, Gracely RH, Baraniuk JN, Clauw DJ: Central neuromodulation in chronic migraine patients with suboccipital stimulators: a PET study. Brain 2004;127: 220–230.
47 Moisset X, Bouhassira D: Brain imaging of neuropathic pain. Neuroimage 2007;37(suppl 1):S80–S88.
48 Pascual-Marqui RD, Michel CM, Lehmann D: Low resolution electromagnetic tomography: a new method for localizing electrical activity in the brain. Int J Psychophysiol 1994;18:49–65.
49 Apkarian AV, Hodge CJ: Primate spinothalamic pathways. I. A quantitative study of the cells of origin of the spinothalamic pathway. J Comp Neurol 1989;288:447–473.
50 Mullan S, Hekmatpanah J, Dobben G, Beckman F: Percutaneous, intramedullary cordotomy utilizing the unipolar anodal electrolytic lesion. J Neurosurg 1965;22:548–553.
51 Rosomoff HL, Brown CJ, Sheptak P: Percutaneous radiofrequency cervical cordotomy: technique. J Neurosurg 1965;23:639–644.
52 Hobbs SF, Oh UT, Chandler MJ, Fu QG, Bolser DC, Foreman RD: Evidence that C1 and C2 propriospinal neurons mediate the inhibitory effects of viscerosomatic spinal afferent input on primate spinothalamic tract neurons. J Neurophysiol 1992; 67:852–860.
53 May A: Neuroimaging: visualising the brain in pain. Neurol Sci 2007;28(suppl 2):S101–S107.
54 May A: A review of diagnostic and functional imaging in headache. J Headache Pain 2006;7:174–184.
55 Martinez-Lavin M, Hermosillo AG: Autonomic nervous system dysfunction may explain the multisystem features of fibromyalgia. Semin Arthritis Rheum 2000:29:197–199.
56 Ulas UH, Unlu E, Hamamcioglu K, Odabasi Z, Cakci A, Vural O: Dysautonomia in fibromyalgia syndrome: sympathetic skin responses and RR interval analysis. Rheumatol Int 2006;26:383–387.
57 Cohen H, Neumann L, Shore M, Amir M, Cassuto Y, Buskila D: Autonomic dysfunction in patients with fibromyalgia: application of power spectral analysis of heart rate variability. Semin Arthritis Rheum 2000;29:217–227.
58 Buskila D: Fibromyalgia, chronic fatigue syndrome, and myofascial pain syndrome. Curr Opin Rheumatol 2001;13:117–127.
59 Cohen H, Neumann L, Alhosshle A, Kotler M, Abu-Shakra M, Buskila D: Abnormal sympathovagal balance in men with fibromyalgia. J Rheumatol 2001; 28:581–589.
60 Chandler MJ, Zhang J, Foreman RD: Vagal, sympathetic and somatic sensory inputs to upper cervical (C1-C3) spinothalamic tract neurons in monkeys. J Neurophysiol 1996;76:2555–2567.
61 Chandler MJ, Hobbs SF, Bolser DC, Foreman RD: Effects of vagal afferent stimulation on cervical spinothalamic tract neurons in monkeys. Pain 1991; 44:81–87.
62 Chandler MJ, Qin C, Yuan Y, Foreman RD: Convergence of trigeminal input with visceral and phrenic inputs on primate C1-C2 spinothalamic tract neurons. Brain Res 1999;829:204–208.

63 Leone M, Proietti Cecchini A, Mea E, Tullo V, Curone M, Bussone G: Neuroimaging and pain: a window on the autonomic nervous system. Neurol Sci 2006;27(suppl 2):S134–S137.

64 Boly M, Balteau E, Schnakers C, Degueldre C, Moonen G, Luxen A, Phillips C, Peigneux P, Maquet P, Laureys S: Baseline brain activity fluctuations predict somatosensory perception in humans. Proc Natl Acad Sci USA 2007;104:12187–12192.

65 Wood PB, Schweinhardt P, Jaeger E, Dagher A, Hakyemez H, Rabiner EA, Bushnell MC, Chizh BA: Fibromyalgia patients show an abnormal dopamine response to pain. Eur J Neurosci 2007;25:3576–3582.

66 Wood PB, Patterson JC 2nd, Sunderland JJ, Tainter KH, Glabus MF, Lilien DL: Reduced presynaptic dopamine activity in fibromyalgia syndrome demonstrated with positron emission tomography: a pilot study. J Pain 2007;8:51–58.

67 Wood PB, Glabus MF, Simpson R, Patterson JC 2nd: Changes in gray matter density in fibromyalgia: correlation with dopamine metabolism. J Pain 2009;10:609–618.

68 Berridge KC: The debate over dopamine's role in reward: the case for incentive salience. Psychopharmacology (Berl) 2007;191:391–431.

69 Berridge KC, Kringelbach ML: Affective neuroscience of pleasure: reward in humans and animals. Psychopharmacology (Berl) 2008;199:457–480.

70 Smith KS, Berridge KC: Opioid limbic circuit for reward: interaction between hedonic hotspots of nucleus accumbens and ventral pallidum. J Neurosci 2007;27:1594–1605.

71 Harris RE, Clauw DJ, Scott DJ, McLean SA, Gracely RH, Zubieta JK: Decreased central mu-opioid receptor availability in fibromyalgia. J Neurosci 2007;27:10000–10006.

Dirk De Ridder, MD, PhD
Brai^{2}n, TRI and Department of Neurosurgery
University Hospital Antwerp, Antwerp University
Wilrijkstraat 10, 2650 Edegem (Belgium)
Tel. +32 3821 3336, Fax +32 3821 4425, E-Mail dirk.de.ridder@neurosurgery.be

Slavin KV (ed): Peripheral Nerve Stimulation.
Prog Neurol Surg. Basel, Karger, 2011, vol 24, pp 147–155

'Hybrid Neurostimulator': Simultaneous Use of Spinal Cord and Peripheral Nerve Field Stimulation to Treat Low Back and Leg Pain

Eugene G. Lipov

Advanced Pain Centers S.C., Hoffman Estates, Ill., USA

Abstract

Treatment of chronic back and leg pain in patients with failed back surgery syndrome (FBSS) remains problematic as none of the currently available approaches are universally successful in achieving lasting pain control. Spinal cord stimulation (SCS) is very effective for controlling radicular pain but rarely provides adequate control of pain in the lower back. Recently, a technique of peripheral nerve stimulation (PNS) was introduced to control pain in a group of patients for whom back pain dominated the clinical picture. Because PNS does not control neuropathic pain due to lumbosacral radiculopathy involving the lower extremities, we developed a hybrid technique of SCS and PNS that offers potential control of both axial pain in the lumbar area and radicular pain to the lower extremities. This chapter presents our results and the possible mechanisms of action.

The management of chronic persistent low back and leg pain is one of the most difficult challenges for the pain physician. This is especially true among patients with chronic pain due to failed back surgery syndrome (FBSS). Many times it is associated with or presents as postlaminectomy syndrome (PLS), a vague term defined clinically as persistent or recurrent pain following otherwise anatomically successful surgery on the lumbar spine. Over 300,000 spinal fusions are performed annually in the United States, 10–40% of which result in PLS [1]. Possible pathophysiologic causes for PLS are myriad and may include, but are not limited to, epidural scarring, dural sac deformity, arachnoiditis, or persistent spinal instability [1].

Spinal cord stimulation (SCS) has been used to treat the above conditions for many years. However, significant limitations have been encountered with the application of SCS in these patients. The main limitation of SCS use has been an inability to provide long term relief for axial back pain; this is likely due to the difficulty in obtaining low back paresthesia without also causing intervening chest or abdominal wall stimulation [2]. Thus, it seemed possible to improve the control of back and leg pain by combining SCS, known to be effective for radicular pain, and peripheral neurostimulation (PNS), a new approach for axial pain treatment.

In the application of the SCS technique, the leads are placed in the epidural space, and electrical stimulation is applied to the large myelinated fibers of the dorsal column/medial lemniscal system. This approach has been used for many years for treatment of chronic pain, particularly in the lower extremities [3–5].

In 2007, PNS emerged on the treatment horizon and recent studies have shown great promise in the treatment of axial pain. In PNS, the leads are placed subcutaneously in the area of pain (as opposed to the epidural space for SCS) to stimulate the region of the affected nerves (cutaneous afferents). Success using PNS has been reported in many clinical settings, originally in the head and cervical regions [6–8]. The success of PNS has also been reported for chronic pain in the abdominal viscera due to chronic pancreatitis [9, 10]. The technique was then successfully used for patients with chronic low back pain refractory to other treatments in 2007 [11] followed by another report of similar effect in 2008 [12]. We also reported successful use of PNfS in the neck for axial pain secondary to cervical discogenic pain [13]. Success has also been reported in combination with the SCS for radicular and axial pain in postlaminectomy syndrome [14]. At the same time, we reported the use of a 'hybrid neurostimulator' (a combination of a single SCS lead with two PNS leads [15]).

We found that patients with chronic low back pain due to PLS or FBSS were very responsive to PNS in terms of reduction in axial pain and associated functional improvements, whereas SCS worked similarly for radicular pain. This approach was only used when the patient was experiencing intractable low back and leg pain and had already failed nerve blocks, neuroablation, transcutaneous electrical nerve stimulation (TENS), and traditional medical management. In our 2008 report, all 8 patients had FBSS, and each had one epidural SCS lead (an 8-contact electrode) and two subcutaneous PNfS 4-contact electrodes. The SCS and PNfS were trialed simultaneously in our pilot study [15].

Hybrid Stimulation Pilot Study Details

Eight patients with chronic, medically intractable pain due to FBSS were treated with the newly described 'hybrid technique'. Each patient satisfied basic inclusion criteria in terms of pain severity and medical intractability. A successful trial of stimulation (over 50% relief from back and leg pain) was necessary for permanent implantation.

Phase I: Trial Implants. The leads were implanted in the subcutaneous tissues of the low back region with neurostimulator leads, two 4-contact leads (3888–45 Quad Plus Pisces, Medtronic, Minneapolis, Minn., USA) as well as a single 8-contact epidural lead (Octad, Medtronic) in the thoracic spine. During phase I of the operation, the number and placement of PNS leads was guided by consultation with the patient to

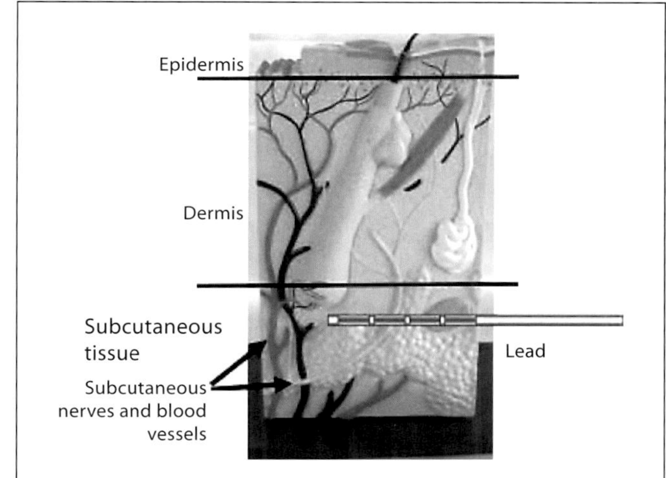

Fig. 1. Skin cross-sectional view depicting the desired location of the subcutaneous peripheral nerve stimulator lead, parallel and just deep to the dermal layer. Modified from Krutsch et al. [12]. Reprinted with permission.

identify the region of maximum pain; depth of the electrode placement was discussed in a previous publication [12] (fig. 1). Epidural and subcutaneous leads were placed percutaneously without incisions. We chose this method because our previous trials were complicated by the patient's inability to discern between relief from new incisional pain and the familiar chronic pain for which we were treating them.

The SCS lead was placed in the area of maximal paresthesia affecting the lower extremities; locations varied between T9 and T11. The placement of the subcutaneous leads was determined by a careful review of the location of pain per patient report (fig. 2a). Since our 2008 publication [15], we have further refined the technique to routinely place one 4-contact lead array in the epidural space and three subcutaneous leads as needed (Pisces Quad Plus, Medtronic). Coverage of the lower extremities seems to be at least as good with this approach compared to an 8-contact lead. The authors found that standard-spaced 8-contact electrodes were unnecessary and 4-contact wide-spaced electrodes worked best, as they seem to give maximal coverage and maximal flexibility in both subcutaneous and epidural placement. If the patient reported pain relief over 50% of the time during the trial implant, the leads were removed and phase 2, the implantation of permanent stimulation system, was performed.

Phase II: Permanent Implants. During electrode placement as a part of phase 2, incisions are made prior to placement of the subcutaneous needles, thus giving the surgeon a better angle of placement for the subcutaneous leads and improving the coverage. The epidural lead is placed via needle first allowing maximal flexibility in the epidural access; once proper placement has been achieved, an incision is made on either side of the needle. Following the wake-up test, confirmation of the epidural and subcutaneous lead coverage is performed before the patient is sedated again. The epidural lead

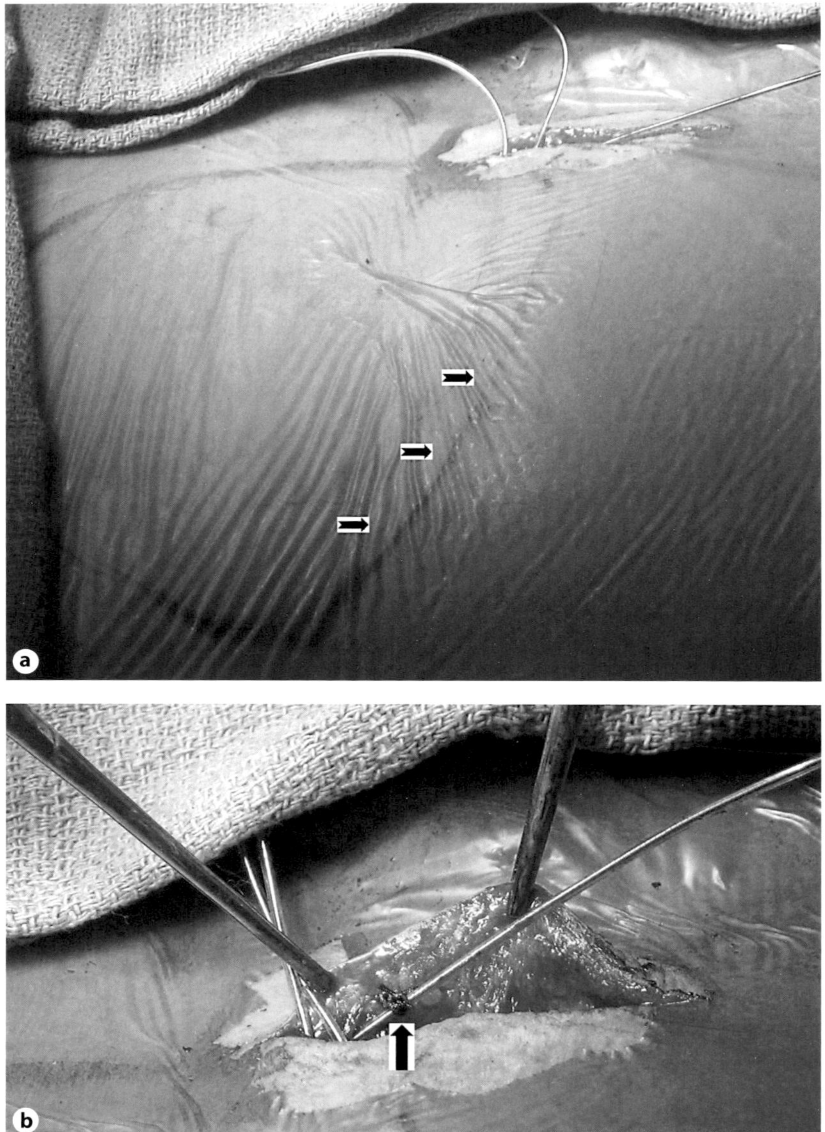

Fig. 2. a Intraoperative picture of the subcutaneous lead placement with arrows demonstrating how location of pain is ascertained during phase I. **b** Intraoperative placement of the Ethibond suture at the dermal/subcutaneous fat junction during phase II.

is secured with a Titan anchor (Medtronic) which holds the lead; then a 0-Ethibond suture (Ethicon, Somerville, N.J., USA) is placed to secure the lead before suturing it to the interspinous ligament. The subcutaneous leads are then secured by a 3–0 Ethibond (Ethicon) nonabsorbable suture placed in subcutaneous fat at the dermis junction and then looped around the lead (see intraoperative pictures for details; fig. 2).

Ethibond sutures are used due to their flexibility vs. prolene (Ethicon) which is not as flexible and had to be removed surgically following skin erosion in 1 patient. The rest of the connections were completed in the usual fashion, utilizing appropriate connectors, extensions, tunneling and the like. The implantable pulse generator (IPG) is placed in the back above the posterior superior iliac spine. The epidural lead placement is far easier in the prone position which dictates the location of IPG. The following are the typical stimulation parameters used for the subcutaneous and epidural leads in our hybrid systems:

- Programming parameters for the subcutaneous leads are usually with end contacts (0 and 3) negative (–) and positive (+).
- Middle contacts (1 and 2) remain in the 'off' position.
- Subcutaneous leads use a pulse width of 450 μs and start with a rate of 60 Hz.
- Give patients the ability to adjust amplitude and rate.
- Epidural leads use same pulse width and rate parameters as subcutaneous leads.
- Generally use a bi-pole or guarded cathode combination to achieve optimal coverage for the leg pain.

The fluoroscopic images in figure 3 depict a typical hybrid approach in our recent implant with a quadripolar lead in the epidural space and three quadripolar leads in the subcutaneous locations.

Results

Of the 10 patients selected for the 'hybrid technique' treatment, 8 completed the trial and underwent permanent implantation. At the time of latest follow-up, an average of 16 months after implantation, the mean reduction in pain intensity was 70% for back pain and 80% for leg pain. Two patients experienced 100% relief of both back and leg pain. The patients were noted to have over 50% reduction of pain medication use, and significant functional improvement. There were no surgical complications.

Overall, a total of 65 trials have been completed as of publication; of 56 hybrid systems placed to date, two have been removed due to infections and the remaining 54 are still in place.

Theoretical Mechanisms of Action

The mechanism of action for subcutaneous PNS remains unknown. It is presumed that the mechanism is similar to that believed responsible for SCS: the stimulation of large diameter A-fibers modulates neuropathic afferents from smaller A- and C-fibers. Regardless of the mechanism, it is commonly believed that neuromodulation is most effective for treating neuropathic conditions as opposed to nociceptive pain, although there is some evidence supporting the notion that it can treat both

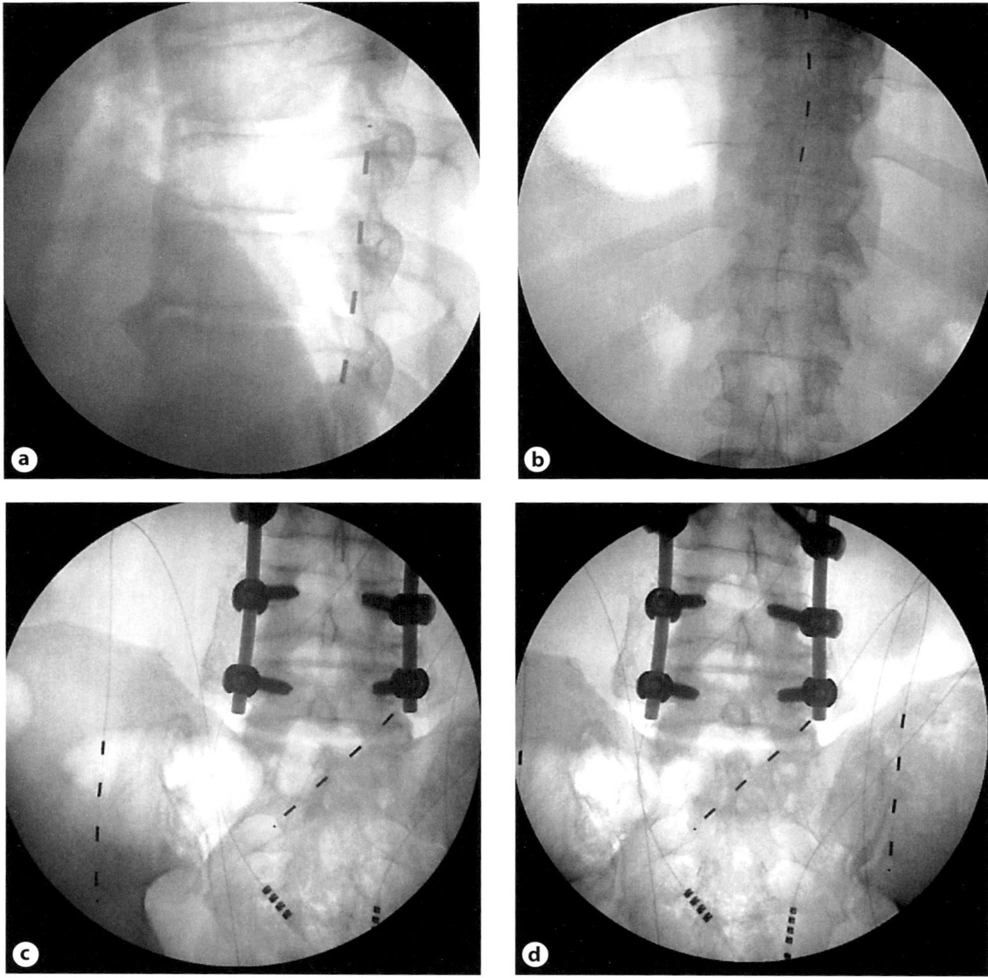

Fig. 3. Hybrid electrode placement. **a** SCS electrode: lateral view. **b** SCS electrode: AP view. **c** Left and midline PNS electrodes. **d** Midline and right PNS electrodes.

[13, 16]. We turn now to the author's hypothesis describing the possible mechanism which explains the effect of both PNS and SCS leading to relief of both nociceptive and neuropathic pain.

The author noted that the spinal cord has to be intact for SCS to be effective as demonstrated by a reduced effect below the spinal cord lesion [17]. This is only partially consistent with the gait theory of pain processing which is reliant on spinal mechanisms instead of cortical connections or central mechanisms. The ability to examine central mechanisms is now possible through the use of functional MRI (fMRI). This technique has demonstrated the activation of the insular cortex when SCS is being used [18]. The activation of the insular cortex, a structure positively correlated with sensing the intensity and unpleasantness of pain [19], is believed to be involved in processing neuropathic pain [18].

While the study of cortical activation using fMRI has only been conducted for SCS and not PNS, it is reasonable to assume that same mechanism is involved in both types of stimulation – epidural and subcutaneous – following insertion of a hybrid implant. Thus, the author believes that the insular cortex is activated by neurostimulation, leading to inhibition of transmission to higher cortical centers and thereby reducing perception of pain.

Discussion

Chronic back and leg pain due to FBSS and other causes can be challenging to treat and many therapies have been utilized with mixed results. Analgesic medications, including opiate and non-opiate drugs, may be effective in alleviating pain, but have significant adverse effects and frequently contribute to the continued disability of individuals who require them for long-term use.

The optimal therapy for chronic low back and leg pain is one that is minimally invasive, easily reversible, safe, effective, and one that allows patients to return to an active lifestyle with minimal interruption of activities and minimal need for ongoing medical interventions. Since its advent in the 1970s, SCS has been used with moderate success in treating chronic back pain. Improvements in the design of hardware have enabled minimally invasive percutaneous placement of multi-contact leads; the development of totally implantable systems with rechargeable batteries and patient-controlled devices has provided many chronic back pain patients with effective pain control and improved quality of life. The SCS helps enabling an active lifestyle without external apparatus or the need for frequent office visits or interruptions in activity (that may be required in use of TENS).

Further, the use of multi-contact leads has increased the options for programming parameters to target precise areas of pain allowing patients to independently modify the location and degree of stimulation in response to changes in activity or positioning, or fluctuations in pain severity. However, as described in the past, the success of SCS has been primarily in the treatment of the radicular pain in the lower extremities and buttocks, while achieving long-term relief in the back has remained disappointing, despite the considerable improvements in hardware [3].

The use of PNS as an adjunct to SCS may overcome the limitations of SCS, and may be a valid option for the treatment of patients whose pain is severe both in the axial back and legs. The SCS component can target the radicular pain while the PNS may more directly and completely relieve the lower back pain. The stimulation directly overlaps the area of pain, and the use of multichannel lead arrays allows for flexibility in programming. Coverage can be easily adjusted over time according to variations in pain.

Conclusions

Using an initial trial of a hybrid approach to stimulation described here among patients with a mixed neuropathic pain syndromes may be a safe and effective way of assessing candidates for combination therapy, giving the patients an opportunity to directly compare their response to both approaches (SCS and PNS) prior to committing to a permanent implant. Simultaneous use of SCS with PNS during a 5- to 7-day trial period for the treatment of chronic low back and leg pain allows comparison of the two methods and of the combination itself, through a single minimally invasive procedure.

Based on our experience, we suggest that a combination trial may be the best way to assess response to stimulation and to select the most effective modality for patients with chronic low back and leg pain. Our experience shows that PNS used in combination with SCS appears to be effective among select patients in relieving lower back and leg pain refractory to conventional management. Our findings in this small group are encouraging, suggesting that the combination of SCS and PNfS may be a valuable therapeutic tool for relieving both localized lower back and radicular lower extremity pain.

References

1 Aldrete JA: Postlaminectomy syndrome; in Waldman SD (ed): Pain Management, ed 1. Philadelphia, Saunders, 2006, p 818.

2 Barolat G, Massaro F, He J, Zeme S, Ketcik B: Mapping of sensory responses to epidural stimulation of the intraspinal neural structures in man. J Neurosurg 1993;78:233–239.

3 North R, Kidd D, Olin J, Sieracki F, Petrucci L: Spinal cord stimulation for axial low back pain: a prospective controlled trial comparing 16-contact insulated electrodes with 4-contact percutaneous electrodes. Neuromodulation 2006;9:56–67.

4 Cameron T: Safety and efficacy of spinal cord stimulation for the treatment of chronic pain: a 20-year literature review. J Neurosurg 2004;100(suppl 3 spine):254–267.

5 Van Buyten J-P, Van Zundert J, Milbouw G: Treatment of failed back surgery syndrome patients with low back and leg pain: a pilot study of a new dual lead spinal cord stimulation system. Neuromodulation 1999;2:258–265.

6 Oh MY, Ortega J, Belotte JB, Whiting DM, Alo K: Peripheral nerve stimulation for the treatment of occipital neuralgia and transformed migraine using a C1–2–3 subcutaneous paddle style electrode: a technical report. Neuromodulation 2004;7:103–112.

7 Slavin KV, Wess C: Trigeminal branch stimulation for intractable neuropathic pain: technical note. Neuromodulation 2005;8:7–13.

8 Johnstone CS, Sunderaj R: Occipital nerve stimulation for the treatment of occipital neuralgia: eight case studies. Neuromodulation 2006;9:41–47.

9 Paicius RM, Bernstein CA, Lempert-Cohen C: Peripheral nerve field stimulation in chronic abdominal pain. Pain Physician 2006;9:261–266.

10 Khan YN, Raza SS, Khan AE: Application of spinal cord stimulation for the treatment of abdominal visceral pain syndromes: case reports. Neuromodulation 2005;8:14–27.

11 Paicius RM, Bernstein CA, Lempert-Cohen C: Peripheral nerve field stimulation for the treatment of chronic low back pain: preliminary results of long term follow-up – a case series. Neuromodulation 2007;10:279–290.

12 Krutsch JP, McCeney MH, Barolat G, Al Tamimi M, Smolenski A: A case report of subcutaneous peripheral nerve stimulation for the treatment of axial back pain associated with postlaminectomy syndrome. Neuromodulation 2008;11:112–115.

13 Lipov EG, Joshi JR, Sanders S, Slavin KV: Use of peripheral subcutaneous field stimulation for the treatment of axial neck pain: a case report. Neuromodulation 2009;12:292–295.

14 Bernstein CA, Paicius RM, Barkow SH, Lempert-Cohen C: Spinal cord stimulation in conjunction with peripheral nerve field stimulation for the treatment of low back and leg pain: a case series. Neuromodulation 2008;11:177–123.
15 Lipov EG, Joshi JR, Slavin KV: Hybrid neuromodulation technique: use of combined spinal cord stimulation and peripheral nerve stimulation in treatment of chronic pain in back and legs. Acta Neurochir (Wien) 2008;150:971.
16 Ellrich J, Lamp S: Peripheral nerve stimulation inhibits nociceptive processing: an electrophysiological study in healthy volunteers. Neuromodulation 2005;8:225–232.
17 Foreman RD, Beall JE, Coulter JD, Willis WD: Effects of dorsal column stimulation on primate spinothalamic tract neurons. J Neurophysiol 1976; 39:534–546.
18 Stancák A, Kozák J, Vrba I, Tintera J, Vrána J, Polácek H, Stancák M: Functional magnetic resonance imaging of cerebral activation during spinal cord stimulation in failed back surgery syndrome patients. Eur J Pain 2008;12:137–148.
19 Lorenz J, Minoshima S, Casey KL: Keeping pain out of mind: the role of the dorsolateral prefrontal cortex in pain modulation. Brain 2003;126:1079–1091.

Eugene G. Lipov, MD
Advanced Pain Centers S.C., 2260 W. Higgins Rd., Ste. 101
Hoffman Estates, IL 60169 (USA)
E-Mail elipovmd@aol.com

Slavin KV (ed): Peripheral Nerve Stimulation.
Prog Neurol Surg. Basel, Karger, 2011, vol 24, pp 156–170

Stimulation of the Peripheral Nervous System for the Painful Extremity

W. Porter McRoberts[a] · Kevin D. Cairns[b] · Timothy Deer[c]

[a]Holy Cross Hospital, and [b]Florida Spine Specialists, Fort Lauderdale, Fla., and
[c]Center for Pain Relief, Inc., Charleston, W. Va., USA

Abstract

Peripheral nerve stimulation and, recently, peripheral nerve field stimulation are excellent options for the control of extremity pain in instances where conventional methods have failed and surgical treatment is ruled inappropriate. New techniques, ultrasound guidance, smaller generators, and task-specific neuromodulatory hardware and leads result in increasingly safe, stable and efficacious treatment of pain in the extremities. Peripheral nerve stimulation has shown to be an increasingly viable option for many painful conditions with neuropathic and possibly nociceptive origins. This chapter focuses on the historical use of neuromodulation in the extremities, technical tasks associated with implant, selection of candidates, and potential pitfalls of and solutions for implanting devices around the peripheral nervous system for extremity pain.

Stimulation of the peripheral nervous system for the treatment of pain has enjoyed renewed interest over the past several years as the modalities of delivery have become more robust and techniques have emerged that not only provide increased safety and ease of delivery but also improved success for the patient. While peripheral nerve stimulation (PNS) has been more common in the periphery, new techniques surrounding peripheral nerve field stimulation (PNfS) have recently emerged. Good outcomes have been demonstrated in the treatment of many painful conditions such as inguinal neuralgia, chronic regional pain syndrome, intercostal neuralgia, carpal tunnel syndrome, the painful postsurgical knee, traumatic and entrapment injury and focal pain of neuropathic and possibly nociceptive origins. The relatively early works of Weiner, Hassenbusch and Stanton-Hicks and others demonstrated that neuromodulation of the peripheral nerve resulted in paresthesia of the sensory distribution of the distal neural territory. However placement required great technical skill in the dissection to the target, and then in the placement of the neural electrodes in manner that provided good sensory stimulation, often in a mixed nerve, as well as considerations of fascial and flap grafting to guard against neural injury. Additionally, the procedures were time consuming and poorly reimbursed. New, percutaneous placement of electrodes, however, has led to an improved level of access for patients, and provided a safe, easy and relatively swift procedural option for the long-term treatment of extremity pain.

This chapter will focus on the historical use of neuromodulation in the extremities, technical tasks associated with implant, selection of candidates, and potential pitfalls and solutions of implanting devices in the peripheral nervous system for extremity pain.

Review of the Literature

Some 40 years ago, Wall and Sweet [1] inserted an electrode into the infra-orbital foramen and found diminution in neuropathic pain. They then successfully treated neuralgias using partially implanted percutaneous PNS [2–4]. Later, Sweet and Wepsic stimulated the median and ulnar nerves for the treatment of causalgia [5]. Variable success was reported in subsequent case series, 58% [6] and 52.6% for upper extremity pain relief and 31% relief for lower extremity pain [7, 8]. Difficulty with foreign body reaction related to the direct contact of the electrode on the exposed nerve limited the therapy until surgical technique utilizing fascial flap from nearby intermuscular septa was used to create a barrier between the nerve and the exposed electrode [9]. Stanton-Hicks suggested the following four criteria for patient selection: neuropathic pain in the nerve distribution, demonstration of pain relief by up to 3 targeted nerve blocks, exclusion of confounding psychosis, and positive response to transcutaneous electrical nerve stimulation (TENS) [10]. Over the ensuing decades of the 1970s, 1980s and early 1990s, many small series were published utilizing a variety of electrodes and techniques for direct nerve stimulation, or implantation in the vicinity of the peripheral nerve proximal to the region of pain to generate paresthesia distal to the implanted electrodes. Reports of long-term success were elusive, and results complicated by erosion, injury from the electrode insertion, and fibrosis in the peri-electrode area made the appeal of PNS largely wane in comparison to the success and ease of dorsal column stimulation [11]. However, by the late 1990s with improving technique, Long [12] produced a quite favorable meta-analysis showing positive effect in the reduction of pain in 82.5% of patients including sufferers of neuroma pain, painful diabetic neuropathy and post traumatic neuropathy [4, 13, 14]. Weiner, Reed, Slavin and Burchiel were credited with renewing interest in PNS as they introduced percutaneous approaches to electrode implantation for remediation of greater occipital neuralgia and craniofacial pain syndromes [15–17]. Additionally, in the late 1990s, following Racz's publication refocusing PNS on CRPS [9], Hassenbusch et al. [18] published a prospective series of consecutive patients with chronic regional pain syndrome in the distribution of a single major peripheral nerve. He and his team implanted paddle electrodes on the affected nerves and tested them for 2–4 days, followed by generator implant if 50% or more pain reduction was achieved during the trial. Two thirds of the patients, followed for 2–4 years, reported good or fair relief and pain was reduced from 8.3 to 3.5 on the numeric pain rating scale at follow-up. Eisenberg et al. [19] published a large retrospective analysis looking at long-term follow-up (3–16 years) of patients with PNS for nerve lesion reporting 'good' results in 78% of patients and an average drop in VAS from 6.9 preoperatively to 2.4 postoperatively. Mobbs et al. [20] retrospectively studied 45 patients with pain as result of nerve trauma. At a mean follow-up of 31 months the pain relief judged as good (>50% improvement) by about 60% of patients, and fair or poor in the remaining 40%. About half of patients reported increased activity levels. Long-term clinical outcomes of peripheral nerve stimulation for peripheral neuropathic pain were investigated by Van Calenbergh et al. [21] showing good clinical outcomes in 5 patients who underwent implantation of the Avery circumferential electrode in the upper extremity.

Historically, most implanters have described dissection to a named nerve and direct application of either a ring or paddle lead in the vicinity of the nerve; this technique is technically demanding, has significant complication rate and requires a considerable amount of operative time, and so recently interest in percutaneous trialing and permanent implantation has arisen. Speaking to that need, Monti [22] described percutaneous placement of electrodes for stimulation of the brachial plexus in the interscalene space. The rise of ultrasound-guided injections and interventions has recently turned attention to the use of ultrasound to negate the need for direct dissection for peripheral nerve visualization as ultrasound can effectively characterize the peripheral nerve by density. Narouze et al. [23] have described ultrasound-guided placement of percutaneous electrodes next to the femoral nerve, and Huntoon and colleagues [24–26] in a series of papers, have quite elegantly described a host of approaches for ultrasound-guided deployment of percutaneous PNS electrodes for neuropathic pain of the extremities.

While the organization of the peripheral nervous system allows direct named nerve stimulation for extremity pain, peripheral nerve field stimulation shows early promise for localized extremity pain. While described by many authors for stimulation of focal and radiating pain in the head, neck and trunk, McRoberts and Roche [27] illustrated successful PNfS in the knee for localized chronic knee pain following knee arthroplasty. Other localized pain in the extremity, and especially that which crosses the sensory fields of multiple nerves may also be amenable to PNfS.

Mechanism of Action

While long observed that pain responded to touch, Melzack and Wall's 1965 introduction of the gate control theory of pain changed the paradigm of pain epistemology, and opened the door for new ideas about the modulation of pain [28]. Their theory supported the concept of activation of A-beta fibers which conduct the innocuous stimuli of vibration and position, and activate inhibitory interneurons within the substantia gelatinosa in the apex of the posterior horn and subsequently influence the wide dynamic range neuron onto which both the large and small pain fibers synapse. When activated, it is theorized, the gate closes and inhibits the cephalad conduction of pain. Although some recent evidence has questioned interneuronal inhibition, the concept of early large fiber recruitment inhibiting small fiber conduction remains the basis of the theory of electrical stimulation and subsequent pain inhibition. Electrical stimulation of A-beta fiber afferents within peripheral nervous system is postulated to inhibit transmission of A-delta and C fibers, but applicability of this concept to stimulation remains somewhat controversial. However, recently Ellrich and Lamp [29] showed the ability of PNS to suppress the somatosensory evoked potentials, and subjective complaints of pain associated with noxious laser induced nociception. They additionally found and subsequently postulated that the much lower sensory threshold of A-beta fibers allows selective activation of those fibers in sensory nerves without excitation of A-delta or C fibers. Their study of direct stimulation of the nerve in vivo demonstrated objective evidence of suppression of nociceptive propagation to the central nervous system. This study provided objective and promising evidence for the antinociceptive effects of PNS and may steer future studies regarding peripheral neuromodulation for pain.

As, it has been at times difficult to stimulate mixed sensory and motor nerve without motor recruitment, PNfS, while in its infancy, may be an effective option for local generation of paresthesia. When correctly deployed, PNfS leads in the extremity allow for selective activation of terminal sensory nerve fibers without muscle activation in the gross majority of patients as the subcutaneous adipose tissue insulates the superficial muscle from recruitment. While the exact mechanism of action is still unknown, the dense population of the subcutaneous layer with terminal A-beta fibers and similarity of this to direct peripheral nerve stimulation suggest that the presence of electrical field depolarizes those terminal sensory afferents.

Patient/Candidate Selection

Generally speaking, PNS is indicated if the pain lies in the distribution of the peripheral nerve to be stimulated. Peripheral nerve lead deployment has historically placed the patient at higher risk of complication than spinal cord stimulation, and in those difficult situations, SCS is preferred. However, SCS is not without out its own limitations. Placement of an SCS electrode over the dorsal column does present the very serious risk of injury to the cord and infection. Paddle lead placement in the spinal canal is yet more invasive and requires permanent changes to the spinal anatomy and its own attendant surgical and general anesthetic risks. Other limitations to SCS include lead migration, reduction of effect over time, as well as density and amplitude of paresthesia that is variably dependent upon posture and position. Central stimulation may additionally have difficulty covering many of the 'high value' target areas of chronic pain like the feet, craniofacial pain, and in the groin and inguinal region [30]. Complex regional pain syndrome type II, and other specific localized pains also remain difficult to capture with SCS. SCS, and many PNS systems, require placement of an internalized pulse generator or RF receiver and so consideration should be given to the planned placement of the energy source. Placement far from the ultimate neural target requires significant tunneling with associated pain to the patient, risk of infection and in time possible lead strain and fracture especially if crossing a joint or area of stress. Although current implantable pulse generators (IPGs) have diminished in size from their predecessors, they still are large and do require careful planning for placement, and, as such, discussion with the patient should take into account activity level, body habitus to house the IPG, and the ability of the patient to charge and manipulate the system. Further reduction in the size of the IPG will contribute to surgical ease and patient safety. Weiner [31] detailed logical patient selection criteria for PNS below, and much can be extrapolated to the candidate for PNfS:

1 a demonstrated injury for the pain complaint,
2 failure of more conservative treatments and therapies, including surgery (if appropriate),
3 absence of significant drug dependence issues,
4 adequate patient motivation and intelligence,
5 clear understanding that PNS neuromodulation is designed to help control chronic pain but not to cure underlying disease processes,
6 successful trial stimulation,
7 identification of the specific injured and painful nerve using selective nerve/root-blocking techniques.

Nerve root blocks may lack the fidelity of named peripheral nerve, and so when the pain lies wholly in the distribution of a smaller peripheral tributary, a distal local nerve infiltration is preferred. If peripheral nerve field stimulation is to be attempted, blocks may be attempted at the local site at which paresthesia is to be directed. Once the patient has been deemed an appropriate candidate for trialing, significant consideration must be given to the planning of the neuromodulatory array.

Selection of Neuromodulation System

The improved and still improving plasticity of available arrays and generators allows the implanter great fidelity in planning for stimulation, not only in terms of the variety of available neural targets, upstream from the pain, but also the ability of the systems to provide complex programming, steering energy to various electrodes for neuromodulation of subelements of the patient's individual montage of pain. For example, a patient with a deeply achy postsurgical knee complaining of concomitant neuropathic anterior leg pain may benefit from a hybrid system providing overlapping paresthesia from any of the following: SCS, L4 nerve root stimulation, direct femoral nerve stimulation or PNfS around the knee or in the region of the infrapatellar branch of the saphenous nerve and the articular branch of the peroneal nerve. Montages of pain change over time and so it is also important to take into account the possibility of pain plasticity as much as possible as revision surgeries add additional cost and risk. Ultimately, it is becoming increasingly common for implanters to meld various elements of the implanted system to meet the various complaints of the patient. PNS was born out of a need to address very specific pain complaints, and hybridization furthers that possibility.

Again it should be the aim of the implanter to provide the densest concordant paresthesia possible via the safest method possible, and so if the pain is readily treatable with spinal cord stimulation, it is preferred, since at present SCS remains the safest modality in most cases. However, if SCS cannot provide adequate coverage or pain relief, or is unsafe or impossible to perform, then PNS or PNfS become reasonable trialing options for the painful extremity. In situations where there is an area of local and definable pain then PNfS may be a consideration. Additionally it should be noted that PNfS, and possibly direct nerve stimulation may provide a degree of additional nociceptive pain relief as opposed to the typical neuropathic pain relief seen in central neuromodulation [27, 29].

Of late, much interest has been directed at possibly increasing limits of electrical field generation by spreading the corresponding electrodes of a circuit across leads as opposed to within the lead. As the corresponding anodal terminal moves away from the cathode it is clear from virtually all electrical modeling research that the anodal and cathodal fields resume independent spherical shapes with little influence upon each other as influence is inversely proportional to the radius to the third power. Little is known about the electrophysiological responses of A-beta sensory terminal afferents to electrical fields at present, but patients routinely report that 'cross-talking' generates much larger areas of perceived paresthesia. This may occur because of local effects of the charge in the tissue across wide areas, or it may be a function of cortical mapping and the way the brain understands paresthesia. Lastly, stimulation may influence local hemodynamics, affect neurotransmitter release, increase endorphins and inhibit neuronal depolarization [32].

Neuromodulation Trial

It is rare in the surgical realm to be able to reversibly test a proposed modality without significant risk or resources from either the patient or physician, but the percutaneous trial offers this unique ability. The purpose of the trial is multifold. It is a not only a test of the modality and the proposed montage but also of the patient in terms of their ability to understand, use and psychologically adapt to the final proposition that their pain is chronic and unremitting but possibly well treated by electricity. While all neuromodulatory trialing should be limited to the minimum amount of time to come to a reasonable conclusion about the therapy's effectiveness, considerations such as fibrosis (and thus future difficulty in later lead placement) and possible epidural abscess are less of a concern when trialing in the periphery, outside of the spinal canal, and so longer trials may be possible. Longer trialing may be desirous if post-procedural pain clouds the patient's ability to asses the therapy. Additionally, a longer trial may afford the patient the option to try multiple different electrical stimulation patterns and see how they work. While direct dissection may have up until recently been the standard, ultrasound guidance and nerve stimulation for the insertion of percutaneous electrodes near a peripheral nerve will likely eliminate the need for most open trialing.

For trialing of the patient using both PNfS as well as PNS it is useful for the patient to mark the areas of pain on their own skin with a permanent marker. Dermatographic maps of pain may further inform the surgeon about the type of pain and the intensity of pain from which the patient suffers influencing the selection of neural target. Preoperative planning should additionally include planned skin entry as well as ultimate lead location, and for PNS this may require a sonographic survey of the anatomy.

For PNfS, the size and shape of the area of pain has enormous implications on lead placement, and in the trunk the aim may simply be to bracket the pain. In the periphery, the areas of pain may fall over joints or areas of stress and so lead placement should avoid possible lead strain. This may obviously be a challenge. The lead array should not be placed over the joint line, and the lead should be placed so that the lead body experiences the least tension and repetitive stress with normal skeletal movement. On occasion, strain relief loops placed at the apex of rotation may distribute the stress of repeated flexion and extension over a longer section of lead body. Although during the trial there will be no lead tunneling, the array location and position can only be considered if the planned lead course supports that ultimate array location.

If a small area exists, less than or equal to the area of a credit card, then one lead may be sufficient. If the area of pain is greater, more leads may be required. At present, four leads may be used per generator. The planned incision should be influenced by the axis of the painful area – generally the lead going through the long axis (unless the area of pain is allodynic or has anesthesia dolorosa in which lead placement lies outside the pattern), and so insertion is outside the area of pain. Additionally, the entry should utilize essentially the entire length of the needle available, so that skin entry site and painful area are as far away from each other as possible, as the incision may greatly increase the intensity of the chronic pain and confound the results of the trial. Octopolar arrays provide little additional benefit over quadripolar arrays, and using more contacts per array may limit further montage development. If the area of pain is large or irregular in shape, then the montage requires even more complexity. As noted earlier, the prospect of 'cross-talking' electrodes may provide extended areas of coverage in these situations [33]. Leads should generally be placed on the periphery of the pain, certainly if the area is much greater than the aforementioned credit card, the leads should exist within the peripheral boundaries, and the cross talking will cover the area of pain between leads. Three- and 4-lead arrays have been shown to be effective with this 'cross-talk' approach.

Once the array has been planned, the patient is brought to the operating theatre and draped in customary sterile fashion. Fluoroscopy is used to document the location of the underlying structures and at the conclusion of the case to document lead placement. A universal protocol to all cases in regards to angle (such as true anterior-posterior and/or true lateral) is suggested to simplify replication of lead placement later when planning and performing the permanent implant. Anesthesia varies based on implanter's preference, but most procedures are easily performed with light sedation and a small amount of short acting local anesthesia at the planned incision only. A puncture incision with an 11-blade scalpel is performed prior to introduction of the lead introducer needle. The curvature of the skin and the underlying anatomy have to be appreciated and the needle can be slightly curved to approximate that curvature. Once the needle is ready, it is inserted steeply through the incision and then quickly flattened to parallel the skin. Needle depth is debated among implanters, however there appears to be an overall agreement that too superficial placement will produce cutaneous pain at low amplitudes, and erroneous depth will either require amplitudes too high to produce useful stimulation, or if placed in the muscle, painful muscle recruitment. In some newer devices, a nerve stimulator can help identify the exact target location. When the shaft of the needle is elevated in plane under the skin the needle is easily palpable and the skin tents over the needle and if depressed the skin should barely dimple. If the needle is too superficial then depression will tug on the dermis and dimple it inward. Once the needle has been sufficiently advanced, the stylet is removed and the lead is deployed and the needle withdrawn using a push-pull method analogous to SCS lead deployment. Then intra-operative trialing ensues. Painful stimulation is first addressed by changing electrical configuration and stimulation amplitude. Often the initial sensation is painful, but with increasing amplitude, paresthesia overcomes the painful stimulus. If pain persists, or lack of paresthesia exists, the lead location must be changed. Type of pain informs the correction – deeper or shallower. If the implanter has used too much local anesthetic at the stab wound there is the potential that the needle has pulled the anesthetic deeper and anesthetized the target neural fibers. Occasionally blood or swelling around the lead array will insulate it and on-table trialing becomes impossible. One must simply wait and retest the array, often swelling abates and good paresthesia is felt without lead repositioning. Effort should be made to limit repeat deployments, as increased tissue damage will spoil the trialing results. Programming may vary, but the authors found a simple bipole not only adequate but also sparing in energy use compared to multiple electrode activation with approximately the same results. Different electrodes may be activated and the lead may be withdrawn or carefully advanced as is the authors' experience that small movements (known as trolling in SCS) may improve the field's location in respect to larger branches of terminal sensory fibers, thus activating nerves that supply larger territories of skin. Fluoroscopic and radiographic images should document final lead placement. Once the nerves or fibers are appropriately stimulated, the lead is fixed to the skin by direct suturing, silastic anchor, tape or a dermal adhesive. Similar to SCS, care is taken to attend to the patient's sleeping preferences so as to minimize the impact of the lead on the patient's body while in repose. The patient is then taken to recovery and reprogramming is undertaken. As mentioned, if swelling or local anesthetic thwarts immediate postplacement programming, one must simply wait for the situation to abate for reattempts. Regardless, the patient will likely need to return the following day as the limits and stimulation parameters will have changed significantly necessitating reprogramming.

Patients who suffer from pain in an extremity within the distribution of a single or possibly two nerves may be better candidates for direct PNS than PNfS. In cases that necessitate direct peripheral nerve stimulation, the deployment of the lead is technically more demanding. Needle stimulators, ultrasound guidance, or both may be used. Prior to consideration of trialing, the patient should undergo appropriate workup and screening. Huntoon and colleagues have spent considerable effort detailing several methods for trialing and implanting peripheral nerves with sonographic guidance. The reader is referred to those papers for additional information [24–26]. Each nerve has preferred loci for stimulation that diminish lead migration and movement. Common neural targets include, but are not limited to the median, ulnar, radial, axilary, suprascapular, brachial plexus, lateral femoral cutaneous, saphenous, sural, peroneal, tibial, sciatic and femoral. Patients should initially undergo trial blockade proximal to the pain with local anesthetic demonstrating at least 80% relief. If surgical intervention is indicated, referral to an orthopedic or neurologic surgeon with familiarity with peripheral nerve surgery must be considered.

Again, preoperative planning is essential as direct nerve stimulation is more complex. Whereas PNfS is concerned with a uniform and single tissue plane and invariable and stationary neural target, PNS arrays and leads cross planes, traveling close to sensitive and often highly mobile structures including the nerves themselves. The patients should only have leads placed while awake and aware and very careful needle advancement is warranted with strict attention to patients' reports of pain or paresthesia. Delivering uniform charge fields to a nerve is much more challenging in PNS. Whereas intra-electrode resistance is generally static in PNfS and even SCS due to the uniformity of tissue types and relative stability of lead placement, with PNS the presence of multiple tissue types and thus multiple resistances as well as lead movement and dynamic field generation raise the importance of system selection. In situations where impedance is highly variable it may be worthwhile to have systems which provide constant current and variable voltage as they may more readily adapt to the ever changing resistance of the environment. However, understanding the multitude of challenges to the system it is a surprise that most are and remain relatively stable over time. As in PNfS the skin should be marked prior to trialing, mainly to force the surgeon run through the technical considerations of the case. Additionally, the process involves the patient in decision-making as well. Ultrasound, being particularly adept in identifying tissue types and fascial planes should be used to identify the nerve as well as the optimal location for lead array and lead body placement. Generally the nerve should be as relatively superficial and as stable as possible. The array location is often best when placed perpendicular to and deep to the nerve, or between the nerve and bone if the nerve closely follows bone as it adds stability to the placement. By placing the array so that it bisects the nerve course in perpendicular fashion the effect of eventual lead migration is minimized. Additionally, needle tract and lead should avoid large vascular branches as well as muscle. Similar to PNfS, considerations are given to lead movement: tunneling and suturing must also be made in PNS even during the trialing phase, as if successful, the permanent implantation must be able to support the lead placement. For example, it may be easy to deploy a small lead to stimulate interdigital nerves but ultimately connecting that lead to a power source may be presently infeasible or quite difficult.

Permanent PNS/PNfS Implantation

Once significant success in capturing and relieving pain with PNS or PNfS is demonstrated with trial lead placement, planning for the permanent implantation of the neuromodulation system ensues. It may be relatively easy to deploy peripheral leads compared with design of and implantation of a PNS system that is both dynamic enough to respond to the movements of the extremities yet durable enough to withstand repeated movement. Most equipment was initially designed to be placed in the central neuroaxis where relatively little movement occurs over time comparing to the often repetitive and extreme movements in the extremities, and so great consideration must be given to reduce the strain on the implanted system.

Body habitus, specifically the amount of adipose tissue available in the extremity, helps determine if the IPG can be implanted there. The patient may lose weight with the additional pain relief as well, and so one must be concerned with changes over time. By peripheral implantation, the surgeon negates the need to cross the shoulder or hip, and this adds to system stability over time; however, if little adipose is available then one defaults to central implantation, either the buttock, lower quadrant of the abdomen, shoulder, pre-cordial region or mid-scapular line/mid-clavicular line. If forced to cross a joint line then one must give consideration not only to the degree of range encountered in the joint, e.g. shoulder greater than elbow, but also to the likelihood of movement and the overall length of the system – array to generator. Sufficient strain relief loop size must be made to allow for incomplete loop closure with ranging movement of the extremity. Extreme extension and or flexion should not tighten the loop to such a degree that a kink appears – if so then all lead flexion will occur at that one point as opposed to the lead loop length in unison and lead fracture will result. Loop size is inversely proportional to loop strain. Additionally, the loop must fold in the plane of movement, not against it, so that increasing the acuity of flexion angle tightens as opposed to loosens the loop.

While loops allow for freedom of movement, the electrode array must move as little as possible in relation to the neural target. In PNfS, the lead is tied to subcutaneous tissue, often the superficial most fascial plane. If a large anchor is selected, and there is little subcutaneous adipose to protect the skin from the new underlying anchor, the anchor may be buried deep to the first fascial layer, and the fascia closed over the anchor. Erosion may occur if the anchor is too superficial. The implanter has a myriad of choices available for anchoring. Direct ligation-like suturing to the lead is often best. Nurolon (Ethicon Inc.) braided nylon or similar suture is suggested for high strength and integrity over time. With this method, the lead is well secured, the anchor is flat, strong and low-profile, and in a short period of time scar tissue fills the crevices in the stitch and further secures the lead. The suggested method of suturing is the 'drain stitch,' similar to that used to secure a chest tube. Challenge may arise, however, if in the event lead revision requires anchor revision, great care must be taken in dissection of the lead from the suture, and this may lengthen the operative time. Low incidence of migration seen with this technique, however, makes up for the increased complexity of the less frequent revisions. Caution must be used to avoid over-tightening the suture on the lead as this may break or deform the lead wires or insulation. To further limit the possibility of migration, the lead should be anchored close to the proximal portion of the array.

Once the lead array is deployed and secured, attention is turned to tunneling over the joint and thus the lead flexion point. At the axis of rotation, dissection to subcutaneous adipose permits the burial of a strain relief loop as described above. The lead loop should not be anchored with permanent suture as unwanted strain may develop in the long term. The lead can be tacked into position using absorbable suture to hold it there while scaring occurs and associated integrity develops. Additionally, in planning the tunneling, it is best to avoid placing the lead over anatomical bony prominences as erosion may occur. Good prior planning, preoperative marking, and attention to detail reward the implanter and patient with stability of the system and thus lasting efficacy.

Common Neural Targets and Treatable Syndromes for PNfS and PNS

Lateral Femoral Cutaneous Nerve and Meralgia Paresthetica

The lateral femoral cutaneous nerve arises from the dorsal roots of L2 and L3, courses through the lateral psoas major muscle, descends into the pelvis crossing the ventral iliacus muscle obliquely and follows the interior of the pelvic girdle anteriorly. It then dives under the inguinal ligament about 1 cm medial and inferior to the anterior superior iliac spine then passes inferiorly arising superficial to the hip flexors and then innervates the anterolateral skin of the thigh. Trauma, compression and metabolic disease can injure the nerve. Often well treated by oral or transdermal medical management of pain and or steroid nerve block, occasionally the pain is unremitting and one must consider neuromodulation. Often SCS works well, but the use of PNS has also been shown effective with leads placed based on tissue mapping and or direct nerve stimulation. Ultrasound guidance may be very effective in inserting the electrode in close proximity to the nerve.

Infrapatellar Branch of the Saphenous Nerve and Articular Branch of the Peroneal Nerve at the Knee

Postoperative knee pain is commonly associated with entrapment injuries to the peripheral nerves as they innervate the anterior knee. Durable pain relief has been demonstrated with placement of electrodes in the lateral tissues surrounding the knee. It has been hypothesized that due to the relative superficiality of the nerves, subcutaneous deployment actually depolarizes the nerve in some cases. Care is made not to cross the joint line with the arrays and deployment of four quadripolar leads is best as the electrodes can 'cross-talk' to each other generating fields across the knee joint itself. The systems are relatively stable over time. Strain relief is at the knee and tunneling carries leads to the IPG pocket either in the thigh or abdomen. If tunneled to the abdomen, care is taken to avoid crossing the inguinal crease near the lateral femoral cutaneous nerve, so leads are usually lateral to the anterior superior iliac spine.

Tibial Nerve

Involved frequently in entrapment at the tarsal tunnel, crush injuries or trauma, the tibial nerve is easily stimulated at the bifurcation, posterior and proximal to the knee, or better yet, if pain is contained to the foot, at the distal medial calf, posterior to the tibialis posterior tendon and deep to the flexor hallucis longus tendon sheath using an anterior to posterior approach. The tarsal tunnel may be a tempting location as the nerve is easily located, but due to the frequency of entrapment syndromes as a function of tight compression and ligamentous movement the addition of a lead there may be problematic. Multiple mobile structures are in close proximity: in addition to the tibial nerve, there are the posterior tibial artery, tibialis posterior, flexor digitorum longus, and flexor hallucis longus.

Peroneal Nerve

Like the tibial nerve, the peroneal is vulnerable to similar insults. In addition to compression injuries and trauma, chronic peroneal neuropathy can result from peripheral neuropathy, surgical insult from fibular harvest, and athletic conditioning. The peroneal nerve can be stimulated at the sciatic bifurcation immediately proximal to the popliteal fossa, or just below the knee posterior to the fibular head itself. It descends from the bifurcation obliquely along the lateral popliteal fossa to the fibular head and close to the medial biceps femoris muscle before descending and winding around the fibular neck next to the peroneus longus before dividing into the superficial and deep divisions. At the sciatic bifurcation, it may be difficult to selectively stimulate the peroneal division, and so better exposure and the option of selective stimulation may exist at the fibular head. The superficial peroneal nerve can be stimulated at the dorsum of the foot.

Sciatic Nerve

As described above, the bifurcation point of the peroneal and tibial presents a good site for stimulation. Direct stimulation has additionally been reported at the greater sciatic notch, dissection to nerve and stabilization of array is difficult however. It is important to place the array proximal to the insult zone of the nerve. More studies are needed to evaluate treatment possibilities.

Median, Radial and Ulnar Nerves

Trauma and entrapment of the sensory nerves of the hand and forearm often result in difficult to treat painful neuropathies. The use of peripheral neuromodulation to treat the sensory nerves is promising. Median neuropathy may be among the most common peripheral nerve disorders. The median nerve is easily stimulated at the carpal tunnel, and new, investigational devices are aimed at this prospect [unpubl. data]. Additionally the median nerve is found in the antecubital fossa medial to the brachial artery; more proximally it runs with the brachial artery between the biceps brachii and brachialis muscles. Distal to the crease of the forearm it passes between the two heads of the pronator teres. The radial nerve can be easily stimulated if a lead is passed posterior and slightly lateral to the humerus proximal to the elbow, at the distal radial groove. This may prove to be a stable location. The ulnar nerve is accessed superior to the medial epicondyle. Again placements deep to the nerve may be more stable over time. Further research needs to explore lead location and long-term stability.

Axillary and Suprascapular Nerves and the Brachial Plexus

Shoulder hand syndrome and a host of other neuropathic and painful disorders affect the distributions of the axilary and suprascapular nerves. Regional blocks often provide excellent but only temporary relief to these areas, and so the prospect of neuromodulation as a long-term treatment of pain remains hopeful. Current studies are evaluating the viability of various treatment options.

Conclusions

PNS and, recently, PNfS are excellent options for the control of extremity pain in instances where conventional methods have failed and surgical treatment is ruled inappropriate. New techniques, ultrasound guidance, smaller generators, task-specific neuromodulatory hardware and leads all add to the burgeoning interest in PNS and PNfS for the long term treatment of pain in the extremity. While much research still needs be done, currently there are safe and effective stimulation options for extremity pain. Prospective science is needed to further evaluate the potential success in broader population categories. Attention to detail, proper planning and good patient selection is required in PNS and PNfS. Despite the need for more clinical investigation, peripheral neuromodulation is an important and effective tool in the interventionalist's compendium of treatment options.

References

1 Wall PD, Sweet WH: Temporary abolition of pain in man. Science 1967;155:108–109.

2 Sweet WH: Control of pain by direct electrical stimulation of peripheral nerves. Clin Neurosurg 1976; 23:103–111.

3 Day M: Neuromodulation: spinal cord and peripheral nerve stimulation. Curr Rev Pain 2000;4: 374–382.

4 White PF, Li S, Chiu JW: Electroanalgesia: its role in acute and chronic pain management. Anesth Analg 2001;92:505–513.

5 Sweet WH, Wepsic JG: Treatment of chronic pain by stimulation of fibers of primary afferent neuron. Trans Am Neurol Assoc 1968;93:103–107.

6 Waisbrod H, Panhans C, Hansen D, Gerbeshagen HU: Direct nerve stimulation for painful peripheral neuropathies. J Bone Joint Surg (Br) 1985;67:470–472.

7 Nashold BS Jr, Goldner JL, Mullen JB, Bright DS: Long-term pain control by direct peripheral-nerve stimulation. J Bone Joint Surg Am 1982;64:1–10.

8 Hunt JL: Electrical injuries of the upper extremity. Major Probl Clin Surg 1976;19:72–83.

9 Racz GB, Lewis R, Heavner JE, Scott J: Peripheral nerve stimulator implant for treatment of RSD; in Stanton-Hicks M, Janig W, Boas RA (eds): Reflex Sympathetic Dystrophy. Boston, Kluwer Academic Publishers, 1989, pp 135–141.

10 Stanton-Hicks M: Transcutaneous and peripheral nerve stimulation; in Simpson BA (ed): Electrical Stimulation and the Relief of Pain. Amsterdam, Elsevier, 2003, pp 37–55.

11 Slavin KV: Peripheral nerve stimulation for neuropathic pain. Neurotherapeutics 2008;5:100–106.

12 Long DM: The current status of electrical stimulation of the nervous system for the relief of chronic pain. Surg Neurol 1998;49:142–144.

13 Campbell JN, Long DM: Peripheral nerve stimulation in the treatment of intractable pain. J Neurosurg 1976;45:692–699.

14 Loeser JD, Black RG, Christman A: Relief of pain by transcutaneous stimulation. J Neurosurg 1975;42: 308–314.

15 Weiner RL, Reed KL: Peripheral neurostimulation for control of intractable occipital neuralgia. Neuromodulation 1999;2:217–221.

16 Slavin KV, Burchiel KJ: Peripheral nerve stimulation for painful nerve injuries. Contemp Neurosurg 1999;21:1–6.

17 Slavin KV, Burchiel KJ: Use of long-term nerve stimulation with implanted electrodes in the treatment of intractable craniofacial pain. J Neurosurg 2000;92:576.

18 Hassenbusch SJ, Stanton-Hicks M, Schoppa D, Walsh JG, Covington EC: Long-term results of peripheral nerve stimulation for reflex sympathetic dystrophy. J Neurosurg 1996;84:415–423.

19 Eisenberg E, Waisbrod H, Gerbershagen HU: Long-term peripheral nerve stimulation for painful nerve injuries. Clin J Pain 2004;3:143–146.

20 Mobbs RJ, Nair S, Blum P: Peripheral nerve stimulation for the treatment of chronic pain. J Clin Neurosci 2007;14:216–221.

21 Van Calenbergh F, Gybels J, Van Laere K, Dupont P, Plaghki L, Depreitere B, Kupers R: Long term clinical outcome of peripheral nerve stimulation in patients with chronic peripheral neuropathic pain. Surg Neurol 2009;72:330–335.

22 Monti E: Peripheral nerve stimulation: a percutaneous minimally invasive approach. Neuromodulation 2004;7:193–196.

23 Narouze SN, Zakari A, Vydyanathan A: Ultrasound-guided placement of a permanent percutaneous femoral nerve stimulator leads for the treatment of intractable femoral neuropathy. Pain Physician 2009;12:E305–E308.

24 Huntoon MA, Burgher AH: Ultrasound-guided permanent implantation of peripheral nerve stimulation (PNS) system for neuropathic pain of the extremities: original cases and outcomes. Pain Med 2009;10:1369–1377.

25 Huntoon MA, Hoelzer BC, Burgher AH, Hurdle MF, Huntoon EA: Feasibility of ultrasound-guided percutaneous placement of peripheral nerve stimulation electrodes and anchoring during simulated movement: part two, upper extremity. Reg Anesth Pain Med 2008;33:558–565.

26 Huntoon MA, Huntoon EA, Obray JB, Lamer TJ: Feasibility of ultrasound-guided percutaneous placement of peripheral nerve stimulation electrodes in a cadaver model: part one, lower extremity. Reg Anesth Pain Med 2008;33:551–557.

27 McRoberts WP, Roche M: Novel approach for peripheral subcutaneous field stimulation for the treatment of severe, chronic knee joint pain after total knee arthroplasty. Neuromodulation 2010;13: 131–136.

28 Melzack R, Wall PD: Pain mechanisms: a new theory. Science 1965;150:971–979.

29 Ellrich J, Lamp S: Peripheral nerve stimulation inhibits nociceptive processing: an electrophysiological study in healthy volunteers. Neuromodulation 2005;8:225–232.

30 Aló KM, Holsheimer J: New trends in neuromodulation for the management of neuropathic pain. Neurosurgery 2002;50:690–703.

31 Weiner RL: Peripheral nerve neurostimulation. Neurosurg Clin N Am 2003;14:401–408.

32 Hamza MA, White PF, Craig WF, Ghoname ES, Ahmed HE, Proctor TJ, Noe CE, Vakharia AS, Gajraj N: Percutaneous electrical nerve stimulation: a novel analgesic therapy for diabetic neuropathic pain. Diabetes Care 2000;23:365–370.

33 Falco FJE, Berger J, Vrable A, Onyewu O, Zhu J: Cross talk: a new method for peripheral nerve stimulation: an observational report with cadaveric verification. Pain Physician 2009;12:965–983.

Timothy Deer, MD
Center for Pain Relief, Inc.
400 Court Street, Suite 100
Charleston, WV 25301 (USA)
Tel. +1 304 347 6141, Fax +1 304 347 6855, E-Mail DocTDeer@aol.com

Slavin KV (ed): Peripheral Nerve Stimulation.
Prog Neurol Surg. Basel, Karger, 2011, vol 24, pp 171–179

Sphenopalatine Ganglion Interventions: Technical Aspects and Application

Chima O. Oluigbo[a] · Girma Makonnen[a] · Samer Narouze[b] · Ali R. Rezai[a]

[a]Department of Neurological Surgery, Ohio State University Medical Center, Columbus, Ohio, and [b]Center for Pain Medicine, Summa Western Reserve Hospital, Cuyahoga Falls, Ohio, USA

Abstract

Recent research has highlighted the important role of the sphenopalatine ganglion (SPG) in cerebrovascular autonomic physiology and in the pathophysiology of cluster and migraine headaches as well as conditions of stroke and cerebral vasospasm. The relatively accessible location of the SPG within the pterygopalatine fossa and the development of options for minimally invasive approaches to the SPG make it an attractive target for neuromodulation approaches. The obvious advantage of SPG stimulation compared to ablative procedures on the SPG such as radiofrequency destruction and stereotactic radiosurgery is its reversibility and adjustable features. The on-going design of strategies for transient and continuous SPG stimulation on as needed basis using implantable SPG stimulators is an exciting new development which is expected to expand the clinical versatility of this technique.

The sphenopalatine ganglion (SPG) is the largest of the peripheral parasympathetic ganglia and is located in the pterygopalatine fossa (fig. 1). Although it is primarily considered a parasympathetic ganglion, it also conveys both sensory and sympathetic fibers which – unlike parasympathetic fibers – only pass through the ganglion without synapsing.

Recent research is defining the sphenopalatine ganglion's key role in the pathophysiology of different headache syndromes including cluster headaches, migraines, and trigeminal autonomic cephalalgias (TACs) [1–3]. The effectiveness of electrical stimulation of the SPG for acute treatment of intractable migraine and cluster headaches has recently been demonstrated [4, 5]. SPG has also been implicated in other autonomic cerebrovascular phenomena. SPG stimulation has been shown to result in increased regional cerebral blood flow [6–8] in animal models as well as reversal of cerebral vasospasm in a dog model of SAH [9].

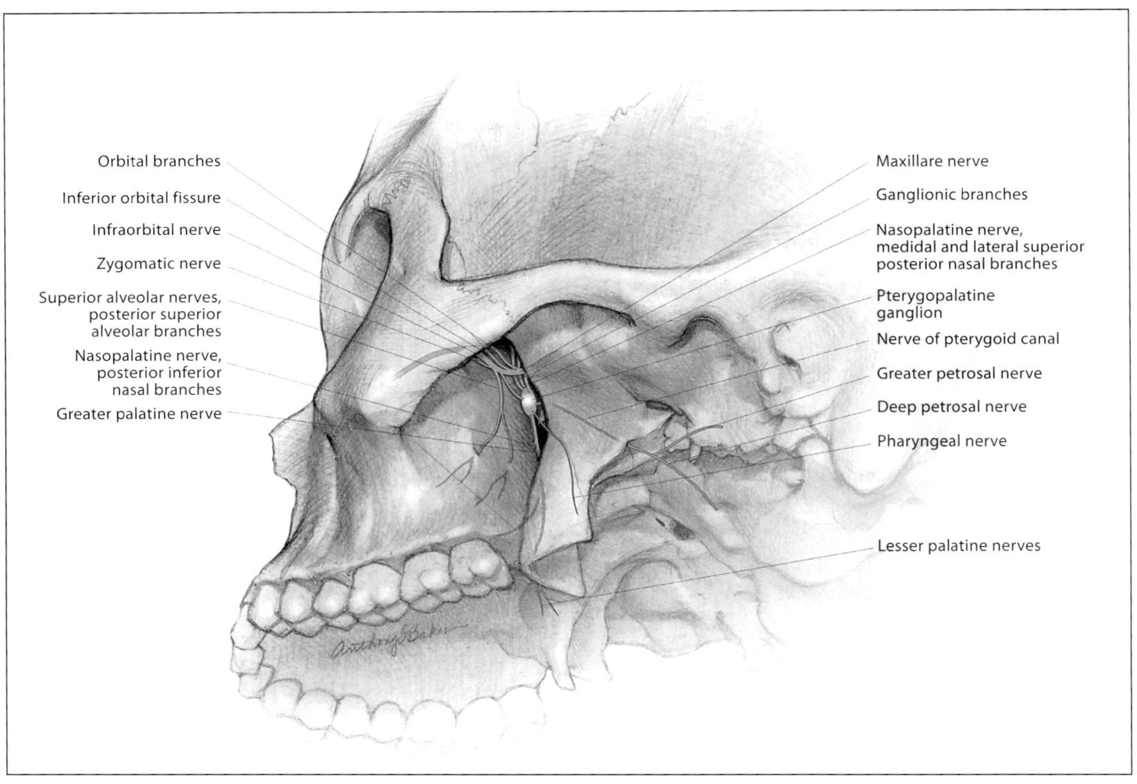

Fig. 1. Anatomy of the sphenopalatine ganglion and pterygopalatine fossa. Original drawing by OSU Medical Illustration.

This increasing body of evidence of the role of the SPG in cluster headaches, migraines and autonomic cerebrovascular phenomena, the relatively accessible location of the SPG within the pterygopalatine fossa and the development of options for minimally invasive approaches to the SPG make it an attractive target for neuromodulation approaches. This chapter will review the underlying anatomic and physiologic considerations, technical aspects of SPG targeting and stimulation as well as novel strategies for chronic stimulation of the SPG.

Anatomic and Physiologic Considerations

The SPG, otherwise known as the ganglion of Meckel is an autonomic extracranial ganglion located within the pterygopalatine fossa (PPF) (fig. 1). The PPF is an inverted pyramidal space located behind the posterior wall of the maxillary sinus and communicates laterally with the infratemporal fossa. The PPF contains the internal maxillary artery and its branches, the maxillary nerve and the SPG with its afferent and efferent branches.

The SPG is situated below the maxillary nerve as it crosses the PPF. The SPG has sensory and autonomic components. The autonomic components are particularly relevant to its effects on cerebrovascular physiology and consist of both parasympathetic and sympathetic components.

The parasympathetic component consists of efferent preganglionic fibers which arise from cell bodies in the superior salivary nucleus of the pons, travel within the nervus intermedius of the facial nerve and then branch out at the geniculate ganglion to become the greater petrosal nerve. Postganglionic sympathetic fibers (second-order neurons arising from the upper thoracic spinal cord and synapsing mainly in the superior cervical ganglia) run within the deep petrosal nerve and then join the greater petrosal nerve to form the vidian nerve. The preganglionic parasympathetic fibers within the vidian nerve synapse with second order parasympathetic cell bodies located within the SPG, and the postganglionic parasympathetic fibers run with branches of the maxillary nerve to reach their target orbital, palatine, posterior superior nasal and pharyngeal structures.

Meanwhile the postganglionic sympathetic neurons within the vidian nerve only pass through the SPG without synapsing on any cell bodies and go on to provide sympathetic innervations to blood vessels.

Physiologic Considerations and Applications

Cluster Headaches and Migraines

Research on the pathophysiology of trigeminal autonomic cephalgias has progressed significantly since Sluder [10] first described the syndrome of sphenopalatine neuralgia in 1909. His description consisted of unilateral facial pain associated with mucosal congestion, rhinorrhea and lacrimation. The type of headaches he described are now referred to as trigeminal autonomic cephalalgias (TACs). They are primary headaches which are characterized by trigeminal distribution of pain, cranial autonomic features and an episodic pattern of attacks [11]. The three main types of TACs are cluster headaches, paroxysmal hemicrania, and short-lasting unilateral neuralgiform headache attacks with conjunctival injection and tearing (SUNCT).

With regard to the major pathways involved in TACs, pain fibers from the trigeminovascular system pass through the ophthalmic division of the trigeminal nerve, carrying signals from the cranial vessels and dura mater. These inputs synapse in the trigeminocervical complex (TCC) [3] and then project to the thalamus and cortex where they are interpreted as pain. Concurrently, there is activation of the parasympathetic reflex through the outflow from the superior salivary nucleus, predominantly involving the sphenopalatine ganglion, which dilates blood vessels and activates trigeminal nerve endings. This autonomic activation results in lacrimation, reddening of the eyes and nasal congestion. In addition to the above, this autonomic activation also causes meningeal vasodilatation and neurogenic inflammation which then sensitizes meningeal nociceptors carrying pain signals centrally [2]. Studies also show that the autonomic symptoms may be generated through the hypothalamus which plays a role in controlling the cycling aspects of the TACs [12]. The central role of the SPG and its anatomical accessibility makes it an important target for modulation of these neural pathways which are involved in the pathophysiology of migraines and cluster headaches.

Augmentation of Cerebral Blood Flow in the Treatment of Acute Ischemic Stroke
Sphenopalatine ganglion stimulation has been shown to increase regional blood flow independent of glucose utilization in cats [6] and reversed cerebral vasospasm in a dog model of subarachnoid hemorrhage [9]. This effect on cerebral blood flow is due to the SPGs connections with parasympathetic cerebrovascular innervation, and the main neurotransmitters involved in this pathway are vasoactive intestinal peptide (VIP) and nitric oxide [13, 14].

The results from the experiments on animal models on the effect of SPG stimulation on cerebral blood flow is now being translated to human clinical studies. Recently, a clinical trial protocol for a pilot study to evaluate the safety and effectiveness of a SPG stimulator implant (the Ischaemic Stroke System 500) to augment cerebral blood flow in the treatment of acute ischemic stroke was published [15].

Sphenopalatine Ganglion Interventional Procedures

Numerous ablative and nonablative procedures directed at the SPG have been used in the past including intranasal local anesthetic drops [16], transnasal nerve blocks [17], radiofrequency ablation [18], surgical ganglionectomy [19], gamma knife radiosurgery [20] and more recently SPG stimulation [4, 5, 21]. The overall trend has however been towards nonablative approaches to the SPG in view of the important functions of the ganglion.

Sphenopalatine Ganglion Stereotactic Radiosurgery
Stereotactic radiosurgery is a minimally invasive option for SPG ablation [20, 22]. Stereotactic techniques are employed in targeting the SPG. CT imaging delineates the walls of the PPF while the contents of the fossa are well visualized on MRI. Radiosurgical dose to the SPG ranges from 75 to 80 Gy [20, 22, 23]. Lasting control of medically refractory cluster headaches with stereotactic radiosurgery is about 60% but high rates of facial sensory disturbance have been reported [20, 23].

Sphenopalatine Ganglion Radiofrequency Ablation
Radiofrequency ablation of SPG requires a minimally invasive percutaneous approach. As described by Narouze et al. [18], once PPF is accessed with a radiofrequency

needle (see detailed description of percutaneous approach to the SPG below), sensory stimulation is performed to produce deep paresthesias behind the nose and then 2 radiofrequency lesions are carried out at 80°C for 60 s each.

Approaches to the Sphenopalatine Ganglion

The relatively superficial location of the SPG in PPF lends it accessible with infrazygomatic (IZ) approaches as well as transnasal approaches.

Lateral Infrazygomatic Approaches

The IZ approaches could be performed percutaneously or transorally (will be discussed under strategies for chronic stimulation). Ruskin first described transoral and lateral injection approaches to SPG [24].

Percutaneous Infrazygomatic Approach

This percutaneous infrazygomatic approach could be either anterior to the mandible or through the coronoid notch of the mandible. The technique is well described by Narouze [25] and it is the same technique that has been used for SPG blocks as well as SPG ablation by other authors [5, 18]. The targeting may be guided with fluoroscopy or CT [5, 18, 25, 26].

The patient is positioned supine on the surgical table and the PPF is identified using fluoroscopic technique (fig. 2). After prepping and draping, local skin and subcutaneous anesthesia is achieved by infiltration of local anesthetic. Subsequently a 22-gauge needle is inserted at the entry point of the zygomatic arch in the appropriate side with a projected course through the coronoid notch on to the pterygoid plate. The needle is then moved anteriorly on the pterygoid plate to the PPF under fluoroscopic guidance. At this point, the needle stylet is removed and a contact stimulation electrode is inserted and advanced through the tip of the needle. The stimulation electrode is connected to an external stimulator. Sensory stimulation at typical parameters of 50 Hz and 30 μs and varying intensities is applied to induce paresthesias in order to verify the location of the needle within the PPF. Optimal location is confirmed by simulation causing paresthesias in the posterior nasopharynx.

Transnasal Approaches

Sluder [27] first proposed transnasal blockade of the SPG using topical cocaine applied transnasally. The transnasal approach to the SPG ganglion is based on the fact that the SPG in the pterygopalatine fossa lies posterior to the middle nasal turbinate under a 1.5 mm layer of connective tissue and mucous membrane. Thus, topical application of anesthetic solutions such as lidocaine applied to the posterior wall of the nasopharynx in the region of the middle turbinate can diffuse across the mucosa to alter activity within the SPG.

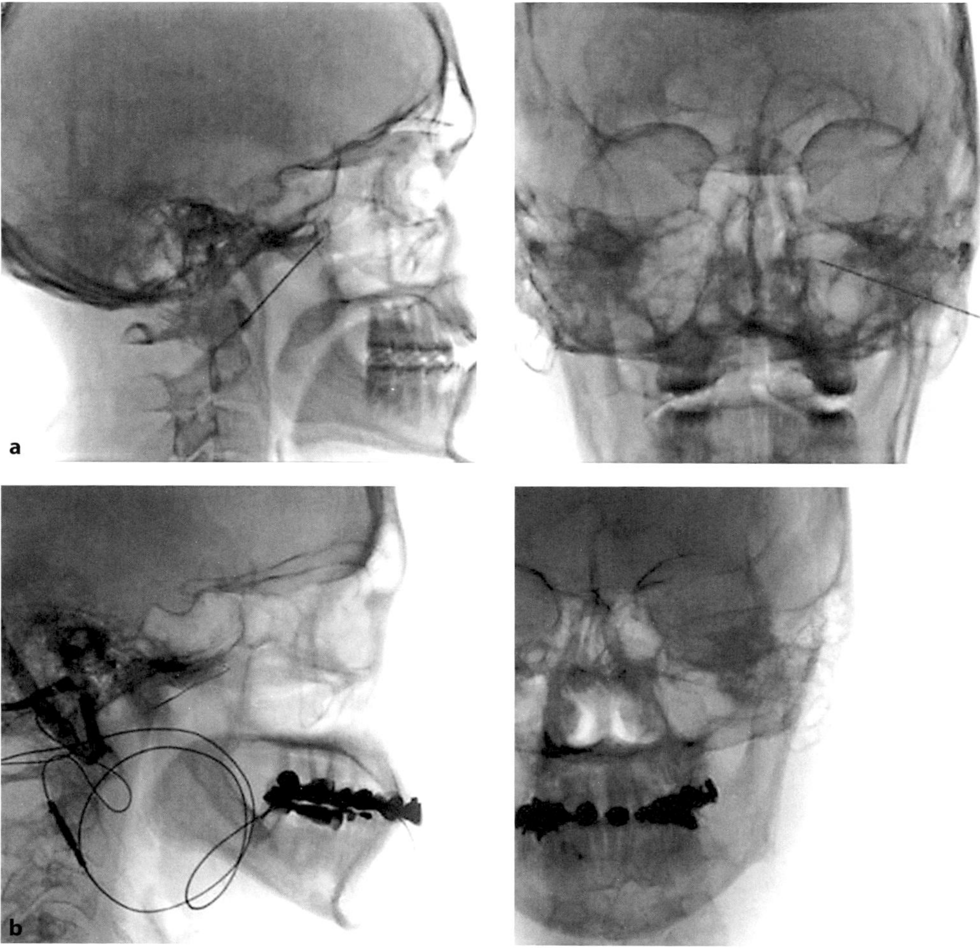

Fig. 2. Percutaneous infrazygomatic approach to the pterygopalatine fossa. From Ansarinia et al. [5], published by Wiley Periodicals; reproduced with permission. **a** Radiographs of needle insertion. **b** Radiographs of final electrode position.

Procedure: The patient is placed supine with the neck extended. The posterior nasal pharynx is anesthesized and lubricated by asking the patient to inhale a small amount of 2% viscous lidocaine instilled into the nares. For topical block of the sphenopalatine ganglion, a sterile 10-cm cotton tipped applicator dipped in 4% lidocaine and slowly advanced along the superior border of the middle turbinate until it reaches the posterior wall of the nasopharynx. The applicator is usually left in place for approximately 20–30 min to diffuse across the mucosa and take effect.

Another transnasal approach to the SPG involves endoscopic techniques for transnasal injection and blocks of the SPG. This technique was first described by Prasanna and Murthy [28] in 1993. The use of an endoscope allows visualization and identification of the relevant anatomical region and precise injection of the anesthetic medication for prolonged pain relief. In this procedure, as described by Felisati et al. [29], a 4-mm 0° endoscope is use to locate the nasal mucous membrane immediately behind and over the middle turbinate tail. A long 20-gauge needle is then inserted into the inferior portion of the sphenopalatine foramen, while avoiding the sphenopalatine artery, and a mixture of triamcinolone acetonide (40 mg), 1% bupivacaine and 2% mepivacaine with 1/100,000 adrenaline is injected directly into the fossa.

Sphenopalatine Ganglion Stimulation and Outcomes

Cluster Headache and Migraines

Tepper et al. [4] and Ansarinia et al. [5] reported that acute stimulation of the SPG can alleviate migraine and cluster headaches, respectively. This technique employed transient neurostimulation with a temporary electrode using the standard lateral infrazygomatic approach described by Narouze [25]. The stimulation parameters of the SPG that most commonly resulted in a favorable outcome during acute treatment of cluster headaches were intensities of up to 2 V, frequency of 50 Hz and pulse width of 300 μs. In 18 distinct cluster headache attacks, acute SPG stimulation resulted in complete resolution of the headache in 11, partial resolution (>50% reduction in VAS) in 3 and no relief in 4 instances. In 10 migraine headache trials, acute SPG stimulation resulted in complete relief in 2, partial in 2 and no relief in 6 instances. SPG stimulation also resulted in resolution of the associated autonomic features of cluster and migraine headaches such as nasal congestion and periorbital swelling in all cases. Acute SPG stimulation did not alter hemodynamic parameters such as blood pressure, heart rate, heart rhythm, respiratory rate, oxygen saturation or neurological status. Ibarra [21] used an infrazygomatic approach with a permanent SPG stimulator, and demonstrated long-term benefits in a patient with cluster headaches.

Trigeminal autonomic cephalgias characteristically produce symptoms intermittently. An emerging approach under current investigation is the use of intermittent SPG stimulation on an as needed basis using a minimally invasive intra-oral approach and a small inductive coupled SPG stimulator implant that will be activated by an external energy delivery control device [unpubl. data].

Conclusion

The growing understanding of the role of the SPG in cerebrovascular autonomic physiology and conditions such as cluster and migraine headaches, as well as cerebral blood flow and stroke, has resulted in an increasing interest in interventional procedures aimed at SPG. SPG stimulation with its inherent reversible and adjustable feature, coupled with emerging minimally invasive and intermittent stimulation approaches, will facilitate the growth of SPG neuromodulation approaches.

References

1 Goadsby PJ: Pathophysiology of cluster headache: a trigeminal autonomic cephalgia. Lancet Neurol 2002;1:251–257.

2 Akerman S, Holland PR, Lasalandra MP, Goadsby PJ: Oxygen inhibits neuronal activation in the trigeminocervical complex after stimulation trigeminal autonomic reflex, but not during direct dural activation of trigeminal afferents. Headache 2009; 49:1131–1143.

3 Bartsch T, Goadsby PJ: The trigeminocervical complex and migraine: current concepts and synthesis. Curr Pain Headache Rep 2003;7:371–376.

4 Tepper SJ, Rezai A, Narouze S, Steiner C, Mohajer P, Ansarinia M: Acute treatment of intractable migraine with sphenopalatine ganglion electrical stimulation. Headache 2009;49:983–989.

5 Ansarinia M, Rezai A, Tepper SJ, Steiner CP, Stump J, Stanton-Hicks M, Machado A, Narouze S: Electrical stimulation of sphenopalatine ganglion for acute treatment of cluster headaches. Headache 2010;50:1164–1174.

6 Goadsby PJ: Sphenopalatine ganglion stimulation increases regional cerebral blood flow independent of glucose utilization in the cat. Brain Res 1990; 506:145–148.

7 Suzuki N, Hardebo JE, Kahrstrom J, Owman C: Selective electrical stimulation of postganglionic cerebrovascular parasympathetic nerve fibers originating from the sphenopalatine ganglion enhances cortical blood flow in the rat. J Cereb Blood Flow Metab 1990;10:383–391.

8 Toda N, Tanaka T, Ayajiki K, Okamura T: Cerebral vasodilatation induced by stimulation of the pterygopalatine ganglion and greater petrosal nerve in anesthesized monkeys. Neuroscience 2000;96: 393–398.

9 Yarnitsky D, Lorian A, Shalev A, Zhang ZD, Takahashi M, Agbaje-Williams M, Macdonald RL: Reversal of cerebral vasospasm by sphenopalatine ganglion stimulation in a dog model of subarachnoid hemorrhage. Surg Neurol 2005;64:5–11.

10 Sluder G: The anatomical and clinical relations of the sphenopalatine ganglion to the nose. NY State J Med 1909;90:293–298.

11 Headache Classification Committee of the International Headache Society: The International Classification of Headache Disorders, ed 2. Cephalalgia 2004;24(suppl 1):1–160.

12 Bolay H, Reuter U, Dunn AK, Huang Z, Boas DA, Moskowitz MA: Intrinsic brain activity triggers trigeminal meningeal afferents in a migraine model. Nat Med 2002;8:136–142.

13 Goadsby PJ, Macdonald GJ: Extracranial vasodilatation mediated by VIP (vasoactive intestinal polypeptide). Brain Res 1985;329:285–288.

14 Goadsby PJ, Uddman R, Edvinsson L: Cerebral vasodilatation in the cat involves nitric oxide from parasympathetic nerves. Brain Res 1996;707: 110–118.

15 Khurana D, Kaul S, Bornstein NM, ImpACT-1 Study Group: Implant for augmentation of cerebral blood flow trial 1: a pilot study evaluating the safety and effectiveness of the Ischaemic Stroke System for treatment of acute ischaemic stroke. Int J Stroke 2009;4:480–485.

16 Kittrelle JP, Grouse DS, Seybold ME: Cluster headache – local anesthetic abortive agents. Arch Neurol 1985;42:496–498.

17 Yang IY, Oraee S: A novel approach to transnasal sphenopalatine ganglion injection. Pain Physician 2006;9:131–134.

18 Narouze S, Kapural L, Casanova J, Mekhail N: Sphenopalatine ganglion radiofrequency ablation for the management of chronic cluster headache. Headache 2009;49:571–577.

19 Meyer JS, Binns PM, Ericsson AD, Vulpe M: Sphenopalatine ganglionectomy for cluster headache. Arch Otolaryngol 1970;92:475–484.

20 McClelland S 3rd, Tendulkar RD, Barnett GH, Neyman G, Suh JH: Long-term results of radiosurgery for refractory cluster headache. Neurosurgery 2006;59:1258–1262.

21 Ibarra E: Neuromodulacion del ganglio esfenopalatino para aliviar los sintomas de la cefalea en racimos: reporte de un caso. Boletin El Dolor 2007; 64:12–18.

22 Donnet A, Valade D, Regis J: Gamma knife treatment for refractory cluster headache: prospective open trial. J Neurol Neurosurg Psychiatry 2005;76: 218–221.

23 Kano H, Kondziolka D, Mathieu D, Stafford SL, Flannery TJ, Niranjan A, Pollock BE, Kaufmann AM, Flickinger JC, Lunsford LD: Stereotactic radiosurgery for intractable cluster headache: an initial report from the North American Gamma Knife Consortium. J Neurosurg 2010 Apr 30 [Epub ahead of print].
24 Ruskin SL: Techniques of sphenopalatine therapy. Eye Ear Nose Throat Mon 1951;30:28–31.
25 Narouze SN: Role of sphenopalatine ganglion neuroablation in the management of cluster headache. Curr Pain Headache Rep 2010;14:160–163.
26 Vallejo R, Benyamin R, Yousuf N, Kramer J: Computed tomography-enhanced sphenopalatine ganglion blockade. Pain Pract 2007;7:44–46.
27 Sluder G: Role of the sphenopalatine (Meckel's) ganglion in nasal headaches. NY State J Med 1908; 87:989–990.
28 Prasanna A, Murthy PS: Sphenopalatine ganglion block under vision using rigid nasal sinuscope. Reg Anesth 1993;18:139–140.
29 Felisati G, Arnone F, Lozza P, Leone M, Curone M, Bussone G: Sphenopalatine endoscopic ganglion block: a revision of a traditional technique for cluster headache. Laryngoscope 2006;116:1447–1450.

Ali R. Rezai, MD
Department of Neurological Surgery
Ohio State University Medical Center
N1043 Doan Hall, 410 West 10th Avenue, Columbus, OH 43210 (USA)
Tel. +1 614 366 2420, Fax +1 614 293 4281, E-Mail Ali.Rezai@osumc.edu

Slavin KV (ed): Peripheral Nerve Stimulation.
Prog Neurol Surg. Basel, Karger, 2011, vol 24, pp 180–188

Spinal Nerve Root Stimulation

Christopher P. Kellner · Michael A. Kellner · Christopher J. Winfree

Department of Neurological Surgery, Columbia University Medical Center, New York, N.Y., USA

Abstract

Spinal nerve root stimulation (SNRS) is a neuromodulation technique that is used to treat chronic pain. This modality places stimulator electrode array(s) along the spinal nerve roots, creating stimulation paresthesias within the distribution of the target nerve root(s), thereby treating pain in that same distribution. There are several different forms of spinal nerve root stimulation, depending upon the exact electrode positioning along the nerve roots. SNRS combines the minimally invasive nature, central location, and ease of placement of spinal cord stimulation with the focal targeting of stimulation paresthesias of peripheral nerve stimulation. This hybrid technique may be an effective alternative for patients in whom other forms of neurostimulation are either ineffective or inappropriate.

Since the first use of a spinal cord stimulator (SCS) for the treatment of neuropathic pain 43 years ago, neuromodulation in the spinal cord has established itself as a standard of care for a number of indications [1]. Although incompletely understood, SCS was born out of the theory proposed in 1965 by Melzack and Wall [2] in which paresthesias perceived by the brain in the same region as a painful sensation, can dull and even alleviate pain. Over time, the indications for SCS have broadened and now include failed back syndrome [3], radiculopathy [4], peripheral neuropathy [5], peripheral vascular disease [6], chronic unstable angina [7], and complex regional pain syndrome [8].

Although indications for SCS have expanded and a few randomized trials have shown its efficacy, there are a number of limitations. These problems include electrode migration, durability, and variable efficacy depending on patient posture and activity [9]. The anatomy of the spinal cord itself limits SCS in that deeper tracts are more difficult to stimulate, and therefore it is difficult to stimulate certain dermatomes, such as the sacral dermatomes.

Given these limitations of SCS and the development of novel electrodes, other forms of neurostimulation have gained traction throughout the neuro-axis. Peripheral nerve stimulation (PNS) in particular has found application in a number of pain syndromes that involve single nerves or discreet regions of the body. The most common syndromes treated with this modality include occipital neuralgia [10], trigeminal neuropathic pain [11], and other neuropathies due to individual nerves such as the ilioinguinal, iliohypogastric, and genitofemoral nerves [12]. Drawbacks to PNS include limited and/or complicated surgical access to some nerves, nerve mobility leading to electrode migration or malfunction, and restricted pain relief that covers only the distribution of a single nerve.

Spinal nerve root stimulation (SNRS) for the treatment of pain was born out of the limitations of both SCS and PNS. The techniques were adapted from both SCS and PNS. SNRS involves direct electrical stimulation of specific nerve roots either within or adjacent to the spinal canal [13]. The patient thus experiences stimulation parasthesias within the dermatomal distributions of the stimulated nerve roots. Depending upon the electrode configuration, single or multiple nerve roots can be stimulated simultaneously. In most cases, paresthesias can be restricted to these nerve roots, with little to no unwanted stimulation elsewhere. Given the reliability of the dermatomal sensory distributions, SNRS can direct stimulation to very specific and reproducible regions of the body that are sometimes inaccessible to SCS or PNS. SNRS employs electrodes that are located within the spinal column, which may protect them to some degree from the migration seen in the more mobile peripheral nervous system [14].

Clinical Evidence and Indications for Spinal Nerve Root Stimulation

There currently exists no class I or class II data on the efficacy of SNRS. Management decisions today are based on reviews [13, 15], case reports, and case series describing the indications, effects, and complications associated with SNRS. This literature will be described below after the introduction of each of the four specific surgical SNRS techniques (table 1). Here we describe the recent efforts to evaluate SNRS in prospective and/or randomized trials.

Spinal nerve root stimulation has been inadequately evaluated in most indications and especially neuropathic pain in general. A prospective trial was recently undertaken to evaluate the efficacy of SNRS in the treatment of patients with neuropathic pain refractory to medical treatment [16]. Although all patients had a successful stimulation test, the therapeutic effects dwindled to zero over the period of a few months despite stimulator adjustment. The study, which only included three patients, was stopped due to the loss of a beneficial effect as well as side effects such as pain attacks or motor phenomena.

There are a limited number of ongoing trials specifically evaluating the clinical benefits of spinal nerve root stimulation in the treatment of pain. A trial in Singapore is examining the use of magnetic stimulation versus placebo to treat chronic neuropathic pain and

Table 1. Categories of spinal nerve root stimulation with respective appropriate spinal cord levels and advantages

Category	Appropriate levels	Advantages
Intraspinal	C2-coccygeal	can target multiple roots per electrode
Transforaminal	caudal thoracic-sacral	less likely to undergo migration than intraspinal placement
Extraforaminal	sacral	least invasive technique for targeting bladder roots
Trans-spinal	C2-S1	unaffected by epidural scarring, stenosis, or fusion at adjacent levels

has recently completed its enrollment but not yet published the results (NCT00443469). Another clinical trial was undertaken to compare intraspinal nerve root stimulation with dorsal column stimulation, but according the clinicaltrials.gov, the trial was terminated due to slow enrollment (NCT00370773). This is an essential question that needs a randomized, blinded clinical trial to properly compare the two options. Further studies are needed to evaluate this form of neuromodulation in various pain syndromes.

Intraspinal Nerve Root Stimulation

Intraspinal nerve root stimulation describes a procedure in which the entire stimulator electrode array is located within the spinal canal. Advantages of this technique are that because the electrode array is oriented cranial-caudally, it can cover multiple nerve roots with a single lead, and the technique is quite similar to dorsal column stimulation, except that the electrodes are placed more laterally in the spinal canal (fig. 1). Thus, most practitioners will readily adapt to its technique. Unlike SCS, intraspinal SNRS targets the exiting dorsal rootlets as they coalesce to form the dorsal spinal nerve root. This intraspinal location also permits its application at any level throughout the spinal axis.

Although the original article describing intraspinal nerve root stimulation utilized a laminectomy to access the spinal cord [17], current procedures are performed almost entirely percutaneously. The introducer needle is advanced into the epidural space at a distance from the level or levels of interest. Once the epidural space is entered, the electrode is steered along the midline until about one spinal segment away from the target level. At that point the electrode is steered laterally, and guided so that it lies just medial to the pedicle(s) associated with the target nerve root(s).

The cervical, thoracic, and rostral lumbar nerve roots are targeted using this anterograde approach [17, 18]. For access to the caudal lumbar and sacral levels, the

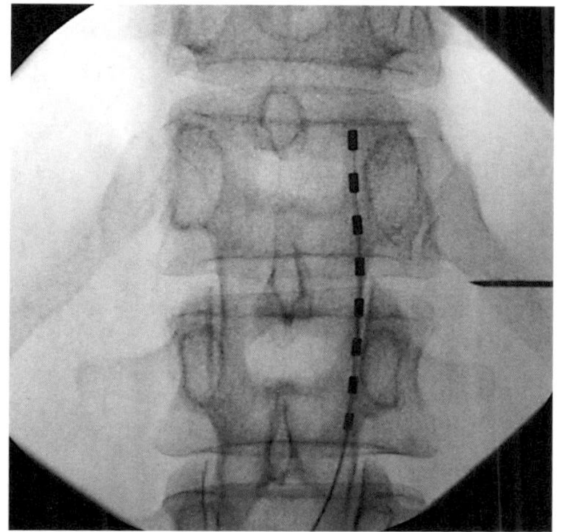

Fig. 1. Intraoperative fluoroscopy showing an intraspinal nerve root stimulator electrode at the right T12-L1 levels. Note that the electrode is immediately medial to the T12 and L1 pedicles, providing selective stimulation to those nerve roots. Note that the electrode is passed up the midline epidural space and then steered laterally within 1–2 segments of the target level to minimize the risk of the electrode passing ventral to the thecal sac.

needle is introduced at a lumbar level and advanced caudally and laterally, in a retrograde fashion, such that it lies parallel spinal roots as they travel within the canal [19]. This retrograde percutaneous approach is contraindicated, or is at least difficult in patients with anatomical abnormalities in the lumbosacral spine, such as epidural fibrosis, spina bifida occulta, lateral and central stenosis, spondylosis, and spondylolisthesis [9]. In some cases an anterograde approach through the sacral hiatus may be used to access the sacral and caudal lumbar levels. The length of the electrode array will determine the number of nerve roots covered.

Clinical Evidence and Indications

The intraspinal technique can target essentially any spinal level. Thus, dermatomal pain of almost unimaginable variety can potentially be treated with this technique [9, 13, 15]. Standard, compact, or subcompact electrode arrays can provide stimulation to single levels, whereas a pair of 'stacked' octapolar leads can cover up to five levels and still require only a single implantable pulse generator (fig. 2).

Transforaminal Nerve Root Stimulation

Transforaminal nerve root stimulation entails placing an electrode first within the spinal epidural space and then directing it out through the neural foramen (fig. 3). Direct stimulation to a single nerve root and dorsal root ganglion is therefore made possible [13]. Initially, transforaminal nerve root stimulator implantation mimics retrograde intraspinal stimulator placement [18, 19]. The electrode is directed into the spinal canal in a retrograde fashion, and then steered out of the neural

2 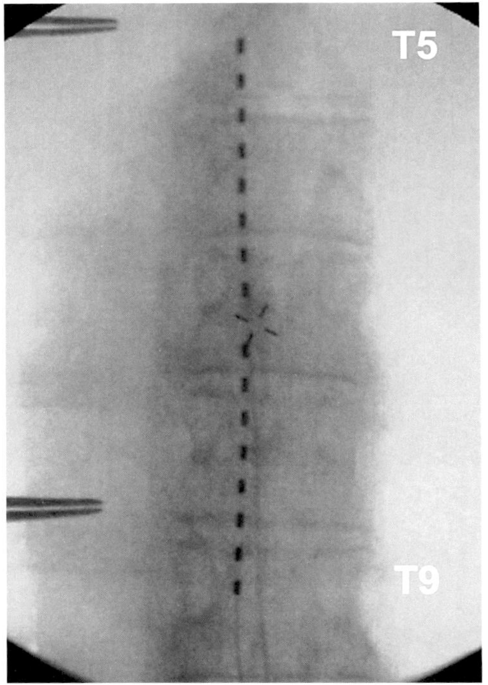

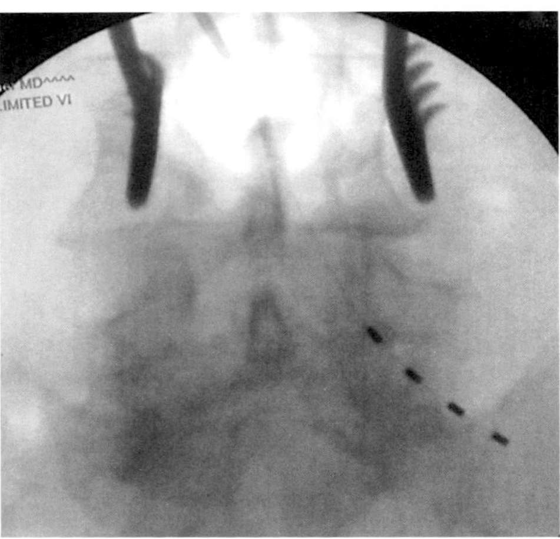 3

Fig. 2. Intraoperative fluoroscopy showing two 8-contact intraspinal nerve root stimulation electrodes spanning the right T5-T9 levels. This patient has postherpetic neuralgia that regionalized to these five levels, and was treated successfully with this electrode array.
Fig. 3. Anteroposterior radiograph showing L-5 and S-1 transforaminal spinal nerve root electrodes.

foramina at the level of interest. Isolation and stimulation of individual nerve roots is facilitated by this procedure. To stimulate multiple nerve roots or dorsal root ganglia, it is necessary to insert multiple electrode arrays. Caudal thoracic, lumbar and sacral nerve roots can be targeted with this approach. The cervical and rostral thoracic nerve roots exit the spinal canal at an essentially 90° angle, too sharp a turn to reliably steer currently available electrodes out of the spinal canal along the nerve root.

Clinical Evidence and Indications
In the transforaminal technique, electrode placement varies according to the pain and paresthestic pattern of the patient and can be adjusted for individualized treatment course. Studies have demonstrated that the technique can be used to alleviate symptoms associated with ilioinguinal neuralgia, discogenic back pain, peripheral neuropathy, failed back surgery syndrome, and interstitial cystitis [13, 18, 19]. The complications associated with this approach are similar to those associated with the

intraspinal approach, which include CSF leakage and inappropriate electrode placement in the intrathecal sac. Nerve root damage, however, is also a possibility with this approach due to the location of the electrode placement.

Extraforaminal Nerve Root Stimulation

This technique involves insertion of the electrode directly into the neural foramina from a posterior or lateral approach without going through the spinal canal. Similar to transforaminal approach, this approach requires one electrode for each individual nerve root. The extraforaminal approach is most often used in the stimulation of the sacral nerve roots, predominantly for urologic dysfunction. The sacral nerve roots are technically easier to access directly than through the intraspinal or transforaminal approaches that both pass retrograde through the spinal canal [20]. Common technique involves electrode insertion into the S-3 foramen using a posterior approach. Addition of fluoroscopy and improvement in secure leads have made this procedure less invasive and more reliable [21].

Application of the extraforaminal approach to other locations of the spine is uncommon and therefore, should be considered in patients who are no candidates for other technique. Patients with evidence of stenotic foramen and obesity may be at increased risk of operative morbidity. When performing a cervical nerve root stimulation extraforaminally, posterolateral introduction of the needle allows electrode insertion parallel to the nerve root [22]. This is important for minimizing injury to the adjacent neurovascular structures.

Clinical Evidence and Indications

Both ventral and dorsal sacral nerve root stimulation with the extraforaminal technique have been reported with satisfactory results. A wide gamut of indications has been tested, such as bladder dysfunction, urge incontinence, urinary retention, and fecal incontinence. In addition, patients with paraplegia and quadriplegia have been treated with satisfactory results [23]. The dorsal route for insertion of electrodes is preferred because it carries less risk for complications such as CSF leak, neurovascular injury, and infection.

Extraforaminal nerve root stimulation has played a major role in the treatment of urologic disease, both through ventral and dorsal stimulation. Dorsal stimulation, however, has been shown to be preferred to ventral stimulation due to a lower side effect profile. This urologic pathology includes urinary urge incontinence [9, 24], urgency-frequency syndromes [25], urinary retention [26], pelvic floor muscle overactivity [25], Fowler syndrome [26], fecal incontinence [27], and interstitial cystitis [26–31]. Extraforaminal nerve root stimulation is particularly suited for the treatment of bladder dysfunction because this clinical manifestation often results from lack of coordination between the reflexes of the bladder, its sphincter, and pelvic floor

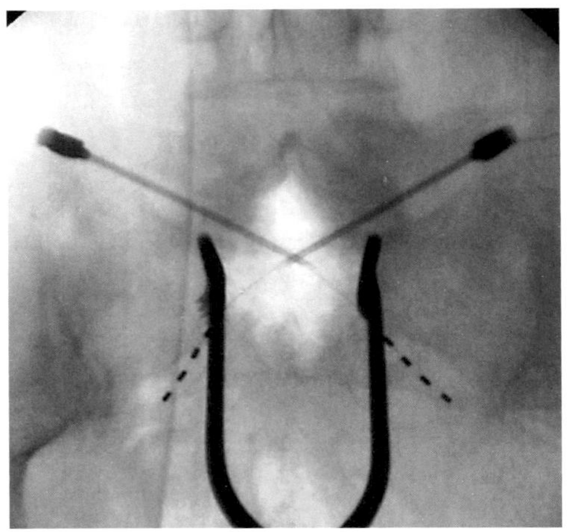

Fig. 4. Intraoperative fluoroscopic image during placement of bilateral trans-spinal nerve root electrodes at the S1 level. The epidural space was accessed through a small midline laminectomy. Each electrode was placed through a small stab incision on the contralateral side, aiming in the direction of the target nerve root foramen. Note the placement of the electrodes within the neural foramen, in a position overlying both the spinal nerve root and the dorsal root ganglion. This may be done through either a percutaneous or an open approach. Also, this technique may be used when previous surgery, scarring, or fusion mass at adjacent levels prevent the use of other nerve root stimulation approaches.

muscles. A multicenter trial with 177 patients was conducted to evaluate the benefit of extraforaminal SNRS for urinary retention and showed improvement in both the rate of symptoms and the rate of self-catheterization [26].

There exists a paucity of reports in the literature regarding extraforaminal SNRS specifically for the treatment of pain in the cervical spine. In one case report, the patient presented with paresthesias and burning unilaterally due to a herniated disk and cervical spinal stenosis. Fusion did not produce improvement and a conventional SCS could not be used due to the stenosis, so an electrode was placed through the extraforaminal technique, which led to pain relief [22].

Trans-Spinal Nerve Root Stimulation

In the trans-spinal technique, the electrode is directed from the side opposite of the target nerve root, passed across the midline at the level of the epidural space, and sent into the target neural foramen (fig. 4). There is a paucity of literature and evidence on this technique, which was first reported in 1982 [32] and is rarely used in clinical practice [15, 33]. The technique may be advantageous over other approaches in that it allows for electrode insertion in regions that are particularly challenging, such as the upper thoracic and cervical spine [15]. In these areas, the spinal nerve roots exit nearly perpendicular to the neural foramina, making it nearly impossible to adequately angle the electrode into the neural foramina from the caudal direction. In addition, the usual transforaminal technique is contraindicated above C-5 due to the proximity of the vertebral artery to the nerve roots at foraminal level. The authors have also found this technique useful for targeting nerve roots immediately adjacent to previously operated, scarred, or fused spinal levels. Since the electrode is directed immediately into the contralateral neural foramen at the desired level, without requiring guidance through several levels of epidural space, as in the transforaminal or intraspinal techniques, adjacent scarring or fusion mass is not usually a problem if present.

Conclusion

Spinal nerve root stimulation is an effective neuromodulatory treatment for chronic pain conditions. This technique combines the advantages of spinal cord stimulation, with the ease of placement and stability of the spinal canal for anchoring options, and the specificity of stimulation paresthesias seen with peripheral nerve stimulation. Although these techniques are already useful additions to the armamentarium of interventional pain physicians, future clinical studies will be needed to establish their indications and confirm long-term clinical efficacy.

References

1 Shealy CN, Mortimer JT, Reswick JB: Electrical inhibition of pain by stimulation of the dorsal columns: preliminary clinical report. Anesth Analg 1967;46:489–491.
2 Melzack R, Wall PD: Pain mechanisms: a new theory. Science 1965;150:971–979.
3 North RB, Calkins SK, Campbell DS, Sieracki JM, Piantadosi S, Daly MJ, Dey PB, Barolat G: Automated, patient-interactive, spinal cord stimulator adjustment: a randomized controlled trial. Neurosurgery 2003;52:572–580; discussion 579–580.
4 Burchiel KJ, Anderson VC, Brown FD, Fessler RG, Friedman WA, Pelofsky S, Weiner RL, Oakley J, Shatin D: Prospective, multicenter study of spinal cord stimulation for relief of chronic back and extremity pain. Spine 1996;21:2786–2794.
5 Kumar K, Toth C, Nath RK, Laing P: Epidural spinal cord stimulation for treatment of chronic pain – some predictors of success: a 15-year experience. Surg Neurol 1998;50:110–120; discussion 120–121.
6 Amann W, Berg P, Gersbach P, Gamain J, Raphael JH, Ubbink DT, Group S-ES: Spinal cord stimulation in the treatment of non-reconstructable stable critical leg ischaemia: results of the European peripheral vascular disease outcome study (SCS-EPOS). Eur J Vasc Endovasc Surgery 2003;26: 280–286.
7 Dejongste MJL, Hautvast RWM, Hillege HL, Lie KI: Efficacy of spinal cord stimulation as adjuvant therapy for intractable angina pectoris – a prospective, randomized clinical study. J Am Coll Card 1994;23: 1592–1597.
8 Kemler MA, Barendse GA, van Kleef M, de Vet HC, Rijks CP, Furnee CA, van den Wildenberg FA: Spinal cord stimulation in patients with chronic reflex sympathetic dystrophy. N Engl J Med 2000; 343:618–624.
9 Aló KM, Holsheimer J: New trends in neuromodulation for the management of neuropathic pain. Neurosurgery 2002;50:690–703.
10 Weiner RL, Reed KL: Peripheral neurostimulation for control of intractable occipital neuralgia. Neuromodulation 1999;2:217–221.
11 Slavin KV, Wess C: Trigeminal branch stimulation for intractable neuropathic pain: technical note. Neuromodulation 2005;8:7–13.
12 de Leon-Casasola OA: Spinal cord and peripheral nerve stimulation techniques for neuropathic pain. J Pain Symptom Manage 2009;38:S28–S38.
13 Haque R, Winfree CJ: Spinal nerve root stimulation: Neurosurg Focus 2006;21:E4.
14 Kunnumpurath S, Srinivasagopalan R, Vadivelu N: Spinal cord stimulation: principles of past, present and future practice: a review. J Clin Monit Comput 2009;23:333–339.
15 Stuart RM, Winfree CJ: Neurostimulation techniques for painful peripheral nerve disorders. Neurosurg Clin N Am 2009;20:111–120.

16 Weigel R, Capelle HH, Krauss JK: Failure of long-term nerve root stimulation to improve neuropathic pain. J Neurosurg 2008;108:921–925.
17 Falco FJE, Rubbani M, Heinbaugh J: Anterograde sacral nerve root stimulation (ASNRS) via the sacral hiatus: benefits, limitations, and percutaneous implantation technique. Neuromodulation 2003;6: 219–224.
18 Feler CA, Whitworth LA, Fernandez J: Sacral neuromodulation for chronic pain conditions. Anesthesiol Clin N Am 2003;21:785–795.
19 Aló KM, Yland MJ, Redko V, Feler C, Naumann C: Lumbar and sacral nerve root stimulation (NRS) in the treatment of chronic pain: a novel anatomic approach and neuro stimulation technique. Neuromodulation 1999;2:23–31.
20 Tanagho EA, Schmidt RA, Orvis BR: Neural stimulation for control of voiding dysfunction: a preliminary report in 22 patients with serious neuropathic voiding disorders. J Urol 1989;142: 340–345.
21 Chai TC, Mamo GJ: Modified techniques of S3 foramen localization and lead implantation in S3 neuromodulation. Urology 2001;58:786–790.
22 Falco FJ, Kim D, Onyewu CO: Cervical nerve root stimulation: demonstration of an extra-foraminal technique. Pain Physician 2004;7:99–102.
23 Kutzenberger J, Domurath B, Sauerwein D: Spastic bladder and spinal cord injury: seventeen years of experience with sacral deafferentation and implantation of an anterior root stimulator. Artif Organs 2005;29:239–241.
24 Aló KM, Gohel R, Corey CL: Sacral nerve root stimulation for the treatment of urge incontinence and detrusor dysfunction utilizing a cephalocaudal intraspinal method of lead insertion: a case report. Neuromodulation 2001;4:53–58.
25 Pettit PD, Thompson JR, Chen AH: Sacral neuromodulation: new applications in the treatment of female pelvic floor dysfunction. Curr Opin Obstet Gynecol 2002;14:521–525.
26 Jonas U, Fowler CJ, Chancellor MB, Elhilali MM, Fall M, Gajewski JB, Grunewald V, Hassouna MM, Hombergh U, Janknegt R, van Kerrebroeck PE, Lylcklama a Nijeholt AA, Siegel SW, Schmidt RA: Efficacy of sacral nerve stimulation for urinary retention: results 18 months after implantation. J Urol 2001;165:15–19.
27 Hassouna M, Elmayergi N, Abdelhady M: Update on sacral neuromodulation: indications and outcomes. Curr Urol Rep 2003;4:391–398.
28 Bosch JLHR, Groen J: Sacral nerve neuromodulation in the treatment of patients with refractory motor urge incontinence: long-term results of a prospective longitudinal study. J Urol 2000;163: 1219–1222.
29 Schmidt RA, Jonas U, Oleson KA, Janknegt RA, Hassouna MM, Siegel SW, van Kerrebroeck PE: Sacral nerve stimulation for treatment of refractory urinary urge incontinence: sacral Nerve Stimulation Study Group. J Urol 1999;162:352–357.
30 Shaker H, Hassouna MM: Sacral root neuromodulation in the treatment of various voiding and storage problems. Int Urogynecol J Pelvic Floor Dysfunct 1999;10:336–343.
31 Shaker HS, Hassouna M: Sacral nerve root neuromodulation: an effective treatment for refractory urge incontinence. J Urol 1998;159: 1516–1519.
32 Urban BJ, Nashold BS Jr: Combined epidural and peripheral nerve stimulation for relief of pain: description of technique and preliminary results. J Neurosurg 1982;57:365–369.
33 Aló KM, Yland MJ, Feler C, Oakley J: A study of electrode placement at cervical and upper thoracic nerve roots using an anatomic trans-spinal approach. Neuromodulation 1999;2:222–227.

Christopher J. Winfree, MD, FACS
Department of Neurological Surgery
Columbia University, College of Physicians and Surgeons
710 West 168th Street, 4th Floor, New York, NY 10032 (USA)
Tel. +1 212 342 2776, Fax +1 212 305 3629, E-Mail cjw12@columbia.edu

Slavin KV (ed): Peripheral Nerve Stimulation.
Prog Neurol Surg. Basel, Karger, 2011, vol 24, pp 189–202

Technical Aspects of Peripheral Nerve Stimulation: Hardware and Complications

Konstantin V. Slavin

Department of Neurosurgery, University of Illinois at Chicago, Chicago, Ill., USA

Abstract

Although commonly used in clinical practice, peripheral nerve stimulation (PNS) for treatment of chronic pain is performed mainly with devices developed and marketed for spinal cord stimulation applications. This may be one of the reasons why PNS approach is marked by a very high complication rate, as the anatomy of peripheral nerves and the surrounding soft tissues is quite different from epidural spinal space for which the current devices are designed. The chapter reviews integral components of PNS systems and accessories. It also lists variety of complications observed with PNS approach and points to the ways to minimize their incidence. Based on the literature data and the analysis of the author's experience with PNS procedures it appears that although the rate of complications is relatively high, the morbidity associated with PNS approach is very minor and most problems may be resolved with simple re-operations, usually on outpatient basis. The reduction in complication rate is expected to occur when the hardware used in PNS procedures is appropriately adapted for PNS applications.

Electrical stimulation of peripheral nerves is used in a variety of medical applications. The most common ones include testing neuromuscular conduction in anesthesia and intensive care units; motor stimulation of phrenic nerves in cases of diaphragmal palsy and somatic nerves of the extremities in patients with hemiplegia and paraplegia; vagal nerve stimulation for treatment of intractable epilepsy and refractory depression; autonomic stimulation for urinary and gastrointestinal disorders; carotid sinus stimulation for hypertension and angina pectoris, and, finally, the stimulation of peripheral nerves for control of neuropathic pain [1].

Although peripheral nerve stimulation (PNS) has been a part of the neurosurgical armamentarium in treatment of chronic pain for almost a half of century, the entire approach is still far from perfection. Unfortunately, this includes not only absence of strong scientific evidence of its effectiveness, but also relatively high incidence of technical complications and re-operations, some or even most of which are related to the fact that most of the devices used for PNS today are neither designed nor approved for this application. Although there are some hardware choices that include PNS in its labeling, vast majority of presently used PNS hardware are in fact designed and approved exclusively for spinal cord stimulation (SCS).

Components of Peripheral Nerve Stimulation Systems

In general, neuromodulation devices consist of several distinct components and the terminology that describes them seems to be nonuniform among the implanters and the device manufacturers. Below is an attempt to provide a unified approach to this terminology and then use it for review of technical complications that may be related in one way or another to the hardware choices.

The electrical energy is delivered to the peripheral nerve by small metal contacts that are arranged on a lead, or electrode. The leads come in different shapes and sizes; and the ones that are used today for treatment of pain are generally divided into (a) so-called percutaneous, cylindrical, or wire-like leads, and (b) flat leads, that are also called paddles, surgical leads or laminectomy-type leads.

In the past, before both of these lead types became available, the electrodes were custom made or manufactured in small quantities. First electrodes were essentially wires that were inserted into the nerve or immediately next to it. This kind of electrodes was used by Wall and Sweet when they were testing 'gate control' theory of pain by stimulating their own infraorbital nerves [2]. At about same time, cuff electrodes were created for long-term direct stimulation of the peripheral nerves. This type of electrodes was used by Shelden and colleagues in the early 1960s, even before the 'gate control' theory of pain (that became a theoretical basis for electrical stimulation for pain control) was introduced [3]. At that time, a Silastic ring that included a metal contact for nerve stimulation would be wrapped around the exposed segment of the nerve.

This technique of electrode application, not surprisingly, was associated with scarring around the dissected nerve as well as with development of fibrosis and nerve constriction from the lead itself. In addition to that, there was an issue related to preferential stimulation of only the nerve segment that was located under the metal contact. This was not a problem in case of smaller and homogeneous sensory nerves, but in case of larger mixed nerves, such arrangement might cause predominantly motor effects and, as a result, desired paresthesias might be associated with muscle contractions. To overcome this problem, it was suggested to use 'button'-type electrodes [4]. These small electrodes could then be sutured directly to the perineurium over the part of nerve circumference that corresponded to underlying sensory fascicles. Although time consuming and requiring a great deal of nerve manipulation, this approach was particularly useful when dealing with the sciatic nerve or the brachial plexus.

Neither cuff-type nor button-type leads are used any more in the field of pain surgery, but in the neighboring fields of neuromodulation these wrap-around (cuff) leads are still being used on regular basis. Two best examples of this are vagal nerve stimulators (Cyberonics, Houston, Tex., USA) used for treatment of refractory epilepsy and treatment-resistant depression, and phrenic nerve stimulators (Avery Biomedical Devices, Comack, N.Y., USA) that are implanted for diaphragmal pacing in treatment of respiratory failure.

The use of flat (paddle-type) leads in PNS was introduced in the late 1980s [5]. Here, the lead was implanted under the nerve in a way that all 4 flat metal contacts of that quadripolar lead were facing the nerve. Such innovation made an impact on the consistency and versatility of stimulation as having multiple contacts along the same nerve gave more freedom in terms of stimulation programming. In order to further reduce the incidence of perineural fibrosis, it was then recommended to use a fascial 'padding' between the metal contacts and the nerve, and then, in a logical progression of this approach, a lead with a mesh attached to it was developed specifically for PNS applications (OnPoint, Medtronic, Minneapolis, Minn., USA) [6]. The most commonly used paddle-type leads are listed in table 1.

Introduction of percutaneous PNS technique in the mid-1990s [7] changed the landscape of hardware used for this application. Both quadripolar (4-contact) and octopolar (8-contact) electrode leads have been used for this purpose, initially in occipital nerve stimulation, followed by stimulation of trigeminal branches, and then in peripheral nerves of the trunk and extremities. Percutaneous electrodes from three major neuromodulation manufacturing companies (Medtronic; Advanced Neuromodulation Systems (ANS – currently St. Jude Neuromodulation), Plano, Tex., USA; and Advanced Bionics (currently Boston Scientific), Valencia, Calif., USA) have been successfully used for PNS applications (table 1).

The number of contacts in a lead, as well as the number of leads in a patient has traditionally been limited by another part of each neuromodulation device – electrical generator of stimulation. Early neuromodulation experience was based on radiofrequency (RF)-coupled systems. Here the generator of impulses and all control units are located outside the patient's body. The receiver is implanted subcutaneously and connected to the electrode lead(s) either directly or with special extension cables. The impulses are transmitted through the skin with a special flexible pancake-shaped antenna that is placed (usually with support of tape or adhesive pad) over implanted receiver and the power source/programming module is worn externally. Main advantages of this system are its ability to deliver high-power complex stimulation and extreme ease in replenishing power supply as most external generators are powered by regular household batteries (1.5 or 9 V). Theoretically, RF-coupled devices may serve forever without additional surgical interventions.

Most RF-coupled systems allow operations with two or more independent channels and are capable of covering 4-, 8- or 16-electrode contacts. This has been particularly important in patients with complex pain patterns and in those cases where pain areas

Table 1. Commonly used paddle and percutaneous electrodes

Percutaneous electrodes	Paddle electrodes
Medtronic	***Medtronic***
4 contacts	*4 contacts*
(frequently referred to as Quad)	**Resume II** (3587A)
Pisces Standard (3487A)	**Resume TL** (3986A)
Pisces Plus (3888)	**On-Point** (3987A)
Pisces Compact (3887)	Resume (3986, out of production)
Verify (temporary) (3862)	Symmix (3982, out of production)
8 contacts	*8 contacts*
(frequently referred to as Octad)	Specify (3988, 3998)
1 x 8 Standard (3777, 3898)	2 × 4 Hinged Specify (3999)
1 x 8 Compact (3778)	*16 contacts*
1 x 8 Subcompact (3776)	Specify 2 × 8 (39286)
	Specify 5-6-5 (39565)
St. Jude Medical	***St. Jude Medical***
4 contacts	*4 contacts*
Quattrode 7 mm (3141, 3143, 3146, 3149)	Lamitrode 22 (3222)
Quattrode 10 mm (3151, 3153, 3156, 3159)	**Lamitrode 4** (3240, 3254, 3255)
Quattrode 7 mm trial (3046)	**Lamitrode S4** (3243, 3246, 3266, 3267)
Quattrode wide spaced (3161, 3163, 3166, 3169)	*8 contacts*
Quattrode wide spaced trial (3066)	Lamitrode 44 (3244, 3262, 3263)
Axxess Quad 3/4 (4143, 4146)	Lamitrode 44C (3245, 3264, 3265)
Axxess Quad 3/6 (4153, 4156)	**Lamitrode 8** (3280)
Axxess Quad 3/4 trial (4044)	**Lamitrode S8** (3268, 3269, 3283, 3286)
Axxess Quad 3/6 trial (4054)	Lamitrode Tripole 8 (3210)
8 contacts	Lamitrode Tripole 8C (3208)
Octrode (3181, 3183, 3186, 3189)	Exclaim (3224, 3225)
Octrode trial (3086)	*16 contacts*
	Lamitrode 88 (3288)
	Lamitrode 88C (3289)
	Lamitrode Tripole 16 (3219)
	Lamitrode Tripole 16C (3214)
	Penta (3228)
Boston Scientific	***Boston Scientific***
8 contacts	*16 contacts*
Linear (2108)	**Artesan** (8116)
Linear ST (2208, 2218)	**Artesan** (slotted contact) (8120)
Linear Phase III (2138, 2158)	
Linear 3-4 (2352)	
Linear 3-6 (2366)	

Electrodes used for PNS are in bold, model numbers are in parentheses.

change with time, since in the past implantable generators had very limited power and programming capabilities. On the other hand, RF-coupled systems require a significantly higher degree of patient participation, which may be difficult for some chronic pain patients. Some RF system users develop dermatitis or other local skin reactions that prevent them from wearing the antennas for extended periods of time. Also, some patients stated that having a permanent external device limits their freedom, eliminates ability to maintain stimulation while showering, bathing or swimming, and they were often willing to trade some of the benefits of RF-coupled systems for a completely implantable system [8]. In the past, RF-coupled devices manufactured by Medtronic and ANS were able to provide an alternative to implantable pulse generators (IPG) – and, as a matter of fact, today the RF-coupled systems remain the only devices that are approved for PNS applications. However, it appears that in treatment of chronic pain these systems are hardly ever used any more, and it is conceivable that one of the reasons they are still listed in the product catalogues is to have this indication (stimulation of peripheral nerves for treatment of pain) open for clinical and marketing purposes. The breathing pacemakers (Avery Biomedical Devices), on the other hand, continue using RF-coupled technology. The company that manufactures them was a major pioneer in the field of PNS hardware but left the pain surgery arena to focus exclusively on the diaphragm-pacing products.

The alternative to externally powered RF systems is a completely internalized device. Here, the power source and impulse controller are contained in a pacemaker-like device – an implantable pulse generator (IPG). Fully implantable devices are more convenient for patients because the entire stimulation system is placed inside the patient's body and the need for external attachments is eliminated. Patients can swim or shower without stopping the stimulation and do not have to worry about poor contact between the antenna and receiver. IPG systems, particularly the non-rechargeable ones, have only limited internal battery power, and, therefore, must be replaced every several (usually between 1 and 10) years, depending on the system usage, battery size and stimulation parameters. This obviously increases the long-term cost of the hardware.

The first generation of IPGs accommodated 4 contacts and was routinely limited to using a single quadripolar lead. The first three consecutive models representing this generation were made by Medtronic (ITREL, Itrel II and Itrel 3) and this line of devices is still in production as some patients continue to enjoy benefits of stimulation with a single 4-contact lead. Subsequent generation (Synergy and Synergy Versitrel from Medtronic and Genesis/Genesis XP from ANS) of IPGs accommodated up to 8 contacts and allowed patients to have more than one stimulation program. The latest generation of devices extended this capacity to 16 contacts – and, in the meantime, the rechargeability became a common feature. Introduction of Precision system (Boston Scientific) was followed by other rechargeable 16-contact devices from Medtronic (Restore) and St. Jude (Eon), and soon thereafter smaller devices (Restore Ultra, Medtronic, and Eon Mini, St. Jude) completed the lineup of most commonly

Table 2. Commonly used implantable pulse generators (IPG) and radiofrequency (RF) receivers

Primary cell IPG	Rechargeable IPG	RF receivers
Medtronic *4 contacts* Itrel (out of production) Itrel II (7424 – out of production) ITREL 3 (7425) *8 contacts* Synergy (7427) Synergy Versitrel (7427V) *16 contacts* RestorePrime (37701) PrimeAdvanced (37702)	***Medtronic*** *16 contacts* Restore (37711) RestoreAdvanced (37713) RestoreUltra (37712)	***Medtronic*** *4 contacts* X-trel (3470 – out of production) *8 contacts* Mattrix (3271/3272)
St. Jude Medical *8 contacts* Genesis (3608, 3643) Genesis XP (3609, 3644) *16 contacts* Eon C (3688)	***St. Jude Medical*** *8 contacts* Genesis RC (3708, 3744) *16 contacts* Eon (3716) Eon Mini (3788)	***St. Jude Medical*** *8 contacts* Renew (3408) *16 contacts* Renew (3416)
	Boston Scientific *16 contacts* Precision (1110)	

Model numbers are in parentheses.

used devices (table 2). The rechargeable batteries make it possible to cover larger areas with stimulation using multiple electrode leads, and the usage-limiting issues related to a continuous use of the device (versus cycling or turning it off at night in order to lengthen battery life), higher frequencies and amplitudes of stimulation are not as overwhelming any more as the batteries may be recharged as needed and are expected to last between 7 and 10 years.

The recharging, however, may be an issue for some of the patients, particularly the elderly and those with memory and cognition problems, and for these circumstances there are non-rechargeable (primary cell) IPG choices that maintain same programming capacity (PrimeAdvanced, Medtronic, and EonC, St. Jude).

In addition to electrode leads and generators/receivers, there are multiple additional hardware pieces that are important in assuring lasting benefits from PNS. First are the extension cables (sometimes called simply extensions). With earlier Medtronic models, extensions were an integral part of the stimulation system, but with those devices that are used today, extensions are needed only if the electrode tail does not reach the IPG or if such reach results in tension at rest or during movements. The bulkiness of the connectors on the original extension cables was resolved with lower-profile devices, and in addition to that there are now new contraptions that convert old extensions into more standard in-line multicontact tails.

There is another purpose for the extensions – these days such cables serve not only as true conducting devices, but also as means of connecting two 4-contact electrodes to a single channel in IPG (so-called bifurcated extensions). These are available with both Medtronic and St. Jude Medical devices. Moreover, there are now so-called splitters (Boston Scientific) that reduce the number of used contacts on each electrode lead from 8 to 4 thereby allowing one to use only certain contacts from each lead for active stimulation (these active contacts may be, for example, the distal 4 of 8 or the 1, 3, 6 and 8 contacts – depending on the splitter model). Both standard bifurcated extensions and splitters allow connecting up to four electrode leads to a single generator.

The extension cables, obviously, add to the complexity of the system but one of the benefits in having the extension is the reduction of stress on the electrode lead and the elimination of direct electrode lead manipulation during revisions and replacements of the IPG. In PNS, we prefer not to use extension cables – unless the bifurcated extensions or splitters are needed – primarily to decrease the number of the incisions and to keep lower profile for the relatively superficial (comparing to spinal or cerebral applications) implant.

The last implantable component of PNS system is an anchor – a device that holds the electrode lead in place and prevents its migration. Most electrode leads come with a set of anchors – and since these leads are designed for SCS applications, so are the standard anchors. The anchors are usually made of silicone. They come in several shapes: the cylindrical anchors that have grooves or bumps to prevent sliding of holding sutures, the anchors 'with ears' that have side flaps with suture holes attached to a cylindrical shaft, and the wrap-on anchors that are applied to the electrode lead and sutured to the tissues.

All of these anchors are designed to hold electrode lead in place by virtue of tension created by the ties or sutures that are placed around them. It is routinely recommended to use non-absorbable sutures, and we prefer using synthetic polyfilaments such as Dacron (Surgidac, Ethibond or Ti-Cron), whereas others may prefer natural (silk) or monofilament (prolene) materials. In addition to (but not instead of) the suturing, a medical glue may be used inside the anchor to assure better electrode-anchor coupling.

Recently, more complex anchors have been introduced – with either metal or polyetherethylketone (PEEK) inserts – for better grasp of the electrode lead outer insulation. These anchors – Titan (Medtronic) and Cinch (St. Jude) – have been widely used by the implanters since their introduction. It is important to remember, however, that anchoring technique does not compensate for excessive mobility of the electrode lead. If such mobility exists, loose anchoring will result in electrode lead migration, whereas anchoring that is too tight may result in electrode fracture.

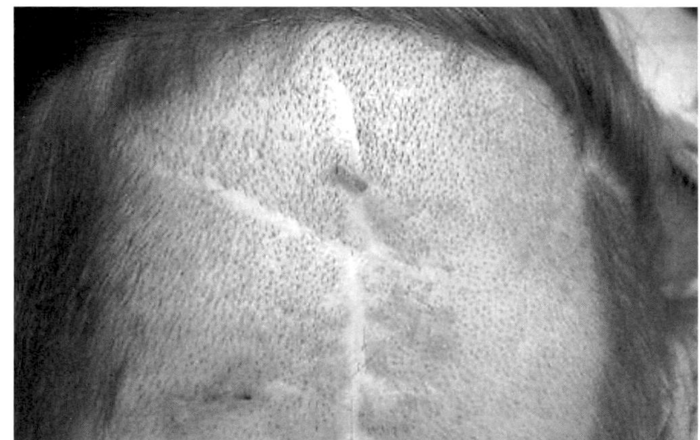

Fig. 1. Erosion of occipital nerve stimulation electrode lead.

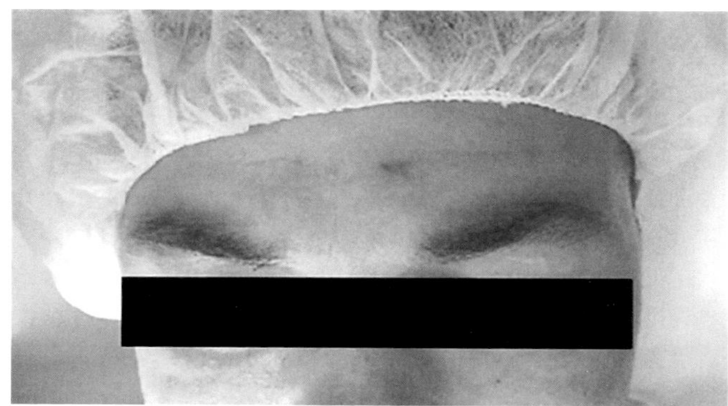

Fig. 2. Erosion of supraorbital nerve stimulation electrode lead.

Peripheral Nerve Stimulation Accessories

In addition to the implantable components, there are multiple important devices that facilitate proper placement of neuromodulation system components. These include insertion needles, stylets, guidewires, introducers, passers/tunnelers, dissecting tools and wrenches. Not all of these accessories are useful for PNS applications as they are designed for SCS – and this presents a major problem that has to be resolved by developing hardware dedicated to PNS use.

For example, straight and curved stylets that facilitate electrode lead advancement in the epidural space and guidewires and introducers that may be used for establishing a path for SCS electrode insertion have very little if any use in PNS applications as the electrodes inserted percutaneously are usually advanced through the needle that is inserted directly toward the target location.

The needles, on the other hand, are integral component of percutaneous PNS electrode lead insertion procedure. Straight shape of these needles is designed for

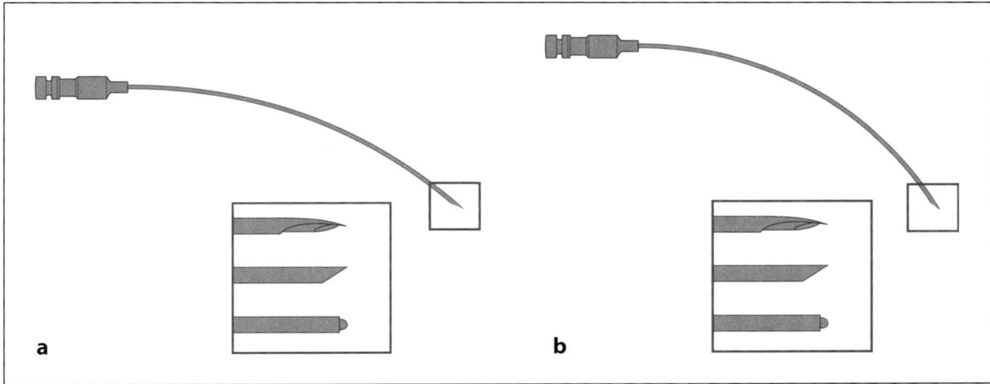

Fig. 3. Curved design of the insertion needle for PNS applications. **a** Needle/stylet assembly with 45° curve and three tip styles (inset). **b** Needle/stylet assembly with 60° curve and three tip styles (inset).

SCS applications – but it does not conform to the body curvature when it comes to PNS procedures. Here the needle straightness may result in bringing electrode tip too close to the surface of the skin thereby increasing the chance of electrode tip erosion (fig. 1, 2). To overcome this, most implanters have been bending the needle prior to its use, although this may be sometimes difficult to do as the needle and its stylet have different mechanical properties and it becomes very challenging to remove the stylet once the needle is positioned. To solve this, we have designed special curved needles with stylets of various configurations – the sharp, oblique and blunt ones – so they can be exchanged at different stages of needle insertion (fig. 3).

The epidural dissectors – the 'hockey-stick' devices and dural separators – may be used for insertion of paddle electrodes in their PNS applications, although in most cases implanters use open dissection with standard dissection instruments for establishing a plane for paddle electrode insertion [9].

Peripheral Nerve Stimulation Complications

In general, complications of neuromodulation are divided into 10 main groups [10]. Some of them occur primarily with intrathecal pumps and other means of chemical neuromodulation; some others are specific to the central nervous system and apply to the electrical stimulators of spinal and cerebral structures. Several categories, however, are applicable to PNS; these include infection, hemorrhage, injury of nervous tissue, placing device into wrong compartment, hardware migration, erosion and malfunction, including fractures and disconnections, and the general category of other issues.

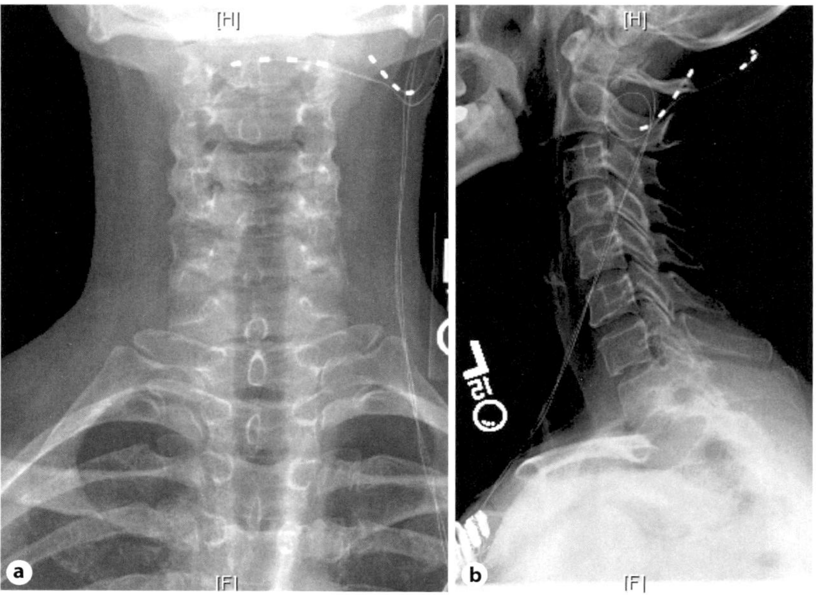

Fig. 4. Migration of occipital nerve stimulation electrode leads – both left and right electrode leads have migrated away from their original position. **a** Anteroposterior radiograph. **b** Lateral radiograph.

Looking at the history of PNS it becomes apparent that some of the technical complications have disappeared with technological advancements, while the others remain essentially unchanged. In the early stages of PNS practice, the electrodes were custom-made. Some wrap-around electrodes had Silastic backing [3] with platinum wire facing the nerve to be stimulated. It turned out that in some circumstances such backing accumulated significant amount of fluid and this phenomenon affected the electrode impedance with subsequent loss of conductivity [3].

Later, such cuff electrodes became more biocompatible, but the main issue became a possibility of nerve injury as a result of fibrosis and possibly ischemia arising from electrode strangling the nerve within soft tissues. Multiple reports of such incidents were one of the main reasons why these devices were abandoned [11–13].

However, even with meticulous dissection and secure suturing of these cuff electrodes some of them ended up becoming displaced, and the only solution for such migration incidents was electrode revision. The migration incidence became higher with introduction of percutaneous PNS technique – here the tissue friction is minimal and the only thing that holds electrode in place is the anchor – along with so-called strain relief loop that is commonly placed next to the anchoring site. Anyone who ever revised or removed percutaneous PNS electrode would agree that these electrodes easily leave their location, and the tissue reaction around them is

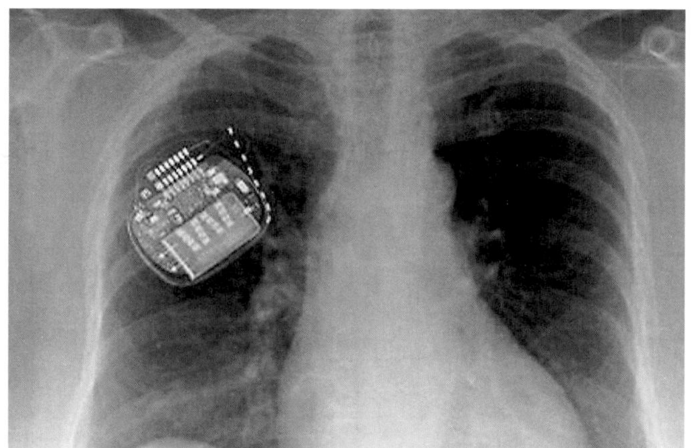

Fig. 5. 'Extreme' migration of occipital nerve stimulation electrode lead – the electrode lead has migrated all the way toward the generator pocket.

rather minimal. The migration is unlikely to happen in lateral (relative to the electrode axis) direction – most of the time it happens as a pullout from the original lead position (fig. 4). Sometimes, if the anchor is completely incompetent, or if the patient presents with hypermobility over the electrode path, this migration may be rather dramatic (fig. 5). In addition to this 'pull-out' phenomenon, the electrode lead may also migrate 'in' shifting more distally along the electrode path (fig. 6). All this, however, is easy to figure out with a simple set of radiographs – and since they have to be compared to the original images, it is important to obtain and save the radiographic image of the electrode lead position at the end of its original implantation. Incidence of migrations varies from series to series ranging from 0 to 100% [14–16].

Functioning malpositioned or migrated electrode leads are easy to re-position. A simple technique allows for such repositioning without re-opening the generator pocket [17, 18]. It is important, however, to have the generator pocket prepped and ready for exploration should the electrode lead turn out to be damaged or otherwise unsuitable for reinsertion.

Electrode leads may break at any time after the implantation. Such breakages (fractures) are usually a result of sharp kink in the electrode lead insulation. The lead insulation or the internal wires may break due to repetitive movement that involves alternating stretching and compression of the device resulting in material fatigue and eventual failure. This issue should be taken into consideration when choosing the path of electrode lead and the location of generator. Crossing large joints and traveling long distances tends to be associated with higher rate of fractures and migrations.

Both infections and hemorrhages have occurred with PNS devices – but both are quite rare. Since most of the devices are placed in superficial locations, the bleeding

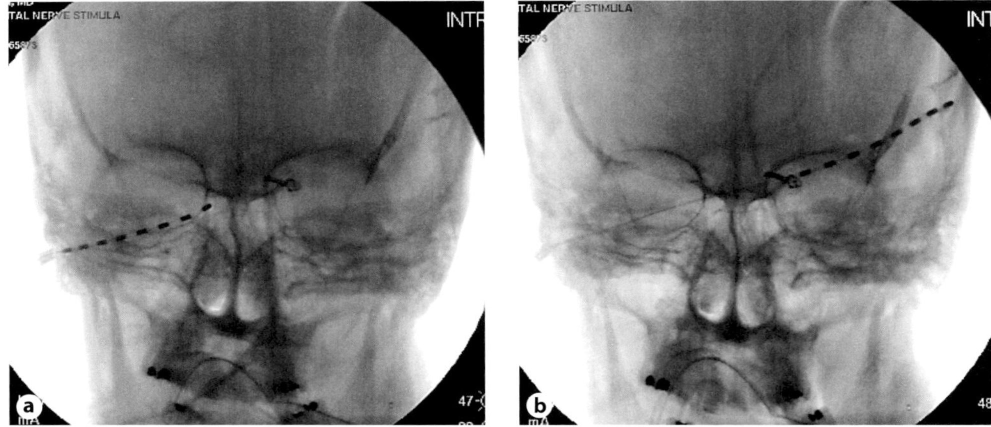

Fig. 6. 'In' migration of the occipital nerve stimulation electrode lead. **a** Original electrode lead position. **b** Electrode position 8 months after insertion with 'in' migration to the contralateral side of the neck.

may be easily controlled and the hematomas are rarely symptomatic. The infections, on the other hand, may occur in both immediate and long-term periods. Surgical infections may be a result of poor surgical technique or an insufficient dissection for the anchors and connectors when the tissue tension prevents adequate wound healing. In our series of 40 patients with PNS implants followed for longer than 30 months, there were 2 infections, and in each case, the device had to be removed. The infection was managed with systemic antibiotics that were adjusted after the microorganisms and antibiotic sensitivities were established. The PNS system may be reimplanted a few months after the infection was eradicated.

Placing the device into a wrong compartment is rather a theoretical concern as most of PNS electrodes are inserted in a subcutaneous epifascial plane. However, since the proximity of electrode lead to the nerve to be stimulated is extremely important in terms of getting adequate paresthesias and keeping stimulation parameters within reasonable range, various techniques have been suggested to improve the placement accuracy. Fluoroscopy is routinely used by most PNS implanters [19], but there are now multiple reports that suggest use of intraoperative ultrasound for localization of the nerve trunk and the surrounding structures [20–22].

Insertion of electrodes too deep into soft tissues tends to cause unpleasant muscle spasms during stimulation [23] whereas placing them too superficially may result in lead tip erosion [24].

Overall, however, most PNS complications are minor and rarely if ever require hospitalization. Recently, we analyzed our institutional experience with PNS [24]. Among almost a hundred of PNS patients operated since April of 2000, we identified 40 patients that had their original PNS trial in our hospital and were followed up for

30 months or longer. The remaining patients had either shorter follow-up or their initial surgery was done in other institutions.

Of 40 patients, 8 did not sufficiently improve during the trial and 32 proceeded with permanent implantation. In a long-term follow-up series of these 32 patients, there was a total of 27 subsequent operations (including 12 battery replacements) but in only one case of infection was hospital admission required. Of 15 re-operations, there were 6 revisions (one for electrode erosion 4 weeks after implantation, 4 for electrode migration at 1, 3, 5 and 9 months after original implantation, and one for device disconnection) and 9 device removals (2 due to infections at 1 and 49 months, 3 due to a loss of effectiveness at 9, 10 and 25 months, and 4 – due to improvement of symptoms at 13, 17, 21 and 56 months after original implantation). This experience illustrates the well-known observation about relatively high rate of complications but, at the same time, very minor morbidity associated with the entire PNS approach [14, 15].

Conclusions

Although commonly used in clinical practice, peripheral nerve stimulation for treatment of chronic pain is performed mainly with devices developed and marketed for spinal cord stimulation applications. This may be one of the reasons why the PNS approach is marked by a very high complication rate, as the anatomy of peripheral nerves and the surrounding soft tissues is quite different from epidural spinal space for which the current devices are designed.

Based on the literature data and the analysis of the author's experience with PNS procedures, it appears that although the rate of complications is relatively high, the morbidity associated with PNS approach is very minor and most problems may be resolved with simple re-operations, usually on outpatient basis. The reduction in complication rate is expected to occur when the hardware used in PNS procedures is appropriately adapted for PNS applications.

References

1 Slavin KV: Peripheral nerve stimulation for neuropathic pain. Neurotherapeutics 2008;5:100–106.

2 Wall PD, Sweet WH: Temporary abolition of pain in man. Science 1967;155:108–109.

3 Shelden CH, Paul F, Jacques DB, Pudenz RH: Electrical stimulation of the nervous system. Surg Neurol 1975;4:127–132.

4 Nashold BS Jr, Mullen JB, Avery R: Peripheral nerve stimulation for pain relief using a multicontact electrode system: technical note. J Neurosurg 1979; 51:872–873.

5 Racz GB, Browne T, Lewis R Jr: Peripheral stimulator implant for treatment of causalgia caused by electrical burns. Tex Med 1988;84:45–50.

6 Mobbs RJ, Blum P, Rossato R: Mesh electrode for peripheral nerve stimulation. J Clin Neurosci 2003; 10:476–477.

7 Weiner RL, Reed KL: Peripheral neurostimulation for control of intractable occipital neuralgia. Neuromodulation 1999;2:217–221.

8 Slavin KV: Epidural spinal cord stimulation: indications and technique; in Schulder M (ed): Handbook of Functional and Stereotactic Surgery. New York, Marcel Dekker, 2002, pp 417–430.

9 Kapural L, Mekhail N, Hayek SM, Stanton-Hicks M, Malak O: Occipital nerve electrical stimulation via the midline approach and subcutaneous surgical leads for treatment of severe occipital neuralgia: a pilot study. Anesth Analg 2005;101:171–174.
10 Slavin KV: Placing neuromodulation in the human body: limiting morbidity; in Arle JA, Shils JL (eds): Essential Neuromodulation. Elsevier, Philadelphia, 2011, pp 303–322.
11 Nielson KD, Watts C, Clark WK: Peripheral nerve injury from implantation of chronic stimulating electrodes for pain control. Surg Neurol 1976;5: 51–53.
12 Kirsch WM, Lewis JA, Simon RH: Experiences with electrical stimulation devices for the control of chronic pain. Med Instrum 1975;9:217–220.
13 Nashold BS Jr, Goldner JL, Mullen JB, Bright DS: Long-term pain control by direct peripheral-nerve stimulation. J Bone Joint Surg Am 1982;64:1–10.
14 Jasper J, Hayek S: Implanted occipital nerve stimulators. Pain Physician 2008;11:187–200.
15 Falowski S, Wang D, Sabesan A, Sharan A: Occipital nerve stimulator systems: review of complications and surgical techniques. Neuromodulation 2010;13: 121–125.
16 Franzini A, Messina G, Leone M, Broggi G: Occipital nerve stimulation (ONS). Surgical technique and prevention of late electrode migration. Acta Neuro chir (Wien) 2009;151:861–865.
17 Slavin KV, Vannemreddy PSSV: Repositioning of supraorbital nerve stimulation electrode using retrograde needle insertion: a technical note. Neuromodulation 2011;14:in press.
18 Mammis A, Mogilner AY: A technique of distal to proximal revision of peripheral neurostimulator leads: technical note. Stereotact Funct Neurosurg 2011;89:65–69.
19 Trentman TL, Zimmerman RS: Occipital nerve stimulation: technical and surgical aspects of implantation. Headache 2008;48:319–327.
20 Huntoon MA, Burgher AH: Ultrasound-guided permanent implantation of peripheral nerve stimulation (PNS) system for neuropathic pain of the extremities: original cases and outcomes. Pain Med 2009;10:1369–1377.
21 Carayannopoulos A, Beasley R, Sites B: Facilitation of percutaneous trial lead placement with ultrasound guidance for peripheral nerve stimulation trial of ilioinguinal neuralgia: a technical note. Neuromodulation 2009;12:296–301.
22 Skaribas I, Aló K: Ultrasound imaging and occipital nerve stimulation. Neuromodulation 2010;13:126–130.
23 Hayek SM, Jasper JF, Deep DR, Narouze SN: Occipital neurostimulation-induced muscle spasms: implications for lead placement. Pain Physician 2009;12:867–876.
24 Trentman TL, Dodick DW, Zimmerman RS, Birch BD: Percutaneous occipital stimulator tip erosion: report of 2 cases. Pain Physician 2008;11:253–256.
25 Eboli P, Aydin S, Colpan ME, Watson KS, Mlinarevich N, Slavin KV: Craniofacial peripheral nerve stimulation – analysis of technical complications. Abstract Book, Biennial ASSFN Meeting, Vancouver, 2008, p 89.

Konstantin V. Slavin, MD
University of Illinois at Chicago
Department of Neurosurgery, M/C 799
912 South Wood Street
Chicago, IL 60612 (USA)
Tel. +1 312 996 4842, Fax +1 312 996 9018, E-Mail kslavin@uic.edu

Slavin KV (ed): Peripheral Nerve Stimulation.
Prog Neurol Surg. Basel, Karger, 2011, vol 24, pp 203–209

Peripheral Nerve Stimulation: Definition

David Abejón[a] · Juan Pérez-Cajaraville[b]

[a]Pain Unit, Hospital Universitario Puerta de Hierro Majadahonda, Madrid, and [b]Pain Unit, Clínica Universitaria de Navarra, Pamplona, Spain

Abstract

Recently, there has been a tremendous evolution in the field of neurostimulation, both from the technological point of view and from development of the new and different indications. In some areas, such as peripheral nerve stimulation, there has been a boom in recent years due to the variations in the surgical technique and the improved results documented by in multiple published papers. All this makes imperative the need to classify and define the different types of stimulation that are used today. The confusion arises when attempting to describe peripheral nerve stimulation and subcutaneous stimulation. Peripheral nerve stimulation, in its pure definition, involves implanting a lead on a nerve, with the aim to produce paresthesia along the entire trajectory of the stimulated nerve.

Before trying to define peripheral nerve stimulation we should make a brief reflection about what we mean with defining something. The classical Aristotelian doctrine provides that, as a general rule, a definition should include the genus as well as the specific difference; that is, on one hand, the class to which it – or the terms associated with it – belongs and, on the other, the features that differentiate it from others in that class. For example, in the definition of pencil (instrument of writing formed by a wood-surrounded graphite bar), the first part (writing instrument . . .) is the ***genus***, and second (. . . formed by a wood-surrounded graphite) is the specific difference. A definition must be clear and exact and as sharp as graphical representation of an image.

The main Aristotle's rules for building a definition are:

- A concept must be defined by means of the closest possible approach to its typification (of sort and species) and by differentiation.
- Differentiation must be an actual characteristic or group of characteristics.

The definition of something takes us to establish a concept. The concept is a graphic representation of the words' representative symbolism; it is the 'mental construction'

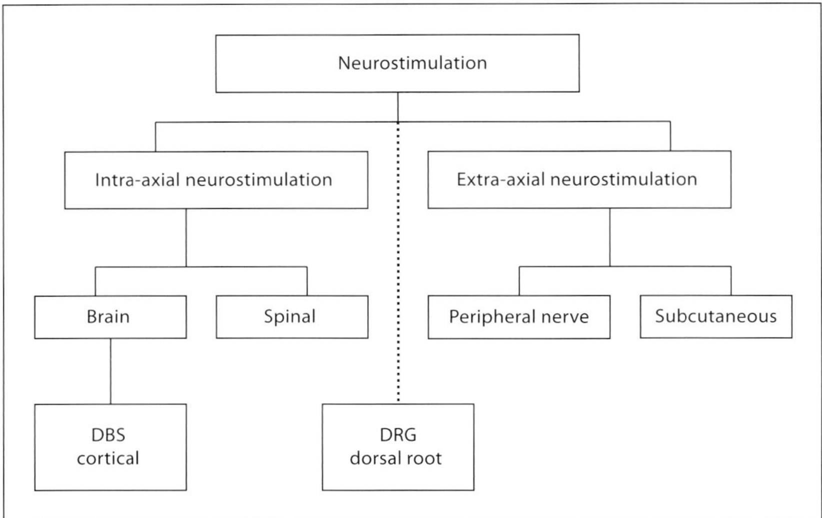

Fig. 1. Neurostimulation classification.

of everything which is around us, which we can perceive, as we effectively do with symbols that define the world that surrounds us. The concept is what makes all of us see things in the same way: for English-speakers, a chair is a device used to sit down, and singing is the action carried out by the singer who performs music. In short, concepts give us the possibility to understand.

To summarize, the definition and the concept of a scientific term is the basic tool used by professionals to understand each other, which is essential from the scientific standpoint.

On the basis of these concepts we will try to develop this chapter and establish a *definition* for peripheral nerve stimulation.

Neurostimulation Classifications

Before attempting to define a type of stimulation it is important to carry out a classification of neurostimulation as a whole (fig. 1). One of the first neurostimulation classifications was developed by Alò and Holsheimer [1], who stressed the need of differentiate between intra-axial (IA) and extra-axial (EA) stimulation. In this work they considered that the first, among other things, will include targeting of specific nerves within the lumbosacral spine and the other will include percutaneous approach that targets the extraspinal nerves.

This classification is too simple but very clarifying. If we try to be more precise, we must carry out a subclassification of both groups. IA may be subdivided in two main groups: one involving cortical, deep brain and thalamic stimulation and the other targeted to spinal stimulation.

Looking at EA, it can also be subdivided into two main groups since some years ago: peripheral nerve stimulation (PNS) and the so-called 'subcutaneous' stimulation (peripheral subcutaneous field stimulation – PSFS) [2]. Some colleagues defend the need to make a more detailed classification, in which dorsal root ganglia stimulation should be considered apart from spinal cord stimulation (SCS) or PNS, since it seems to be an independent kind, both anatomically and functionally.

In deep brain stimulation (DBS), indications and exact stimulation sites seem to be very well-established, as in Parkinson disease (nucleus ventralis intermedius of the thalamus – Vim, internal part of globus pallidus – GPi, sub-thalamic nucleus – STN and zona incerta), dystonia (GPi), tremor (Vim, zona incerta), choreoathetosis (Vim, GPi, zona incerta, nucleus ventro-oralis posterior of the thalamus – Vop) and deafferentation pain (ventro-postero-medial thalamic nucleus – VPM, ventro-postero-lateral thalamic nucleus – VPL, centro-median thalamic nucleus – CM, periaqueductal gray matter – PAG, periventricular gray matter – PVG), as well as in others in experimental phase such as epilepsy, cluster headache, obsessive-compulsive disorders, depression, drug addiction, aggressivity and obesity [3, 4]. Motor cortex stimulation (MCS) has been proposed for patients with post-stroke or post-traumatic pain, as well as in deafferentation facial pain, the latter having demonstrated the best clinical results [5, 6]. The technique involves the insertion of a multi-contact plate electrode epidurally over the motor cortex (precentral gyrus) followed by the electrical stimulation at a less than motor threshold amplitude which results in the analgesic effect [7]. Finally, inside IA we can find SCS. This procedure was initially called dorsal column stimulation (DCS), given the presumption that most of the effects observed (paresthesia and pain relief) were due to the direct stimulation of the dorsal columns. Further advances in the study of its action mechanisms demonstrated that stimulation from the epidural space may activate a larger number of neural structures and, therefore, nowadays this kind of stimulation is called SCS instead of DCS [8]. Stimulated structures include dorsal columns, dorsal horn, dorsal root entry zone (DREZ) and dorsal roots [9, 10]. The best established indications for this type of stimulation are neuropathic pain, whose most typical examples are FBSS and CRPS [11–15]. In Europe, it is also very commonly used for peripheral vascular disease and refractory angina [16, 17].

It seems that limits are very well established in IA, both regarding indications and surgical techniques.

The problem arises when we speak about EA. Today, it seems that, due to the advances performed in EA, we have no other choice but to think carefully about what we are doing, basically in order to make scientific communication precise. At present we can find in the literature cases in which the technique is defined according to the stimulating target or to the surgical technique. This is particularly obvious in occipital nerve stimulation for the management of Arnold's neuralgia [18, 19] and ilioinguinal nerve stimulation for post-herniorrhaphy pain.

Initially, the technique was called peripheral nerve stimulation (e.g. Weiner and Oh) but today we also find references as subcutaneous stimulation [20] or just peripheral stimulation [21], as well as other names to denominate the same technique. The same happens with PSFS: there are multiple different denominations in the literature for this stimulation modality, ranging from subcutaneous stimulation to peripheral field nerve stimulation [22–25]. That is why we think it is absolutely necessary to establish an exact definition of what should be understood as peripheral nerve stimulation.

Definition of Peripheral Nerve Stimulation

The concept of PNS was introduced in the clinical practice in 1967 by Wall and Sweet [26], who applied stimulation on the infraorbital nerve by means of a percutaneous needle, obtaining hypoesthesia and pain relief distal to the stimulation. During the 70's, after demonstrating that in some patients with highly localized pains and very specific nerve involvement SCS was not as effective, it was proposed to use both techniques together. PNS reached its highest peak in the 1980s [27] although, due to different technical problems, lack of systematic investigation and poor patient selection criteria, the initial enthusiasm was lost [28]. From those days to the present, the technique has suffered some ups and downs. Before 1999, only 50 articles had been published, with very uneven results and a high rate of complications [29]. Although there are certainly some clear indications for the use of this neurostimulation modality outside of pain, such as motor stimulation of phrenic nerves in cases of diaphragmal palsy and somatic nerves of the extremities in patients with hemiplegia and paraplegia; vagal nerve stimulation for treatment of intractable epilepsy and refractory depression; autonomic stimulation for urinary and gastrointestinal disorders, it continues to be used for various types of neuropathic pain which is the focus of this review [30–32]. Following Aristotle's classical guidelines for building up a definition, we must establish its genus and specific differentiation. The exact definition of this technique must be addressed to what is used and to where it is used. In this way, PNS is defined as electric stimulation performed on the peripheral nerve system and applied to a specific nerve. It seems to be a very simple definition, although it is a very precise definition as well. Unlike SCS, where electric stimulation is performed on the central nervous system, PNS is applied to a nerve with a specific name.

If we try to compare PNS and PSFS, the difference is quite clear. The latter is also performed on the peripheral nervous system (peripheral stimulation) but not on a specific nerve but on a group of nervous endings at the subdermal level (field stimulation).

The aim of PNS will always be to produce paresthesia along the territory innervated by the stimulated nerve, while PSFS distributes paresthesia as an electric field around the lead's active electrodes without achieving a clearly-defined nervous distribution. This concept can be made very clear with a couple of practical examples.

It is easy to understand which kind of stimulation is performed in a patient with a lesion in the sciatic nerve or in the cubital nerve. In both cases, the lead will be implanted, either by percutaneous or surgical approach, with the aim of producing a paresthesia running along the injured nerve, in order to reach one of the neurostimulation premises: to obtain a constant and complete paresthesia of the painful area. If, on the contrary, the patient refers pain in the lumbar zone or at the junction between the iliac crest and the lumbar spine (L5 region), or in the parascapular zone, if we use peripheral stimulation we will never be able to stimulate a specific nerve in those areas, as it is not a dermatomal pain and does not belong to any specific nerve's territory. It seems very clear that these two types of stimulation are different. As in any other neurostimulation technique, the purpose is to relieve pain by means of producing paresthesia and, depending on the pain location and type, sometimes we need more specificity and sometimes what we pursue is a larger paresthesia coverage. Although the procedure is performed in a very similar way – percutaneously –, it is important to take into account that if we want to give a name to the procedure, what is it that we really seek from the pathophysiologic point of view: if we try to stimulate a peripheral nerve (e.g. the median nerve) we will perform PNS; if we try to stimulate a specific painful area, without a specific nerve, we will be performing PSFS. The need to define each technique is given by the similarity of both surgical approaches.

There are other differences that help understanding the differential concept between both techniques, always referred to what we are trying to obtain when we decide to perform one of these types of extraspinal stimulation. When we choose PNS, we seek a unidirectional paresthesia along the stimulated nerve; when we choose PSFS we seek a concentric stimulation in a specific area without radiation, kept in the patient's precise painful site [33].

This concept should also make us think about the kind of lead to be used in each case. In PNS, although both percutaneous and paddle lead types may be used, the paddle may theoretically produce better results because, when implanted on the targeted nerve, the quality of the stimulation will be higher since it is unidirectionally aimed toward the nerve; in PSFS it may probably be better to use a percutaneous lead, because the concentric stimulation generated around the active electrodes seems to be more appropriate, since the exact location of the target fibers is totally unknown.

The main indication for this kind of stimulation – PNS – is the presence of neuropathic pain in 1 or 2 nerves, in such a way that stimulation is performed specifically in the distribution of the affected nerves [34]. PNS may be performed in two clearly differentiated ways: on one hand, by means of surgical approach, leaving the lead over or inside the epineurium; on the other, by percutaneous introduction. In any case, PNSs purpose is the same. An important advance in the technique was the launch of Resume® On-Point® leads (Medtronic Inc., Minneapolis, Minn., USA) [33]. The use of this technique has relevant advantages over other modalities, as it makes possible to stimulate the affected nerve without propagating the paresthesias to adjacent areas and keeping the stimulation constant, unlike in SCS, where any movement of the spine may cause variations in stimulation.

Conclusion

From the scientific point of view it is important to have a precise denomination of the performed technique. A cholecystectomy is always a cholecystectomy, regardless of whether it is open or laparoscopic: the result is always the extirpation of the gallbladder, and it does not receive a different name for each different technique. If we stimulate a peripheral nerve, it should always be referred to as PNS; if no nerve is stimulated, then we should call it PSFS.

References

1 Aló K, Holsheimer J: New trends in neuromodulation for the management of neuropathic pain. Neurosurgery 2002;50:690–704.

2 Abejón D, Krames ES: Peripheral nerve stimulation or is it peripheral subcutaneous field stimulation; what is in a moniker? Neuromodulation 2009;12: 1–4.

3 Benabid AL, Benazzouz A, Hoffmann D, Limousin P, Krack P, Pollak P: Long-term electrical inhibition of deep brain targets in movement disorders. Mov Disord 1998;13(suppl 3):119–125.

4 Robaina F: Surgical neuromodulation: new frontiers in neurosurgery. Neurocirugía 2008;19:143–155.

5 Nguyen JP, Lefaucheur JP, Decq P, Uchiyama T, Carpentier A, Fontaine D, Brugières P, Pollin B, Fève A, Rostaing S, Cesaro P, Keravel Y: Chronic motor cortex stimulation in the treatment of central and neuropathic pain: correlations between clinical, electrophysiological and anatomical data. Pain 1999; 82:245–251.

6 Rainov NG, Heidecke V: Motor cortex stimulation for neuropathic facial pain. Neurol Res 2003;25: 157–161.

7 Nguyen JP, Lefaucheur JP, Keravel Y: Motor cortex stimulation. Pain Res Clin Manage 2003;15: 197–209.

8 Barolat G: Spinal cord stimulation for chronic pain management. Arch Med Res 2000;31:258–262.

9 Barolat G: Epidural spinal cord stimulation: anatomical and electrical properties of the intraspinal structures and clinical correlations. Neuromodulation 1998;2:63–71.

10 Holsheimer J: Which neuronal elements are activated directly by spinal cord stimulation. Neuromodulation 2002;5:25–31.

11 Barolat G: A prospective study to assess the efficacy of spinal cord stimulation utilizing a multi-channel radio frequency system for the treatment of intractable low back and lower extremity pain: initial considerations and methodology. Neuromodulation 1999;2:179–183.

12 Aló KM, Redko V, Charnov J: Four-year follow-up of dual electrode spinal cord stimulation for chronic pain. Neuromodulation 2002;5:79–88.

13 Turner JA, Loeser JD, Deyo RA, Sanders SB: Spinal cord stimulation for patients with failed back surgery syndrome or complex regional pain syndrome: a systematic review of effectiveness and complications. Pain 2004;108:137–147.

14 North RB, Kidd DH, Olin J, Sieracki JM, Farrokhi F, Petrucci L, Cutchis PN: Spinal cord stimulation for axial low back pain: a prospective, controlled trial comparing dual with single percutaneous electrode. Spine 2005;30:1412–1418.

15 Kemler MA, Barendse GA, van Kleef M, de Vet HC, Rijks CP, Furnee CA, van Der Wildenberg FA: Spinal cord stimulation in patients with chronic reflex sympathetic dystrophy. N Engl J Med 2000; 343:618–624.

16 Amann W, Berg P, Gersbach P, Gamain J, Rápale JH, Ubbicnk D,e SCS-EPOS Study Group: Spinal cord stimulation in the treatment of non-reconstructable stable critical leg ischaemia: result of the European peripheral vascular disease outcome study (SCS-EPOS). Eur J Vasc Endovasc Surg 2003;26: 280–286.

17 Ubbink D, Vermeulen H: Spinal cord stimulation for critical leg ischemia: a review of effectiveness and optimal patient selection. J Pain Symptom Manage 2006;31:S30–S35.

18 Weiner RL, Reed KL: Peripheral neurostimulation for the control of intractable occipital neuralgia. Neuromodulation 1999;2:369–375.
19 Oh MY, Ortega J, Bradley Bellotte J, Whiting DM, Aló K: Peripheral nerve stimulation for the treatment of occipital neuralgia and transformed migraine using a C1–2–3 subcutaneous paddle style electrode: a technical report. Neuromodulation 2004; 7:103–112.
20 Reverberi C, Bonezzi C, Demartini L: Peripheral subcutaneous neurostimulation in the management of neuropathic pain: five case reports. Neuromodulation 2009;12:146–155.
21 Rodrigo-Royo MD, Azcona JM, Quero J, Lorente MC, Acín P, Azcona J: Peripheral neurostimulation in the management of cervicogenic headaches: four case reports. Neuromodulation 2005;4:241–248.
22 Paicius RM, Bernstein CA, Lempert-Cohen C: Peripheral nerve field stimulation in chronic abdominal pain. Pain Physician 2006;9:261–266.
23 Paicius RM, Bernstein CA, Lempert-Cohen C: Peripheral nerve field stimulation for the treatment of chronic low back pain: preliminary results of long term follow-up – a case series. Neuromodulation 2007;10:279–290.
24 Krutsch JP, McCeney MH, Barolat G, Al Tamimi M, Smolenski A: A case report of subcutaneous peripheral nerve stimulation for the treatment of axial back pain associated with postlaminectomy syndrome. Neuromodulation 2008;11:112–115.
25 Stinson LW, Roderer GT, Cross NE, Davis BE: Peripheral subcutaneous electrostimulation for control of intractable postoperative inguinal pain: a case report series. Neuromodulation 2001;4:99–104.
26 Wall PD, Sweet EH: Temporary abolition of pain in man. Science 1967;155:108–109.
27 Stanton-Hicks M: Transcutaneous and peripheral nerve stimulation; in Simpson BA (ed): Electrical Stimulation and Relief of Pain. Pain Res Clin Manage 2003;15:37–57.
28 Stanton-Hicks M: Peripheral nerve stimulation for pain: peripheral neuralgia and complex regional pain syndrome; in Krames ES, Peckham PH, Rezai AR (eds): Neuromodulation. London, Elsevier, 2009, pp 397–409.
29 Gybels JM, Nuttin BJ: Peripheral nerve stimulation; in Loeser J (ed): Bonica's Management of Pain, ed 3. Philadelphia, Lippincott, 2000, pp 1851–1855.
30 Slavin KV: Peripheral nerve stimulation for neuropathic pain. Neurotherapeutics 2008;5:100–106.
31 de León-Casasola OA: Spinal cord and peripheral nerve stimulation for neuropathic pain. J Pain Sympton Manage 2009;38(suppl 2):S28–S38.
32 Stuart RM, Winfree CJ: Neurostimulation technique for painful peripheral nerve disorders. Neurosug Clin N Am 2009;20:111–120.
33 Racz GB, Browne T, Lewis R Jr: Peripheral stimulator implant for treatment of causalgia caused by electrical burns. Tex Med 1988;84:45–50.
34 Law JT, Sweet J, Kirsch W: Retrospective analysis of 22 patients with chronic pain treated by peripheral nerve stimulation. J Neurosurg 1998;52:482–485.

David Abejón, MD, FIPP
Unidad de Dolor
Hospital Universitario Puerta de Hierro Majadahonda
C/Joaquín Rodrigo, 2, ES–28222 Majadahonda, Madrid (Spain)
Tel. +34 91 191 6000, Fax +34 91 373 0535, E-Mail dabejon@telefonica.net

Slavin KV (ed): Peripheral Nerve Stimulation.
Prog Neurol Surg. Basel, Karger, 2011, vol 24, pp 210–217

The Future of Peripheral Nerve Stimulation

Michael Stanton-Hicks[a] · Ioannis G. Panourias[b] · Damianos E. Sakas[b] · Konstantin V. Slavin[c]

[a]Pain Management Department, Center for Neurological Restoration, Cleveland Clinic, Cleveland, Ohio, USA; [b]Department of Neurosurgery, University of Athens Medical School, Evangelismos Hospital, Athens, Greece; [c]Department of Neurosurgery, University of Illinois at Chicago, Chicago, Ill., USA

Abstract

The field of peripheral nerve stimulation (PNS) is now experiencing a phase of rapid growth in number of patients, number of implanters, number of indications, and procedure types. This, however, appears to be only a beginning of major developments that could revolutionize the field of PNS. It is expected that the progress in PNS will continue simultaneously in several directions as new indications, new stimulation targets and new device designs evolve in the foreseeable future. Responding to a major need for safe and effective pain treatments and following a general trend toward less-invasive and nondestructive interventions, PNS has the potential of becoming a premier pain-relieving modality that will be used instead of or in combination with existing more established approaches such as spinal cord stimulation and pharmacological pain control. Recent technological advancements are cause for considerable optimism regarding the development of PNS and are likely to be a beginning of a major overhaul in our perception of PNS approaches. Expanding the number of applications will without question strengthen the field of PNS. The turning point, however, will not occur until sufficient scientific evidence is gathered to unequivocally prove its safety, clinical efficacy and cost-effectiveness, and when PNS applications become officially endorsed through regulatory approval of each indication. Such changes will allow implanters to use approved devices for approved indications – instead of the contemporary 'off-label' use – and at the same time give device manufacturers a chance to market these devices and support education on their appropriate use.

Peripheral nerve stimulation (PNS) is estimated by some to be the most rapidly growing field of neuromodulation. Despite its long history (first introduced in the early 1960s, even before the 'gate control' theory of pain was introduced), PNS has not become a mainstream pain-relieving modality, although many enthusiastic centers continued to use the technique on a regular basis. Currently, there is a significant increase in the number of patients treated with PNS and a corresponding surge in the number of publications dealing with this particular subject.

Current State of PNS: Key Issues

Accumulation of Objective Evidence
PNS, though a very promising methodology for alleviating medically refractory neuropathic pain conditions, is largely performed at present under research protocols or on an 'off-label' basis. In practice, evidence for its effectiveness based on randomized controlled trials (RCTs) is lacking. Mobbs et al. [1] have recognized the difficulty in pursuing such studies; they point out that a study that included randomizing patients to a 'best medical therapy' versus a peripheral nerve stimulator would be ideal, although not feasible as these patients are referred because they have failed the 'best medical therapy' option. In particular, two parameters necessary for conducting fully RCTs, i.e. blinding and sham control, are difficult to achieve in the PNS case. Patients implanted with a PNS system have been 'taught' to recognize associated paresthesias at the offending dermatome as an indicator of good system function; lack of such a sensation, therefore, precludes blinding of the procedure. Furthermore, the high cost of PNS technology renders it unethical and inexpedient to implant such expensive systems for satisfying only the 'sham control' component of a randomized control study without also offering patients the desired therapy. Nevertheless, it becomes obvious that to shape a brighter future for PNS, well-performed prospective RCTs of novel designs are needed to determine the true efficacy, best indications and most appropriate parameters of stimulation.

Understanding the Mechanism of Action
Experimental and basic research into the mechanism of action of PNS will help gain an understanding of its effects on pain and on improving organ function but, so far, such research is rather limited. Multicenter studies are under way to further define its mechanism and pathophysiology. For instance, it is noteworthy that syndromes in which the pain is mainly felt in a specified nerve distribution, e.g. the ophthalmic division of the trigeminal nerve, can be modified by stimulation in the corresponding dermatome. This significant observation implies that the key part of PNS may be closely related to brain function and, particularly, of brain plasticity. Apparently, when such observations are substantiated by research and clinical evidence, they are expected to refine the existing surgical indications of PNS, justify individual tailoring of appropriate treatment approaches, and contribute in optimizing implanted systems for each sufferer.

Cost-Benefit Analyses
In a modern era of medicine, cost containment has evolved as a major concern, the field of PNS being no exception. In this context, evidence-based medical practice increasingly becomes a fundamental issue for acceptance and financial support from third-party payers. Simpler and less-expensive devices will lead to further popularization and expansion of the technique. Moreover, if sufferers are trialed

objectively prior to implantations of the complete system, the cost of unnecessary system implantations will be lowered. In spite of the limitations inherent in conducting RCTs for the evaluation of implantable stimulators and long-term efficacy of PNS treatments, it is apparent that addressing the lack of level 1 and/or level 2 evidence for this neuromodulatory treatment should be a priority in the coming years. Medical industry and neuromodulation practitioners should continue to support relevant research by providing more advanced systems and conducting well-designed studies.

Electrodes and Generators
As mentioned earlier in this book, PNS procedures are currently performed with devices that are not specifically approved for this application. Most of the time, surgeons are using devices designed and approved for spinal cord stimulation (SCS). Those few electrodes such as OnPoint (Medtronic, Minneapolis, Minn., USA) and radiofrequency receivers Mattrix and X-Trel (Medtronic) and Renew (St. Jude Medical Neuromodulation, Plano, Tex., USA) that are approved for PNS are rarely used these days – mainly because of the patients' and practitioners' preference for implantable pulse generators and other electrode types [2]. Electrodes and generators that are dedicated for PNS applications are expected to facilitate surgical procedures, minimize hardware-related complications and maximize confidence of both practitioners and sufferers in using these promising treatment modalities.

Future Prospects of PNS

There is no doubt that PNS will continue to grow and while its future is bright, it is likely to develop in several directions. This account will attempt to review the potential for growth; while predicting the future is always difficult, and it is possible that some of these predictions may never materialize, others may become clinical reality even before this work is published.

New Indications
In the past, PNS has been used for a variety of focal neuropathic pain conditions [3]. The most common indications have been the pain from peripheral nerve injury, complex regional pain syndromes (CRPS) types I and II, postsurgical and post-traumatic neuropathies, pain from neuromas and amputation stumps. More recently, PNS has been successfully used for treatment of occipital neuralgia, trigeminal neuropathy, intercostal neuralgia, post-thoracotomy pain, inguinal and abdominal pain, postherpetic neuralgia in the face and body, cervicogenic headaches, migraines and cluster headaches. Chronic pain in the low back and in the neck, two very common clinical conditions, have also been successfully treated with PNS.

A new trend that may revolutionize the field is an attempt to treat not only focal neuropathic conditions, but also diffuse neuropathic pain. The best example of this is the use of PNS for treatment of pain in fibromyalgia [4, 5] – an idea that came about as a result of the rather serendipitous discovery of 'whole-body' pain relief from upper occipital PNS when it was used to control occipital pain associated with this disorder. The authors called this approach 'C2 area neurostimulation' as their electrodes were placed higher than the usual occipital PNS landmarks. Based on results of this uncontrolled series of patients, a larger randomized prospective study is currently in progress.

As a component of the surgical armamentarium in the field of pain management, PNS is likely to continue being considered for three distinct categories of conditions. The first of them includes focal neuropathies where it may seem intuitive to stimulate the involved nerve rather than attempt stimulation of the nerve roots or the spinal cord. Traumatic neuropathies, CRPS, as well as cases of postherpetic neuralgias and recurrent or persistent nerve entrapment symptoms that do not respond to focal decompressions also fit into this category.

Second would be those conditions in which the neuropathic pain cannot be attributed to a single nerve but which are also known to respond poorly to the 'classical' pain-relieving interventions such as SCS; this category includes low back pain, postherniorrhaphy inguinal pain, post-thoracotomy pain, and other regional, rather than focal, pain syndromes.

The third group of indications includes those for which PNS may be the only neuromodulation option – such as patients with occipital neuralgia who may be considered for some destructive interventions (neurectomies, ganglionectomies) – or for those where surgery is generally not considered an option at all (migraines). Cluster headaches, which have traditionally been treated with medications, should also be included. PNS is essentially a less invasive alternative to recently introduced hypothalamic deep brain stimulation.

A major shift in thinking is the potentially useful PNS application in the treatment of not only chronic neuropathic pain but also nociceptive pain conditions. The recent introduction of PNS for pain of an osteoarthritic nature affecting the neck [6] and extremities [7, 8] may change the way we look at PNS in particular and neuromodulation in general.

The scope and volume of PNS are expected to increase dramatically. While most traditional and some newer applications of PNS are comparatively small in number (peripheral nerve injuries, CRPS, cluster headaches), quite a few of the newer and potential indications are extremely prevalent (migraines, post-herniorrhaphy pain, low back pain, etc.). Even if only a small percent of these patients might qualify for PNS use, the volume of PNS will expand dramatically. Before this can occur, two conditions must be met. One is that scientific data must conclusively demonstrate safety, efficacy and cost-effectiveness of PNS, and the other, related to the first one, is regulatory approval of PNS.

New Targets

In addition to new indications, development of new targets for PNS is expected to add momentum to growth in this field. Currently, PNS applications are focused on large (named) peripheral nerves – so-called 'true PNS' – and on unnamed nerve or nerve endings – so-called 'subcutaneous PNS' or 'peripheral nerve field stimulation'.

Whenever one discusses PNS, the stimulation of peripheral and cranial sensory nerves comes to mind. In addition to this, there is some possibility of getting pain relief from stimulating nerves that are not involved with somatic sensory processing. An example of this may be stimulation of the vagus, and the initial experience with vagal nerve stimulation for treatment of migraines, cluster headaches and other daily headache conditions [9–11] is encouraging.

Since the peripheral nervous system consists of a number of components including large nerves, their divisions into smaller nerve branches, nerve roots and nerve plexuses, PNS targets are not limited to individual nerves. One of these targets has already been explored: implantation of a PNS device over the brachial plexus was recently described [12]. More PNS uses in the treatment of plexopathies (brachial, cervical, lumbosacral) are expected to occur in the future; selective stimulation of targeted parts of the plexus awaits innovated approaches and site- or target-specific technological developments.

Other potential PNS targets are nerve ganglia. It is appealing to consider neuromodulation of sympathetic nerves and their ganglia. While stimulation of sympathetic ganglia or sympathetic chain may at first sight appear theoretical, stimulation of the sphenoplaltine ganglion has already become a target and stimulation of sensory nerve ganglia is already a reality. The gasserian ganglion has been a stimulation target for the treatment of neuropathic pain in the trigeminal distribution for many years [13, 14]. A recent multicenter study of dorsal root ganglia (DRG) stimulation suggests that this modality may provide additional benefits in chronic pain treatment. This will most likely be a frequent target once appropriate devices become available.

The junction between central and peripheral nervous systems – the nerve root – has been subject to PNS. Stimulation of both spinal [15] and trigeminal [16] nerve roots has been undertaken. With development of new hardware and stimulation paradigms, nerve root stimulation may become one of the most promising PNS applications as an alternative to the use of SCS.

One issue that has been addressed in the past, but never resolved, is the use of PNS on mixed nerves. Having the capability of selective stimulation of sensory fascicles or even selective stimulation of certain fiber types, will allow the application to achieve maximal sensory stimulation without associated and unwanted motor stimulation.

Combination of PNS with Other Neurostimulation Methods

Finally, there is a possibility of combining PNS with existing pain-relieving approaches analogous to multimodal pain control. 'Hybrid' techniques that combine PNS and SCS [17–19], the combined use of stimulation of nerve and ganglion, or nerve and nerve root, or the use of PNS in combination with focal or systemic pharmacological interventions is appealing. The latter approach may include both anesthetic drugs and newer agents that may sensitize nerves to the effect of neurostimulation.

New Devices

The most fascinating developments are now occurring in the field of medical technology as companies pursue PNS applications as their primary clinical objective. Not only are there new electrodes and generators, but new devices based on very different principles specifically conforming to the demands of PNS are being developed. Although the conceptual information presented here is derived from the authors' understanding of the current state of affairs, the factual data are provided from publicly available sources in order to obviate any existing confidentiality agreements and intellectual property issues.

A single piece ultra-compact electrode/generator combination (BION®, Boston Scientific, Valencia, Calif., USA) has been used in many clinical studies [20, 21]. Initially developed for stimulation of peripheral nerves as a part of functional electrical stimulation approaches, BION was subsequently employed for chronic pain treatment. Most notably, it was used in the treatment of primary headaches [22] and hemicrania continua [23]. With its very small size and cylindrical shape, implantation is significantly simpler compared to the multicomponent systems, but its single contact setup and mobility within soft tissues have been problematic and prompted a series of technological advancements [24].

Importantly, having an integrated electrode and generator design allows one to eliminate a common problem encountered in PNS cases – the need for extension cables to cross mobile areas such as large joints in the extremities, neck or back. There are, however, other solutions for this issue. The StimRouter® device (Bioness, Valencia, Calif., USA), for example, is based on an integrated electrode and receiver that is powered transcutaneously by an external pulse generator. The electrode used in the published study [25] has an external component used for measurement of received electrical current, but the final version of the device is fully implantable such that three electrode contacts are positioned next to the target nerve while the opposite end of the lead is situated under the skin in order to receive electrical energy from the external pulse transmitter that is attached to the skin surface.

A somewhat similar approach is used by the SAINT® (Subcutaneous Array of Implantable Neural Transponders) system (Microtransponder, Dallas, Tex., USA) where the fully implanted electrode is powered by an external stimulator using an electromagnetic induction principle [26]. In this case, the implanted stimulator is 3.1 mm long, 1.5 mm wide and 0.3 mm thick. In addition to PNS application for treating chronic pain, this device is now being tested for stimulation of the vagal nerve in the treatment of tinnitus and neurological deficits after traumatic brain injury.

Miniaturization and simplification are not the only directions for technological advancement. The development of new stimulation parameters, waveforms and paradigms aimed at PNS applications will be supplemented by the creation of dedicated PNS systems. These, in turn, will have specially designed insertion and anchoring tools, all this will result in the further improvements of safety and efficacy of PNS.

Further, the standard practice of using biologically inert smooth metal surfaces for the current electrode contacts will undoubtedly change – the electrode contacts in the future may be of different texture to change the pattern of material interaction at the device/nerve interface. The contact may be concave instead of flat or convex and it may be supplemented by small 'micro-teeth' that both attach to and partially penetrate the epineurium in order to decrease the chance of migration or, more importantly, improve the device interface with the underlying fascicles. These future electrode contacts may have a special antibiotic coating to reduce the incidence of local infection or incorporate new materials at the terminal electrode contacts to facilitate electrical transmission to potentiate effects of the stimulation.

Conclusion

Given the current trend and increasing popularity of PNS as another means to manage chronic pain, one may expect to see growth in all aspects of this therapeutic modality. The development of new indications, new stimulation targets, and new equipment choices will strengthen PNS as a therapeutic field. The turning point will occur when sufficient scientific evidence is garnered to unequivocally prove safety, clinical efficacy and cost effectiveness of PNS and when PNS applications become officially endorsed through regulatory approval. These developments will allow implanters to use approved devices for approved indications – instead of their contemporary 'off-label' basis – which at the same time will signal to device manufacturers to both market these devices and support education for their rational use.

References

1 Mobbs RJ, Nair S, Blum P: Peripheral nerve stimulation for the treatment of chronic pain. J Clin Neurosci 2007;14:216–221.
2 Slavin KV: Peripheral nerve stimulation for neuropathic pain. Neurotherapeutics 2008;5: 100–106.
3 Stanton-Hicks M, Salamon J: Stimulation of the central and peripheral nervous system for the control of pain. J Clin Neurophysiol 1997;14:46–62.
4 Thimineur M, De Ridder D: C2 area neurostimulation: a surgical treatment for fibromyalgia. Pain Med 2007;8:639–646.
5 Slavin KV: Peripheral neurostimulation in fibromyalgia: a new frontier?! Pain Med 2007;8:621–622.
6 Lipov EG, Joshi JR, Sanders S, Slavin KV: Use of peripheral subcutaneous field stimulation for the treatment of axial neck pain: a case report. Neuromodulation 2009;12:292–295.
7 McRoberts WP, Roche M: Novel approach for peripheral subcutaneous field stimulation for the treatment of severe, chronic knee joint pain after total knee arthroplasty. Neuromodulation 2010;13: 131–136.
8 Yakovlev AE, Resch BE, Karasev SA: Treatment of intractable hip pain after THA and GTB using peripheral nerve field stimulation: a case series. WMJ 2010;109:149–152.

9 Hord ED, Evans MS, Mueed S, Adamolekun B, Naritoku DK: The effect of vagus nerve stimulation on migraines. J Pain 2003;4:530–534.

10 Mauskop A: Vagus nerve stimulation relieves chronic refractory migraine and cluster headaches. Cephalalgia 2005;25:82–86.

11 Cecchini AP, Mea E, Tullo V, Curone M, Franzini A, Broggi G, Savino M, Bussone G, Leone M: Vagus nerve stimulation in drug-resistant daily chronic migraine with depression: preliminary data. Neurol Sci 2009;30(suppl 1):S101–104.

12 Goroszeniuk T, Kothari SC, Hamann WC: Percutaneous implantation of a brachial plexus electrode for management of pain syndrome caused by a traction injury. Neuromodulation 2007;10: 148–155.

13 Taub E, Munz M, Tasker RR: Chronic electrical stimulation of the gasserian ganglion for the relief of pain in a series of 34 patients. J Neurosurg 1997; 86:197–202.

14 Machado A, Ogrin M, Rosenow JM, Henderson JM: A 12-month prospective study of gasserian ganglion stimulation for trigeminal neuropathic pain. Stereotact Funct Neurosurg 2007;85:216–224.

15 Aló KM, Yland MJ, Feler C, Oakley J: A study of electrode placement at the cervical and upper thoracic nerve roots using an anatomic trans-spinal approach. Neuromodulation 1999;2:222–227.

16 Young RF: Electrical stimulation of the trigeminal nerve root for the treatment of chronic facial pain. J Neurosurg 1995;83:72–78.

17 Bernstein CA, Paicius RM, Barkow SH, Lempert-Cohen C: Spinal cord stimulation in conjunction with peripheral nerve field stimulation for the treatment of low back and leg pain: a case series. Neuromodulation 2008;11:116–123.

18 Mironer YE, Hutcheson JK, Satterthwaite JR, LaTourette PC: Prospective, two-part study of the interaction between spinal cord stimulation and peripheral nerve field stimulation in patients with low back pain: development of a new spinal-peripheral neurostimulation method. Neuromodulation 2011;14:in press.

19 Koutsarnakis C, Korfias S, Themistocleous M, Sakas DE: Spinal cord stimulation (SCS), and/or peripheral subcutaneous field stimulation (PSFS) in drug-resistant chronic pain: a single center experience of 72 patients. Program Book XIX Congress of the European Society for Stereotactic and Functional Neurosurgery, Athens, 2010, p 34.

20 Loeb GE, Peck RA, Moore WH, Hood K: BION system for distributed neural prosthetic interfaces. Med Eng Phys 2001;23:9–18.

21 Carbunaru R, Whitehurst T, Jaax K, Koff J, Makous J: Rechargeable battery-powered Bion microstimulators for neuromodulation. Conf Proc IEEE Eng Med Biol Soc 2004;6:4193–4196.

22 Trentman TL, Rosenfeld DM, Vargas BB, Schwedt TJ, Zimmerman RS, Dodick DW: Greater occipital nerve stimulation via the Bion microstimulator: implantation technique and stimulation parameters. Clinical trial: NCT00205894. Pain Physician 2009; 12:621–628.

23 Burns B, Watkins L, Goadsby PJ: Treatment of hemicrania continua by occipital nerve stimulation with a Bion device: long-term follow-up of a crossover study. Lancet Neurol 2008;7:1001–12.

24 Kane MJ, Breen PP, Quondamatteo F, Olaighin G: BION microstimulators: a case study in the engineering of an electronic implantable medical device. Med Eng Phys 2011;33:in press.

25 Deer TR, Levy RM, Rosenfeld EL: Prospective clinical study of a new implantable peripheral nerve stimulation device to treat chronic pain. Clin J Pain 2010;26:359–372.

26 Cho SH, Cauller L, Rosellini W, Lee JB: A MEMS-based fully-integrated wireless neurostimulator. Micro Electro Mechanical Systems (MEMS), 2010 IEEE 23rd International Conference, Wanchai, Hong Kong, 2010, pp 300–303.

Dr. Michael Stanton-Hicks
Cleveland Clinic
9500 Euclid Ave. C-25
Cleveland, OH 44195 (USA)
Tel. +1 216 445 9539, E-Mail STANTOM@ccf.org

Author Index

Abejón, D. 203
Abramova, M.V. 41
Al-Jehani, H. 27
Aló, K.M. 41

Barolat, G. 70
Bartsch, T. 16
Bolognese, P. 118
Burchiel, K.J. IX

Cairns, K.D. 58, 156

De Ridder, D. 133
Deer, T. 58, 156
Dekelver, I. 133
Dodick, D.W. 96

Ellens, D.J. 109

Goadsby, P.J. 16

Jacques, L. 27

Kapural, L. 86
Kellner, C.P. 180
Kellner, M.A. 180

Levy, R.M. 109
Lipov, E.G. 147
Lunsford, L.D. VII

Magis, D. 126
Makonnen, G. 171
McRoberts, W.P. 58, 156
Milhorat, T.H. 118
Mogilner, A.Y. 118

Narouze, S. 171

Oluigbo, C.O. 171

Panourias, I.G. 210
Pérez-Cajaraville, J. 203
Plazier, M. 133

Rezai, A.R. 171
Richter, E.O. 41

Sable, J. 86
Sakas, D.E. 210
Schoenen, J. 126
Slavin, K.V. 1, 189, 210
Stanton-Hicks, M. 210

Thimineur, M. 133
Trentman, T.L. 96

Vadivelu, S. 118
Vanneste, S. 133

Weiner, R.L. 77
Winfree, C.J. 180

Zimmerman, R.S. 96

Subject Index

Abdominal pain
- inguinal neuropraxia and peripheral nerve field stimulation 62, 63
- peripheral subcutaneous stimulation for intractable abdominal pain 70–75

Anchor, leads 195

Anterior cingulate cortex
- greater occipital nerve stimulation effects on brain function 139
- pain processing 22

Arm, *see* Extremity pain

Back surgery, *see* Failed back surgery syndrome

Calcitonin gene-related peptide, pain role 17

Causalgia 27

Chiari malformation
- chronic headache 118
- etiology and clinical features 119
- occipital nerve stimulation for headache
  - complications 123, 124
  - outcomes 120–123, 125
  - patient selection 120, 124
  - surgery
    - percutaneous trial 120, 121
    - permanent implant 121

Cholecystokinin, analgesic tolerance role 21

Chronic neurogenic pain
- conventional management 28
- epidemiology 29
- etiology 27–29
- peripheral neuromodulation
  - complications 38
  - mechanism of action 29, 30
  - outcomes 35–38
  - patient selection 30, 31
  - permanent implantation 35
  - surgical insertion technique 31–34
  - trial of stimulation 35

Cluster headache, *see also* Headache, Sphenopalatine ganglion
- clinical features 126
- conventional treatment 126, 127
- deep brain stimulation 127
- occipital nerve stimulation
  - adverse events 128, 129
  - mechanism of action 129, 130
  - outcomes 128, 131
  - rationale 127
- pathophysiology 173, 174
- supraorbital nerve stimulation 130
- vagus nerve stimulation 130, 131

Complex regional pain syndrome
- peripheral nerve stimulation
  - historical perspective 3, 4, 6–8
  - prospects 212, 213
- types 27

Complications, peripheral nerve stimulation
- occipital nerve stimulation 84, 93, 94, 102–105, 123, 124
- overview 197–201

Cost-benefit analysis, peripheral nerve stimulation 211, 212

Deep brain stimulation, cluster headache 127

Definition, peripheral nerve stimulation
- Aristotle's rules 203, 204
- classification of neurostimulations 204–206
- historical perspective 206
- importance 208
- peripheral subcutaneous field stimulation comparison 206, 207

Electrode placement, peripheral nerve stimulation
accessories 196, 197
anchors 195
axon reflex in branching axons 43, 44
blood supply to peripheral nerves 44, 45
case studies 52–54
fascicular anatomy 44
initial surgical placement overview 42, 43
lead types 190–192
nerve trunk 44
prospects for study 212
subcutaneous peripheral nerve field stimulation 49, 50
subcutaneous targeted peripheral stimulation 50, 51
surgical insertion technique
chronic neurogenic pain 31–34
mapping of painful neural structure 45–47
occipital nerve stimulation
overview 47
paddles 48, 49, 90, 91, 93
wire electrodes 47, 48, 81, 82
Erosion, leads 196
Extremity pain
peripheral nerve stimulation
knee
peroneal nerve 167
saphenous nerve 167
lateral femoral cutaneous nerve 166, 167
literature review 157, 158
mechanism of action 158, 159
median nerve 168
meralgia paresthetica 166
neuromodulation system selection 160, 161
overview 156, 157
patient selection 159, 160
permanent implantation 165, 166
peroneal nerve 167, 168
prospects 168, 169
radial nerve 168
sciatic nerve 168
tibial nerve 167
trial implantation 161–165
ulnar nerve 168
spinal cord stimulation/peripheral nerve field stimulation for leg pain management
mechanism of action 151–153
outcomes 151
permanent implants 149–151
prospects 153, 154
trial implants 148, 149

Failed back surgery syndrome
peripheral nerve field stimulation 60–62
postlaminectomy syndrome 147
spinal cord stimulation/peripheral nerve field stimulation management
mechanism of action 151–153
outcomes 151
permanent implants 149–151
prospects 153, 154
trial implants 148, 149
spinal nerve root stimulation 184
Fascicle, anatomy 44
Femoral cutaneous nerve, stimulation for extremity pain 166, 167
Fibromyalgia
clinical features 133, 134
conventional treatment 134, 135
epidemiology 134
occipital nerve stimulation
mechanism of action 140–143
outcomes 135–138
pathophysiology 134

Ganglia, peripheral nerve stimulation prospects 214
Gate control theory, pain 3, 17, 29, 59
Greater occipital nerve
anatomy 97, 135
pain processing 17, 22
stimulation, *see* Occipital nerve stimulation

Halo peripheral nerve stimulation 82
Headache, *see also* Chiari malformation, Cluster headache, Migraine, Occipital nerve stimulation, Sphenopalatine ganglion
chronic neurogenic pain
conventional management 28
epidemiology 29
peripheral neuromodulation
complications 38
mechanism of action 29, 30
outcomes 35–38
patient selection 30, 31

permanent implantation 35
surgical insertion technique 31–34
trial of stimulation 35
gate control theory of pain 17
mechanism of nerve stimulation analgesia
analgesic tolerance 21
central sensitization and descending inhibition 17, 18
opioid receptors 21
peripheral neurostimulation 21–23
spinal mechanisms 18–20
supraspinal mechanisms 20, 21
Historical perspective, peripheral nerve stimulation
early years 3–5
invention 2, 3
maturation stage 5–7
percutaneous era 7–9
recent advances 9, 10
Hybrid stimulation, *see* Spinal cord stimulation/peripheral nerve field stimulation

Implantable pulse generator 101, 193–195, 215
Inguinal neuropraxia
peripheral nerve field stimulation 62, 63
peripheral subcutaneous stimulation for intractable abdominal pain 70–75

Knee, *see* Extremity pain

Leg, *see* Extremity pain
Lesser occipital nerve, anatomy 97
Liver transplant, peripheral subcutaneous stimulation for intractable abdominal pain 73, 74

Mapping, painful neural structure 45–47
Mechanism of action
chronic neurogenic pain peripheral neuromodulation 29, 30
extremity pain peripheral nerve stimulation 151–153
headache analgesia via stimulation
analgesic tolerance 21
central sensitization and descending inhibition 17, 18
opioid receptors 21
peripheral neurostimulation 21–23
spinal mechanisms 18–20
supraspinal mechanisms 20, 21
occipital nerve stimulation
fibromyalgia 140–143
headache 87–89, 112, 129, 130
peripheral nerve field stimulation for truncal pain 59, 60
prospects for study 211
spinal cord stimulation/peripheral nerve field stimulation 158, 159
Median nerve, stimulation for extremity pain 168
Meralgia paresthetica 166
Migraine, *see also* Headache, Sphenopalatine ganglion
conventional treatment 109, 110
epidemiology 109
occipital nerve stimulation
independent clinical trials 112, 113
industry-sponsored clinical trials 113–115
mechanism of action 112
Northwestern experience 115, 116
surgical technique 110–112
pathophysiology 173, 174
Miniaturization, devices 215

Nerve trunk, anatomy 44
Nucleus raphe magnus, pain processing 18

Objective evidence, accumulation 211
Occipital nerve stimulation
anatomy 97, 135
Chiari malformation headache
complications 123, 124
outcomes 120–123, 125
patient selection 120, 124
surgery
percutaneous trial 120, 121
permanent implant 121
cluster headache
adverse events 128, 129
mechanism of action 129, 130
outcomes 128, 131
rationale 127
complications 84, 93, 94, 102–105
fibromyalgia
mechanism of action 140–143
outcomes 135–138
greater occipital nerve stimulation effects on brain function 138, 139
halo peripheral nerve stimulation 82

Occipital nerve stimulation (cont.)
headache 22, 23, 35, 38
historical perspective 8, 77–80
implantable pulse generator 101
indications 80
mechanism of action 87–89
migraine
independent clinical trials 112, 113
industry-sponsored clinical trials 113–115
mechanism of action 112
Northwestern experience 115, 116
surgical technique 110–112
neuralgia features and treatment 89, 90, 105, 106
outcomes 82, 83, 92, 93
overview 96, 97
programming patterns and parameters 102
prospects 84, 85, 107
surgical insertion technique
anatomy 97
approaches 99, 100
overview 47
paddles 48, 49, 90, 91, 93, 101
permanent implant 99–102
trial implant 81, 97, 98
wire electrodes 47, 48, 81, 82
Opioid receptors, activation in nerve stimulation 21

Pain, gate control theory 3, 17, 29, 59
Pancreatitis, peripheral subcutaneous stimulation for intractable abdominal pain 74
Percutaneous electrical nerve stimulation, historical perspective 6, 9
Periaqueductal gray, pain processing 18, 20, 21
Peripheral nerve field stimulation, *see also* Spinal cord stimulation/peripheral nerve field stimulation
lead placement 49, 50
overview 58, 59, 87
patient selection 51
truncal pain management
failed back surgery syndrome 60–62
inguinal neuropraxia 62, 63
mechanism of action 59, 60
patient selection 60
post-thoracotomy pain 63
postherpetic neuralgia 62
programming 66–68
technical considerations 63–65
Peripheral subcutaneous field stimulation, definition 206, 207
Peroneal nerve, stimulation for extremity pain 167, 168
Plexopathy, peripheral nerve stimulation prospects 214
Postherpetic neuralgia, peripheral nerve field stimulation 62
Postlaminectomy syndrome 147
Pterygopalatine fossa, anatomy 172

Radial nerve, stimulation for extremity pain 168
Radiofrequency coupling 191, 193, 194
Rostroventral medulla, pain processing 18, 21

Saphenous nerve, stimulation for extremity pain 167
Sciatic nerve, stimulation for extremity pain 168
Sphenopalatine ganglion
anatomy 171–173
radiofrequency ablation 174, 175
stereotactic radiosurgery 174
stimulation
cerebral blood flow improvement in stroke 174
cluster headache outcomes 177
migraine outcomes 177
prospects 177, 178
surgical approaches
lateral infrazygomatic 175
percutaneous infrazygomatic 175
transnasal 175, 176
Spinal cord stimulation
historical perspective 6, 7
indications 180
limitations 180, 181
Spinal cord stimulation/peripheral nerve field stimulation
low back pain/leg pain management
mechanism of action 151–153
outcomes 151
permanent implants 149–151
prospects 153, 154
trial implants 148, 149
overview 147, 148

Spinal nerve root stimulation
classification 182
extraforaminal 185, 186
indications 181, 182
intraspinal 182, 183
prospects for study 187
rationale 181
transforaminal 183–185
trans-spinal 186, 187
Stroke, sphenopalatine ganglion stimulation for cerebral blood flow improvement 174
Subcutaneous Array of Implantable Neural Transponders 215
Supraorbital nerve stimulation, cluster headache 130

Thoracotomy, post-thoracotomy pain and peripheral nerve field stimulation 63
Tibial nerve, stimulation for extremity pain 167
Transcutaneous electrical nerve stimulation
analgesia mechanisms 18–21
analgesic tolerance 21
headache 16
historical perspective 2, 6
Triple anode single cathode programming, peripheral nerve field stimulation 66–68

Ulnar nerve, stimulation for extremity pain 168

Vagus nerve stimulation, cluster headache 130, 131

Wide-spaced cross-talk programming, peripheral nerve field stimulation 66